Pancreatitis:
Advances in Pathobiology, Diagnosis and Treatment

FALK SYMPOSIUM 143

Pancreatitis:
Advances in Pathobiology,
Diagnosis and Treatment

Edited by

R.W. Ammann
University Hospital Zürich
Department for Internal Medicine
Zürich
Switzerland

G. Adler
Department of Medicine I
University Clinic Ulm
Ulm
Germany

M.W. Büchler
Department of Visceral Surgery
University Clinic
Heidelberg
Germany

E.P. DiMagno
Gastrointestinal Unit
Mayo Clinic
Rochester, MN
USA

M. Sarner
Wellington Hospital
London
United Kingdom

*Proceedings of the Falk Symposium 143 held in Freiburg, Germany,
October 14–15, 2004*

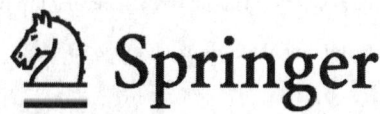

Springer

Library of Congress Cataloging-in-Publication Data is available.

ISBN-10: 1-4020-2895-4
ISBN-13: 978-1-4020-2895-3

Published by Springer,
PO Box 17, 3300 AA Dordrecht, The Netherlands

Sold and distributed in North, Central and South America
by Springer,
101 Philip Drive, Norwell, MA 02061 USA

In all other countries, sold and distributed
by Springer,
PO Box 322, 3300 AH Dordrecht, The Netherlands

Printed on acid-free paper

Contents

CONTENTS

CHRONIC PANCREATITIS II
SECTION VII: CONTROVERSIAL ISSUES OF THERAPY
Chair: P Layer, J Mössner

SECTION VIII: TREATMENT OF COMPLICATIONS AND OUTCOME
Chair: G Adler, PG Lankisch

List of principal contributors

G. Adler
Innere Medizin I
Universitätsklinikum Ulm
Robert-Koch-Str. 8
D-89081 Ulm
Germany

RW Ammann
Universitätsspital Zürich
Departement für Innere Medizin
Gastroenterologie und Hepatologie
Rämistrasse 100
CH-8091 Zürich
Switzerland

MV Apte
Pancreatic Research Group
The University of New South Wales
Room 463, Level 4, Health Services
  Building, Liverpool Hospital
Campbell Street
Liverpool, NSW 2170
Australia

S Bank
Division of Gastroenterology
Long Island Jewish Medical Center
Division of Gastroenterology
270-05 76th Avenue
New Hyde Park, NY 11040-1433
USA

PA Banks
Center for Pancreatic Disease
Brigham and Women's Hospital
Boston, MA
USA

C Beglinger
Division of Gastroenterology
University Hospital of Basel
CH-4031 Basel
Switzerland

D Bimmler
Praxis für Viszeralchirurgie
Rämistrasse 25
CH-8001 Zürich
Switzerland

MW Büchler
Department of General and Visceral
  Surgery
University of Heidelberg
Im Neuenheimer Feld 110
D-69120 Heidelberg
Germany

P-A Clavien
Department of Visceral and
  Transplantation Surgery
University Hospital of Zürich
Rämistrasse 100
CH-8091 Zürich
Switzerland

EP DiMagno
Mayo Clinic
Gastrointestinal Unit
200 First Street SW
Rochester, MN 55905
USA

UR Fölsch
Innere Medizin I
Universitätsklinikum
Schittenhelmstr. 12
D-24105 Kiel
Germany

PC Freeny
Department of Radiology
Box 357115, University of
  Washington School of Medicine
1959 Pacific Avenue
Seattle, WA 98195
USA

LIST OF PRINCIPAL CONTRIBUTORS

B Göke
Department of Internal Medicine
Klinikum Grosshadern
University of Munich
Marchioninistr. 15
D-81377 Munich
Germany

L Gullo
Internal Medicine
PAD 11 - St. Orsola Hospital
University of Bologna
Via Massarenti 9
I-40138 Bologna
Italy

C Imrie
Glasgow Royal Infirmary
Department of Surgery
Glasgow, G4 0SF
UK

JBMJ Jansen
Dept of Gastroenterology and
  Hepatology
Radboud University Medical Center
Geert Grooteplein 8
PO Box 9101
NL-6500 HB Nijmegen
The Netherlands

CD Johnson
University Surgical Unit
Southampton General Hospital
Tremona Road
Southampton, SO16 6YD
UK

V Keim
Medizinische Klinik und Poliklinik II
Universitätsklinikum Leipzig
Philipp Rosenthal Str. 27
D-04103 Leipzig
Germany

G. Klöppel
Allgemeine Pathologie
Universitätsklinikum Kiel
Michaelisstr. 11
D-24105 Kiel
Germany

PG Lankisch
Medizinische Klinik
Städt. Klinikum Lüneburg
Bögelstr. 1
D-21339 Lüneburg
Germany

P Layer
Department of Medicine
Israelitic Hospital
Orchideenstieg 14
D-22297 Hamburg
Germany

MM Lerch
Department of Gastroenterology,
  Endocrinology and Nutrition
Klinikum der Ernst-Moritz-Arndt
Universität Greifswald
Friedrich-Loeffler Str. 23A
D-17489 Greifswald
Germany

AB Lowenfels
Department of Surgery
New York Medical College
Valhalla, NY 10595
USA

J Mössner
Medizinische Klinik und Poliklinik II
Universitätsklinikum Leipzig
Philipp-Rosenthal-Str. 27
D-04103 Leipzig
Germany

JP Neoptolemos
Division of Surgery and Oncology
University of Liverpool
5th Floor, UCD Building
Daulby Street
Liverpool, L69 3GA
UK

M Sarner
University College London Hospitals
25 Grafton Way
London
WC1 6AU
UK

RM Schmid
Innere Medizin II
Klinikum rechts der Isar der
  Technischen Universität
Ismaninger Str. 22
D-81675 München
Germany

MV Singer
II Medizin. Universitätsklinik
Universitätsklinikum Mannheim
Theodor-Kutzer-Ufer 1-3
D-68167 Mannheim
Germany

ML Steer
Department of Surgery
Tufts-New England Medical Center
860 Washington St
Boston, MA 02111
USA

M Stern
University of Tübingen
University Children's Clinic
Hoppe-Seyler-Str. 1
D-72074 Tübingen
Germany

DC Whitcomb
GI Administration
UPMC Presbyterian
Mezzanine Level 2, C Wing
200 Lothrop Street
Pittsburgh, PA 15213
USA

Preface

In the long history of almost 40 years of the traditional Falk Symposia, the Pancreatitis Symposium in Freiburg, Germany in October 2004 was the first 2-day meeting devoted to acute and chronic pancreatitis. The main purpose of the symposium was to provide a state-of-the-art progress report on the pathobiology, diagnosis and treatment of pancreatic inflammatory diseases and to critically review the abundant and often controversial literature on clinically relevant issues. To achieve this goal, the symposium was fortunate in having the cooperation of a group of internationally recognized experts in basic science, gastroenterology, radiology, endoscopy, pathology and surgery, all of whom are active in pancreatic research and members of at least one of the three international leading pancreatic research 'clubs': the EPC (European Pancreatic Club), the APA (American Pancreatic Association), and the IAP (International Association of Pancreatology). This book contains most of the 30 lectures presented at the Pancreatitis Symposium.

Substantial progress in the understanding of the pathobiology of pancreatitis is usually based on animal models but new diagnostic tools – molecular biology and molecular genetics and the advent of new diagnostic imaging methods, e.g. modern CT techniques, magnetic resonance imaging, positron emission tomography or endoscopic ultrasound have opened new perspectives in the elucidation of pancreatic pathology. Despite these technical advances, many clinically relevant issues remain; for example, optimal management of severe necrotizing pancreatitis, chronic pancreatitis, factors that favour or prevent progression from acute to chronic pancreatitis, pathomechanisms of pain and its optimal management in chronic pancreatitis.

At present, and despite the marked progress in knowledge, we seem to be far away from David Whitcomb's plea "of being able to prevent the development of end-stage chronic pancreatitis – that hopeless condition that should be confined to history books" (Chapter 14).

We are grateful to the outstanding scientists who have contributed to the success of this symposium and in particular to thank Dr Dr h.c. H. Falk and the Falk Foundation for the generous support which made this meeting and the production of this book possible.

RW Ammann, G Adler, EP DiMagno, MW Büchler, M Sarner

Acute pancreatitis I

Section I
Pathobiology of acute pancreatitis

Chair: C. IMRIE and R.M. SCHMID

1
Where and how does acute pancreatitis begin?

M. L. STEER, A. SHARMA, X.-H. TAO and G. PERIDES

INTRODUCTION

Acute pancreatitis is most commonly triggered by the passage of a biliary tract stone into or through the terminal biliopancreatic ductal system[1]. Other known causes include exposure to certain drugs, abuse of ethanol, trauma, obstruction of the pancreatic duct, and performance of endoscopic retrotrade pancreatography. The disease is relatively common, sometimes lethal and, in its severe form, it can lead to the consumption of significant medical resources. In spite of these factors the pathogenesis and pathobiology of acute pancreatitis are poorly understood and specific treatment for the disease has not been identified. To a great extent our poor understanding of pancreatitis and its treatment reflect the complex nature of the clinical disease and its many uncontrollable variables, the fact that patients with pancreatitis are usually not identified during the earliest stages of the disease, and our inability to access the human pancreas during the evolution of pancreatitis. As a result, research into the mechanisms underlying clinical pancreatitis has been considerably hampered and students of the disease have been forced to employ models of the disease, in experimental animals, to explore these issues.

Most of the studies dealing with the pathobiology of acute pancreatitis have utilized one or more of the following four types of experimental pancreatitis models (Table 1): diet-induced pancreatitis elicited by feeding young female mice a choline-deficient, ethionine-supplemented diet[2]; secretagogue-induced pancreatitis elicited by exposing rodents or the rodent pancreas to a dose of the cholecystokinin analogue caerulein that is in excess of the dose which elicits a maximal rate of digestive enzyme secretion[3,4]; duct-infusion-induced pancreatitis elicited by retrogradely infusing bile salts and/or trypsin into the rat pancreatic duct[5]; and obstruction-induced pancreatitis elicited by ligating the biliopancreatic ductal system of the American opossum[6]. Each of these models has its own advantages and disadvantages when applied to such studies and each is, to a certain extent, imperfect – i.e. none of the models completely replicates the events that are known to trigger clinical acute pancreatitis. In spite of these limitations, however, studies employing these various models

Table 1 Experimental pancreatitis model

Model	Animal	Severity	Evolution	Lethality	Comments
Diet	Mice	Severe	Days	Yes	Haemorrhage, necrosis
Secretagogue	Rats and mice	Mild to severe	Hours	No	Reproducible and cheap
Duct infusion	Rats	Severe	Minutes	Yes	Hard to control
Duct ligation	Opossums	Severe	Days	Yes	Expensive

have provided potentially important insights into a variety of issues concerning clinical pancreatitis. In this chapter we will review some of the studies that our group and others have performed employing these models to answer two fundamental questions regarding acute pancreatitis – i.e. Where and how does the disease begin?

WHERE DOES ACUTE PANCREATITIS BEGIN?

Gallstone pancreatitis, the most common type of clinical acute pancreatitis, is believed to be triggered by passage of a biliary tract stone into or through the terminal biliopancreatic duct[1,7], and many investigators believe that, in gallstone pancreatitis, the stone triggers pancreatitis by obstructing the ductal system. Over the years, considerable controversy has surrounded the question of where, in the pancreas, pancreatitis begins. Some have suggested that it begins in the perilobular and peripancreatic region as fat necrosis caused by ischaemia[8], while others have suggested that pancreatitis begins in the periductal regions of the gland as a result of ductal disruption and intraparenchymal extravasation of pancreatic juice[9]. Still other investigators have hypothesized that acute pancreatitis might begin within acinar cells as a result of premature activation of digestive enzyme zymogens such as trypsinogen.

The pancreas and the terminal biliopancreatic ductal system of the American opossum and humans are similar. In both species there is a single distal bile duct which is joined by the major pancreatic duct shortly before the combined biliopancreatic duct enters the duodenum. Ligation of the terminal biliopancreatic duct of the American opossum, like passage of a stone into the terminal biliopancreatic duct of humans, triggers severe, necrotizing pancreatitis[6]. Furthermore, the ligation-induced injury in opossums closely resembles, morphologically, the clinical injury in human severe pancreatitis.

These similarities between humans and opossums led us to reason that the American opossum might be an ideal experimental animal for studies designed to explore the question of where human pancreatitis begins. For our studies we ligated the opossum ductal system and sacrificed the animals at varying times over the initial 24 h following duct ligation[10]. As shown in Figure 1, the initial changes that we observed were confined to acinar cells of the pancreas. Three

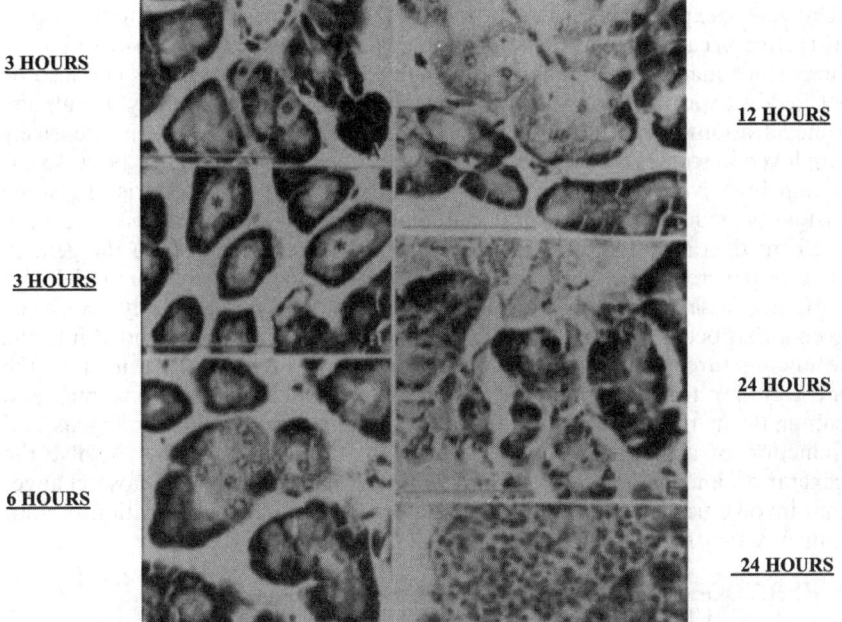

3 HOURS

12 HOURS

3 HOURS

24 HOURS

6 HOURS

24 HOURS

Figure 1 Microscopic changes noted during the initial 24 h of pancreatitis induced by biliopancreatic duct ligation in the opposum

hours after duct ligation the acinar lumina appeared dilated and scattered acinar cells appeared necrotic. Six hours after duct ligation, larger areas of the parenchyma were occupied by necrotic-appearing acinar cells and these areas of acinar cell necrosis appeared even larger by 12 h after duct ligation. At that time, no evidence of perilobular or periductal injury was seen. Those changes, including fat necrosis, intraparenchymal haemorrhage, and inflammation were first observed 24 h after duct ligation.

These studies have led us to conclude that acute pancreatitis begins within pancreatic acinar cells. Periductal and perilobular injury appear to be later events, perhaps reflecting the processes that begin within acinar cells.

HOW DOES PANCREATITIS BEGIN?

Ideally, efforts to prevent and/or treat acute pancreatitis should be based upon a comprehensive knowledge of where, within acinar cells, the disease begins, and upon an understanding of the intracellular derangements that underlie development of acute pancreatitis. The secretagogue-induced model of experimental pancreatitis is ideally suited to studies exploring these issues because it evolves in a rapid and highly reproducible manner, it is easily induced, and it is relatively inexpensive. Furthermore, the secretagogue-induced model is also attractive because it permits studies under easily controllable, *in-vitro* conditions since many of the pancreatitis-related pancreatic alterations can also be elicited by exposing freshly isolated rodent acini to supramaximally stimulating concentrations of caerulein[11]. The diet-induced model has also been extensively employed in studies focused on the pathophysiology of pancreatitis because it is a non-invasive and highly lethal model of severe pancreatitis. In some instances, studies using several different models of pancreatitis have been performed in an attempt to identify changes that are relevant to the general issue of pancreatitis rather than being 'model-specific' for only one model.

Using these approaches we and others have found that the early acinar cell events that occur during the evolution of pancreatitis can be divided into the following three groups: (a) those changes that involve alterations in the intracellular trafficking and secretion of acinar cell-derived enzymes and culminate in the intracellular activation of digestive enzyme zymogens and induction of acinar cell injury/necrosis; (b) those changes that involve the generation and/or action of proinflammatory factors; and (c) those changes that involve triggering of anti-inflammatory events and/or generation of anti-inflammatory factors (Figure 2).

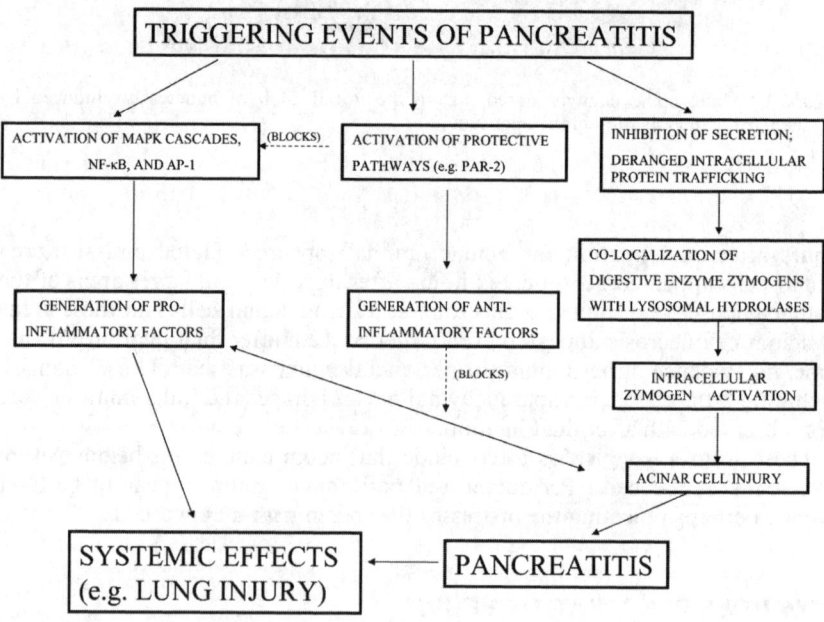

Figure 2   Intracellular events underlying the evolution of acute pancreatitis

Alterations in the secretion and intra-acinar cell trafficking of enzymes during pancreatitis

In health, digestive enzyme zymogens and lysosomal hydrolases are assembled within the cisternae of the rough endoplasmic reticulum and vectorially transported to the Golgi stacks where some, particularly those destined to be transported to lysosomes, are post-translationally modified. Subsequently, lysosomal hydrolases are phosphorylated at the 6-position of mannose residues, bound by mannose-6-phosphate specific receptors, and shuttled to the pre-lysosomal compartment where they function to degrade intracellular proteins. In contrast, digestive enzyme zymogens that are destined for export from acinar cells, pass through the Golgi stacks and are packaged within condensing vacuoles that mature into zymogen granules as they migrate to the lumenal cell surface. There, the limiting membrane of the granule and the apical plasmalemma fuse, allowing the contents of the granule to be discharged into the acinar (i.e. ductal) space[12,13].

We have performed a number of studies using several of the otherwise dissimilar models to evaluate these issues during the evolution of pancreatitis. During the very early stages of the disease, before evidence of acinar cell injury can be detected, digestive enzyme secretion from acinar cells is inhibited and the intracellular trafficking of newly synthesized enzymes is perturbed. The normal events which lead to the segregation of digestive enzyme zymogens from lysosomal hydrolases are altered and, as a result, the two types of enzymes become co-localized within the same intracellular vacuoles. There, cathepsin B, a lysosomal hydrolase, catalytically activates trypsinogen and, we believe, trypsin activates the other digestive enzyme zymogens[11]. Our studies suggest that this premature, intracellular activation of digestive enzymes leads to acinar cell injury and triggers the inflammatory response which is typically observed during pancreatitis[14].

Little is known about the molecular signals which lead to the inhibition of secretion and to the co-localization phenomenon which is observed during the early stages of pancreatitis. A pathological rise in intracellular ionized calcium levels is required[15,16] but, by itself, not sufficient to trigger these changes[15]. Activation of phosphoinositide-3-kinase is also critical[17]. In some of the models, co-localization appears to be the result of defective sorting of lysosomal hydrolases from digestive enzyme zymogens as the two types of enzymes pass through the Golgi stacks[18] but, in other models, co-localization appears to result from the fusion of zymogen granules with lysosomes[19]. Recent studies by Gorelick's group have suggested that elevations of intracellular cyclic AMP levels may sensitize acinar cells to intracellular zymogen activation[20].

Generation of proinflammatory factors by acinar cells during the early stages of pancreatitis

In addition to acinar cell injury, acute pancreatitis is characterized by an intrapancreatic inflammatory process which, in severe attacks, is accompanied by evidence of systemic inflammation and, occasionally, by distant organ failure. The morbidity and mortality of a pancreatitis attack is directly related to the magnitude of these inflammatory events and, therefore, therapies that successfully limit the severity of pancreatitis-associated inflammation could significantly alter the outcome of a clinical attack.

Studies independently performed by several investigative groups, including our own, have shown that proinflammatory processes are activated during the very earliest stages of experimental pancreatitis. The mitogen-activated protein kinase (MAPK) cascade is triggered very shortly after rodents are given supramaximally stimulating doses of caerulein or after rodent pancreatic acini are exposed to supramaximally stimulating concentrations of caerulein[21], and this leads to activation of proinflammatory intracellular protein kinases. At roughly the same time, proinflammatory cytoplasmic transcription factors, including NF-κB and AP-1, are activated within acinar cells[22,23]. Intra-acinar cell activation of MAPK, NF-κB, and AP-1 appears to occur in parallel with the co-localization phenomenon and zymogen activation, and not be to dependent upon intracellular activation of digestive enzyme zymogens[24]. Following their extranuclear activation, these various factors (i.e. the MAPK, NF-κB, AP-1, etc.) are translocated to the nucleus where they regulate transcription of a wide variety of proinflammatory mediators including cytokines, chemokines, adhesion molecules, etc. Acinar cell generation of these factors leads to the activation and chemoattraction of inflammatory cells and to the triggering of a parenchymal pancreatic inflammatory reaction. Systemic release of these factors, from acinar cells as well as from inflammatory cells sequestered within the inflamed pancreas, further accelerates pancreatic inflammation and it also triggers systemic inflammatory changes such as acute lung injury. Some of the proinflammatory factors generated and released from the inflamed pancreas (e.g. GM-CSF[25], P- and E-selectins, ICAM-1[26], cyclo-oxygenase-2[27], TNF-α[28], etc.) appear to primarily up-regulate the severity of pancreatic injury while others (e.g. platelet-activating factor[29], substance P[30], chemokines acting via the CCR-1 receptor[31]) appear to up-regulate the coupling of pancreatitis with acute lung injury.

The inflammatory cells, particularly the polymorphonuclear neutrophils, which are activated and chemoattracted to the pancreas during the early stages of pancreatitis, also play an important role in regulating the severity of both pancreatic and systemic injury. Neutrophil depletion or genetic deletion of the adhesion molecule ICAM-1 interferes with neutrophil sequestration in areas of injury and, as a result, reduces the severity of pancreatitis and pancreatitis-associated lung injury[32]. Genetic deletion of neutrophil NADPH-oxidase has similar effects[33]. However, recent studies suggest that the acinar cell necrosis seen in severe pancreatitis can occur even in the absence of neutrophil sequestration in the pancreas. In those studies neutrophil sequestration was reduced by deletion of the proto-oncogene Tpl2 which regulates TNF-α activity but, even with reduced neutrophil sequestration, pancreatic acinar cell necrosis was not altered (Perides, Sharma, Tao, Tsichlis, Steer, unpublished).

Generation of anti-inflammatory factors during pancreatitis

In addition to proinflammatory changes, a number of recent studies by our group, as well as others, have shown that anti-inflammatory events are initiated during the early stages of experimental pancreatitis and that these anti-inflammatory events may serve to limit the severity of a pancreatitis attack. IL-10 expression is up-regulated during pancreatitis and administration of IL-10 has been shown to reduce the severity of pancreatitis[34,35]. Genetic deletion of IL-11 and complement factor C5a[36] has been shown to worsen the severity of experimental pancreatitis, indicating that these factors act to reduce the severity of an attack. Heat-shock proteins, including HSP70[37], HSP60[38], and HSP27[39], which are generated during the early stages of experimental pancreatitis, have also been shown to exert a protective effect in pancreatitis. The mechanisms by which these anti-inflammatory factors reduce the severity of pancreatitis are not entirely clear, but studies addressing this issue may provide insights into treatments that could reduce the severity of clinical pancreatitis.

Protease-activated receptors (PAR) are a recently recognized family of receptors which are activated by circulating or locally generated proteases including thrombin and trypsin[40]. Proteolytic cleavage of the N-terminal extracellular domain of the receptor releases a tethered ligand which can intermolecularly bind to activate the receptor. Once activated, PAR are phosphorylated, internalized, and degraded, thus terminating their signal until new receptors are inserted into the surface membrane. PAR-2, a member of the PAR family, is widely expressed and its presence on acinar cells has been demonstrated[41]. Trypsin is believed to be the pathophysiological activator of PAR-2 and this suggested to us that PAR-2 might play an important role in regulating the severity of pancreatitis.

To examine this issue we induced pancreatitis in mice genetically modified to lack PAR-2. We found that pancreatitis was markedly worsened by PAR-2 deletion. Furthermore, we found that pharmacological activation of PAR-2, by infusion of the PAR-2-activating peptide, protected mice from pancreatitis[41]. Taken together, these findings indicate that PAR-2 activation during pancreatitis exerts a protective effect on the disease and, from a teleological standpoint, one might hypothesize that PAR-2 provides a survival advantage by protecting animals from the injurious effects of premature, intrapancreatic activation of trypsinogen. The mechanisms by which PAR-2 activation protects mice from pancreatitis and PAR-2 deletion worsens the disease are not entirely clear but, in preliminary studies, we have found that PAR-2 activation may exert this protective effect by interfering with the nuclear translocation (and action) of proinflammatory kinases such as the ERK 1/2[41].

SUMMARY AND FUTURE DIRECTIONS

Over the past two decades, considerable progress has been made in achieving an understanding of where and how acute pancreatitis begins. To a great extent that progress has been made using a variety of acute pancreatitis models. Based on studies using the opossum model of pancreatitis, the disease appears to begin within acinar cells. Studies using several otherwise dissimilar models of pancreatitis, including the secretagogue and diet-induced models, have indicated that digestive enzyme secretion is reduced during the early stages of the disease and intracellular trafficking of newly synthesized proteins (i.e. enzymes) is perturbed. As a result, digestive enzyme zymogens and lysosomal hydrolases become co-localized within acinar cell cytoplasmic vacuoles where the lysosomal hydrolase cathepsin B activates trypsinogen and trypsin activates the other digestive zymogens. This intracellular activation of digestive enzymes leads to acinar cell injury. In parallel with these changes, a number of proinflammatory and anti-inflammatory processes are activated within acinar cells during the earliest phases of pancreatitis, and these inflammation-related events serve to regulate the severity of both the pancreatic and the extrapancreatic injury.

The currently available treatments for acute pancreatitis are purely supportive and non-specific. To date, no specific treatment for the disease has been shown to be effective. With further study our understanding of the pathogenesis of pancreatitis will expand. Hopefully, this greater understanding of the events which trigger the disease and of the processes which regulate the severity of an attack will lead to the development of therapies that can effectively prevent the onset and/or reduce the severity of an attack.

References

1. Acosta JL, Ledesma CL. Gallstone migration as a cause of acute pancreatitis. N Engl J Med. 1974;190:484–7.
2. Lombardi B, Estes LW, Longnecker DS. Acute hemorrhagic pancreatitis (massive necrosis) with fat necrosis induced in mice by dl-ethionine fed with a choline deficient diet. Am J Pathol. 1975;79:465–80.
3. Lampel M, Kern HF. Acute interstitial pancreatitis in rats induced by excessive doses of a pancreatic secretagogue. Virchows Arch A Pathol Anat Histol. 1977;373:97–113.
4. Grady T, Saluja A, Klaiser A, Steer M. Pancreatic edema and intrapancreatic activation of trypsinogen during secretagogue-induced pancreatitis precedes glutathione depletion. Am J Physiol. 1996;271:G20–6.
5. Aho H, Koskensalo SML, Nevalainen TJ. Experimental pancreatitis in the rat. Sodium taurocholate-induced haemorrhagic pancreatitis. Scand J Gastroenterol. 1980;15:411–24.
6. Senninger N, Moody FG, Coelho JC, VanBuren DH. The role of biliary obstruction in the pathogenesis of acute pancreatitis in the opossum. Surgery. 1986;99:688–93.
7. Opie EL. The etiology of acute hemorrhagic pancreatitis. Bull Johns Hopkins Hosp. 1901; 12:182–92.
8. Kloeppel G, Dreyer T, Willemer S, Kern HF, Adler G. Human acute pancreatitis: its pathogenesis in the light of immunocytochemical and ultrastructural findings of acinar cells. Virchows Arch A Pathol Anat Histopathol. 1986;409:791–803.
9. Foulis AK. Histological evidence of initiating factors in acute necrotizing pancreatitis in man. J Clin Pathol. 1980;33:1123–31.
10. Lerch MM, Saluja AK, Runzi M, Dawra R, Saluja M, Steer ML. Pancreatic duct obstruction triggers acute necrotizing pancreatitis in the opossum. Gastroenterology. 1993;104:853–61.
11. Saluja AK, Donovan EA, Yamanaka K, Yamaguchi Y, Hofbauer B, Steer ML. Caerulein-induced *in vitro* activation of trypsinogen in rat pancreatic acini is mediated by cathepsin B. Gastroenterology. 1997;113:304–10.
12. Palade G. Intracellular aspects of the process of protein secretion. Science. 1975;189:347–58.
13. Kornfield S. Trafficking of lysosomal enzymes in normal and disease states. J Clin Invest. 1986;77:1–6.

14. Hofbauer B, Saluja AK, Lerch M et al. Intra-acinar cell activation of trypsinogen during caerulein-induced pancreatitis in rats. Am J Physiol. 1998;275:G352–62.
15. Saluja AK, Bhagat L, Lee HS, Bhatia M, Frossard JL, Steer ML. Secretagogue-induced digestive enzyme activation and cell injury in rat pancreatic acini. Am J Physiol. 1999;276: G835–42.
16. Raraty M, Ward J, Erdemli G et al. Calcium-dependent enzyme activation and vacuole formation in the apical granular region of pancreatic acinar cells. Proc Natl Acad Sci USA. 2000; 97:13126–31.
17. Singh VP, Saluja A, Bhagat L et al. Inhibition of phosphoinositide-3-kinase prevents trypsinogen activation and reduces the severity of acute pancreatitis. J Clin Invest. 2001; 108:1387–95.
18. Saito I, Hashimoto S, Saluja A, Steer ML, Meldolesi J. Intracellular transport of pancreatic zymogens during caerulein supramaximal stimulation. Am J Physiol. 1987;251:G517–26.
19. Koike H, Steer ML, Meldolesi J. Pancreatic effects of ethionine: blockade of exocytosis, crinophagy and autophagocytosis precede cellular necrosis. Am J Physiol. 1982;242:G297–307.
20. Lu Z, Kolodecik TR, Karne S, Nyce M, Gorelick F. Effect of ligands that increase cAMP on caerulein-induced zymogen activation in pancreatic acini. Am J Physiol. 2003;285: G822–8.
21. Dabrowski A, Grady T, Logsdon CD, Williams JA. Jun kinases are rapidly activated by cholecystokinin in rat pancreas both *in vitro* and *in vivo*. J Biol Chem. 1996;271:5686–90.
22. Gukovsky I, Gukovskaya AS, Blinman TA, Zaminovic V, Pandol SJ. Early NF-κB activation is associated with hormone-induced pancreatitis. Am J Physiol. 1998;275: G1402–14.
23. Steinle AU, Weidenbach H, Wagner M, Adler G, Schmid RM. NFκB/Rel activation in cerulein pancreatitis. Gastroenterology. 1999;116:420–30.
24. Hietaranta AJ, Saluja AK, Bhagat L, Singh VP, Song AM, Steer ML. Relationship between NF-κB and trypsinogen activation in rat pancreas after supramaximal caerulein stimulation. Biochem Biophys Res Commun. 2001;280:388–95.
25. Frossard JL, Saluja AK, Mach N et al. *In vivo* evidence for the role of GM-CSF as a mediator in acute pancreatitis-associated lung injury. Am J Physiol Lung Cell Mol Physiol. 2002;283:L541–8.
26. Zaninovic V, Gukovskaya AS, Gukovsky I, Mmouria M. Pandol SJ. Cerulein upregulates ICAM-1 in pancreatic acinar cells which mediates neutrophil adhesion to these cells. Am J Physiol. 2000;279:G666–76.
27. Ethridge RT, Chung DH, Slogoff M et al. Cyclooxygenase-2 gene disruption attenuates the severity of acute pancreatitis and pancreatitis-associated lung injury. Gastroenterology. 2002;123:1311–22.
28. Gukovskaya AS, Gukovsky I, Zaninovic V et al. Pancreatic acinar cells produce, release, and respond to tumor necrosis factor-alpha. Role in regulating cell death and pancreatitis. J Clin Invest. 1997;100:1853–62.
29. Hofbauer B, Saluja AK, Bhatia M et al. Effect of recombinant platelet-activating factor acetyl-hydrolase on two models of experimental acute pancreatitis. Gastroenterology. 1998; 115:1238–47
30. Bhatia M, Saluja AK, Hofbauer B et al. Role of substance P and neurokinin 1 receptors in acute pancreatitis and pancreatitis-associated lung injury. Proc Natl Acad Sci USA. 1998; 95:4760–5.
31. Gerard C, Frossard JL, Bhatia M et al. Targeted disruption of the beta-chemokine receptor CCR1 protects against pancreatitis-associated lung injury. J Clin Invest. 1997;100:2022–7.
32. Frossard JL, Saluj A, Bhagat L et al. The role of intercellular adhesion molecule 1 and neutrophils in acute pancreatitis and pancreatitis-associated lung injury. Gastroenterology. 1999;116:694–701.
33. Gukovskaya AS, Vaquero E, Zaninovic V et al. Neutrophils and NADPH oxidase mediate intrapancreatic trypsin activation in murine experimental acute pancreatitis. Gastroenterology. 2002;122:974–84.
34. Van Laethem JL, Marchant A, Delvaux A et al. Interleukin 10 prevents necrosis in murine experimental acute pancreatitis. Gastroenterology. 1995;108:1917–22.
35. Rongione AJ, Kusske AM, Kwan K, Sahley SW, Reber HA, McFadden DW. Interleukin 10 reduces the severity of acute pancreatitis in rats. Gastroenterology. 1997;112:960–7.

36. Bhatia M, Saluja AK, Singh VP et al. Complement factor C5a exerts an anti-inflammatory effect in acute pancreatitis and associated lung injury. Am J Physiol. 2001;280:G974–8.
37. Bhagat L, Singh V, Hiertaranta A, Agrawal S, Steer M, Saluja A. Heat shock protein 70 prevents secretagogue-induced cell injury in pancreas by preventing intracellular trypsinogen activation. J Clin Invest. 2000;106:81–9.
38. Lee HS, Bhagat L, Frossard JL et al. Water immersion stress induces heat shock protein 60 expression and protects against pancreatitis in rats. Gastroenterology. 2000;119:220–9.
39. Kubisch C, DiMagno MJ, Tietz AB et al. Overexpression of heat shock protein Hsp27 protects against cerulein-induced pancreatitis. Gastroenterology. 2004;127:275–86.
40. Dery O, Corvera CU, Steinhoff M, Bunnett NW. Proteinase-activated receptors: novel mechanisms of signaling by serine proteases. Am J Physiol. 1998;274:C1429–52.
41. Sharma A, Tao X, Gopal A et al. Protection against acute pancreatitis by activation of protease-activated receptor-2. Am J Physiol Gastrointest Liver Physiol. 2005;288:G388–95.

2
Clinical relevance of experimental models of acute pancreatitis

J. MAYERLE, F. U. WEISS and M. M. LERCH

INTRODUCTION

Acute pancreatitis is one of the most common diseases in gastroenterology. The incidence of acute pancreatitis per 100 000 population ranges from 10 to 46 per year; 2% of all patients admitted to hospital are diagnosed with acute pancreatitis. Nevertheless even in the 21st century neither the aetiology nor the pathophysiology of the disease is fully understood and causal treatment options are not at hand. This fact has prompted numerous researchers to study the initial triggering events of acute pancreatitis in order to develop new treatment strategies. Much of our current knowledge regarding the onset of pancreatitis was gained not from studies involving the human pancreas or patients with pancreatitis, but from animal or isolated cell models. There are several reasons why these models have been used. (1) The pancreas is a rather inaccessible organ because of its anatomical location in the retroperitoneal space; unlike the colon or stomach, biopsies of human pancreas are difficult to obtain for ethical and medical reasons. (2) Patients who are admitted to hospital with acute pancreatitis have usually passed through the initial stages of the disease where the triggering early events could have been studied. Particularly the autodigestive process that characterizes this disease has remained a significant impediment for investigations that address initiating pathophysiological events. Therefore, the issue of premature protease activation has mostly been studied in animal models of the disease, before randomized placebo-controlled trials to evaluate new therapeutic concepts in humans could be performed. Experimental models are now irreplaceable tools in studying aetiological factors, pathophysiology, and new diagnostic tools, as well as treatment options in acute pancreatitis. The advantages of animal models are the possibility to isolate specific aspects of a complex and varying disease course, the high degree of standardization and reproducibility, and the reduction of the required sample size eliminating variability in the study population.

Animal models can be grouped into invasive *in-vivo* models, non-invasive *in-vivo* models and *ex-vivo* models. The mode of onset and development, the disease severity, the extent of inflammation and the associated mortality vary considerably among different models.

NON-INVASIVE MODELS

Secretagogue induced pancreatitis

It is generally believed that the morphological changes that characterize acute pancreatitis result from digestion of the gland by enzymes that are normally synthesized and secreted by pancreatic acinar cells[1–3]. Evidence which supports this notion includes the observations that: (a) the morphological changes of severe pancreatitis resemble those that are typical of digestive necrosis[4]; (b) pancreatic acinar cells synthesize digestive enzymes which, when activated, lead to digestive necrosis of the gland[5]; and (c) activated digestive enzymes have been detected within the gland during severe pancreatitis[6]. Most of the potentially harmful digestive proteases of acinar cells are normally synthesized and secreted as inactive zymogens and activated in the duodenum by brush-border enzymes[7].

As early as 1895 Mouret reported that excessive cholinergic stimulation is associated with the development of pancreatic injury determined by acinar cell vacuolization and necrosis[8]. Mouret suggested that the activation of trypsin might be actively involved in the development of acute pancreatitis. This hypothesis was in accordance with the hypothesis of Hans Chiari, who in 1986 proposed autodigestion as the consequence of premature zymogen activation to be the pathomechanism underlying acute pancreatitis[1]. Subsequently experimental animal models employing cholinergic agonists such as carbamylcholine and charbachol, cholesystokinin (CCK) and its analogues, as well as scorpion venom, were shown to induce pancreatic injury in a time- and dose-dependent manner[9–13]. In rodents CCK plays a major role in regulating exocrine pancreatic secretion after stimulation by food ingestion. However, human pancreatic acinar cells do not directly respond to CCK stimulation, but are regulated by cholinergic pathways that involve neurogenic CCK stimulation[14]. In 1977 Lampel and Kern characterized the clinical and biochemical pattern of acute interstitial pancreatitis in rats after administration of excessive doses of pancreatic secretagogue[15]. The most prominent clinical characteristic is the development of excessive oedema as early as 1 h after the onset of the disease[16]. Since that time the model of pancreatitis induced by caerulein (a CCK analogue derived from the Australian tree frog *Litoria caerulea*) in rodents is widely used, and one of the best characterized.

The primary physiological effect of CCK and its analogues on the pancreas is to stimulate protein-rich secretion, and it has a lesser effect on fluid and electrolyte secretion. Doses of CCK that lead to continued maximal stimulation of enzyme secretion are associated with increased rates of both protein synthesis and the movement of newly synthesized proteins through the secretory pathway. The increase in protein synthesis is outpaced by the rate of protein secretion. Thus, following stimulation with maximal secretory doses of caerulein, the enzyme stores of the exocrine pancreas may be reduced by 75% within several hours. Increasing the concentration of CCK by an order of magnitude over the levels that produce maximal secretion is known as supraoptimal stimulation, supramaximal stimulation or hyperstimulation[16]. Compared to maximal stimulation, supramaximal stimulation generates a distinct pancreatic response that includes diminished secretion, accumulation of secretory proteins within the pancreas and pancreatic injury. The route of administration for caerulein that induces acute pancreatitis differs in various rodents, as does the severity of the disease[17-20]. While in rats caerulein can be continuously intravenously infused either via a polyethylene catheter placed either into the external jugular vein or into the tail vein, in mice caerulein is generally injected repeatedly into the peritoneal cavity[21]. The caerulein concentration that results in pancreatic oedema, increased serum levels of pancreatic enzymes, inflammation and necrosis ranges between 5 and 10 µg/kg per h in rats, and thereby exceeds the maximal secretory doses 10–20-fold. Maximal pancreatic injury occurs after 12 h of continuous infusion, but changes can be monitored as early as 15 min after the start of the caerulein infusion and resolve spontaneously after 24–48 h. One of the earliest consequences of hyperstimulation is the formation of pancreatic oedema. This increase in pancreatic fluid, which occurs within the first hour of caerulein hyperstimulation, is probably the result of several factors: increased vascular permeability, increased hydrostatic pressure from the constriction of small vessels and increased tissue oncotic pressure from the interstitial release of pancreatic enzymes and hydrolytic products. At present the exact mechanism which leads to the formation of massive oedema is not fully understood, but from its time-course a primary signalling effect of caerulein, which does not parallel acinar cell damage, is suggested. Under the conditions of supramaximal caerulein stimulation secretion of zymogens into the pancreatic duct is virtually abolished, premature zymogen activation can be observed after a sustained intracellular calcium rise and a breakdown of the actin cytoskeleton[22]. These events lead to a systemic inflammatory response syndrome which eludes extrapancreatic damage such as pancreatitis-related lung injury[23].

The caerulein model of experimental pancreatitis is now widely used for the analysis of intracellular events in the early phase of pancreatitis. The model offers several advantages: it is non-invasive since no surgical intervention affecting the bile duct or pancreatic duct is necessary, it allows easily controlled grades of injury, it is highly reproducible and it is applicable in several animal species such as mice, rats, hamsters and dogs. The most important limitation of this model is that only a mild, self-limited disorder is generated, which is of limited use to study the destructive effects of the disease which confer clinical morbidity and mortality[24-30] (Figure 1).

L -Arginine-induced pancreatitis

Despite medical treatment severe acute pancreatitis is still burdened with a high mortality rate of up to 20–40%[31]. With the aim of establishing a non-invasive animal model burdened with a significant mortality, in 1984 Mizu-

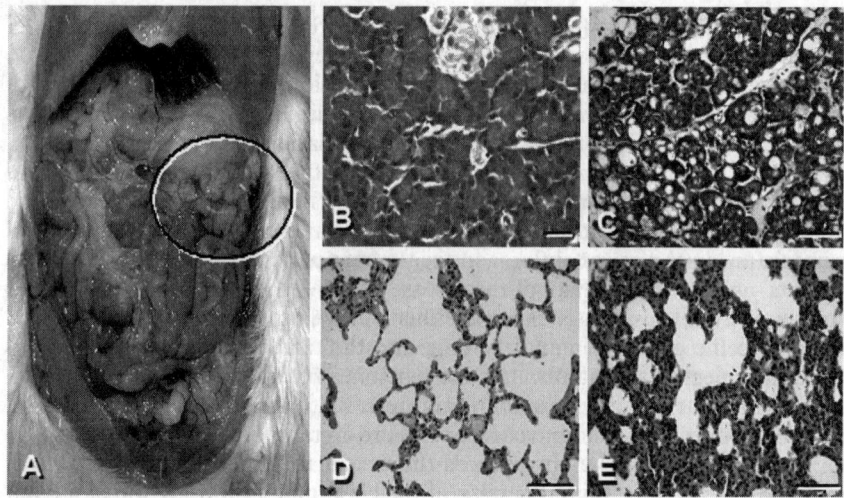

Figure 1 **A**: The macroscopic findings of the pancreas after supramaximal caerulein stimulation in rats. Note the gelatinous mass of the pancreas marked with a black circle, which comprised 90% water content. **B, C**: Light microscopy of pancreatic tissue: pancreatic tissue was fixed, embedded in paraffin wax and haematoxylin–eosin-stained. Note the development of interstitial oedema, the infiltration of inflammatory cells and the development of vacuoles in the animals treated with supramaximal concentrations of caerulein (C). **B**: Tissue section from control animals. **D, E**: Light microscopy of lung tissue. Lung tissue was fixed, embedded in paraffin wax and haematoxylin–eosin-stained. The morphological changes in the lungs of animals with caerulein-induced pancreatitis consisted of alveolar fluid accumulation and a progressive thickening, hyperaemia and neutrophil infiltration of the interalveolar tissue. **D**: Lung tissue from a control animal

numa et al. developed a new type of experimental pancreatitis by intraperitoneal administration of high concentrations of L-arginine in rats[32]. In subsequent studies it was shown that L-arginine leads, in a dose-dependent manner, to acinar cell necrosis of up to 100%. At 24 h after the first intraperitoneal injection the pancreas doubles its weight and ultrastructural examinations reveal partial distension of the endoplasmatic reticulum. At 48 h after the onset of pancreatitis dissociation and necrosis of acinar cells was noted. Subsequently necrotic cells are replaced by interstitial tissue composed of leukocytes and fibroblasts[33–35]. The mechanism by which L-arginine causes pancreatitis is not fully understood, and so far the crucial question of whether excessive concentrations applied intraperitoneally cause premature intracellular zymogen activation is not solved. Several reports suggest that oxygen-free radicals, nitric oxide and inflammatory mediators might play a key role. Long-term administration of L-arginine for 30 days induces pancreatic atrophy with exocrine pancreatic insufficiency resembling the clinical picture of chronic pancreatitis[36].

Choline-deficient/ethionine-containing diet

Acute haemorrhagic necrotizing pancreatitis, first reported in 1939, can be induced by the administration of a choline-deficient/ethionine-supplemented (CDE) diet to young female mice[37,38]. The animals develop haemorrhagic necrosis of the pancreas with a lethal course within 5 days[39]. The mortality rate can be titrated between 0% and 100% by the duration of diet feeding. Oestrogens and/or a reduced capacity to neutralize active pancreatic enzymes probably mediate the sex differences in the response to the dietary regime[40]. Feeding only ethionine in mice, rats and dogs leads to acute oedematous pancreatitis but no signs of necrosis. This variant of the disease usually leads to acinar cell regeneration and the deposition of fibrotic tissue. Similar to the pathophysiological mechanism of caerulein hyperstimulation feeding of a CDE diet leads to blockage of zymogen secretion and the fusion of zymogen granules and lysosomes, which are retained in the cytoplasm[41,42]. This leads to premature intracellular zymogen activation and this supported, for the first time, the hypothesis of autodigestion of the gland put forward by Hans Chiari in 1896 in an animal model[1]. The underlying signalling mechanism was investigated by the group of Steer et al.. Their observations indicated that the CDE diet interferes with stimulus-secretion coupling in mouse pancreatic acini at a step subsequent to hormone-receptor binding and prior to Ca^{2+} release. This conclusion was confirmed by the finding that the hormone-stimulated generation of [^{3}H]inositol phosphates (inositol trisphosphate, inositol bisphosphate, and inositol monophosphate) from acini labelled with [^{3}H]inositol phosphates is markedly reduced in acini prepared from mice fed the CDE diet. This reduction is not due to a decrease in phosphatidylinositol-4,5-bisphosphate[43]. Most interesting for this model is the large extent of acinar cell damage compared to ductal cells and islet of Langerhans. The underlying cause of this phenomenon has so far not been studied in an experimental approach.

In conclusion the CDE diet feeding model of acute necrotizing pancreatitis in young female mice shares similarities with the clinical course of pancreatitis in humans. Diet-induced pancreatitis shows a lengthy time-course which resembles the human disease better than other, usually rapidly progressive, experimental models, and the biochemical course and the gross and histological appearance of pancreatic inflammation correspond closely to the human disease. This model is therefore suitable for studying necrotizing pancreatitis as well as the efficacy of new therapeutic substances by assessing survival, biochemical and histological features.

Immune-induced acute pancreatitis

Animal models which are based on immunological mechanisms are either invasive or non-invasive. In 1954 Thal and Brackney reported that when *Escherichia coli* or meningococcal toxin was injected into the pancreatic duct of goats and rabbits, and 24 h later the same toxin was applied intravenously, a haemorrhagic form of necrotizing pancreatitis interpreted as a local Shwartzman reaction was observed[44]. Subsequently the authors of this study reported on necrotizing and edematous pancreatitis as a result of the Arthus phenomenon[45]. First the animals were sensitized by subcutaneous application of ovalbumin and later ovalbumin was injected into the pancreatic duct. The underlying pathophysiological mechanism which leads to the clinical picture of pancreatitis is most likely determined by vascular factors[46]. Pancreatitis can also be induced by intraperitoneal application of serum samples from different animal species. The clinical picture of a septic shock syndrome characterizes this animal model, and one can speculate that the interaction between serum complement factors and the acinar cell membrane induces a cytotoxic immune response which leads to pancreatitis. Since experiments with these models have a limited specificity, and are mainly based on a generalized immunological response, and they face difficulties inducing a graded response, as well as the fact that induction is technically difficult, they have found limited acceptance. In addition, the high mortality rate in most experiments makes investigations addressing the pathogenesis or treatment difficult. Clinically relevant information can probably only be derived from early drug- or toxin-induced acute pancreatitis. The clinical relevance of this model, however, remains doubtful. Recent advances in our knowledge concerning autoimmune pancreatitis is likely to lead to the development of clinically more relevant models.

INVASIVE MODELS

Invasive animal models of acute pancreatitis mainly mimic biliary pancreatitis. Until today three different hypotheses, which try to explain how the impaction of a gallstone in the common bile duct leads to the development of pancreatitis, have been controversially discussed:

1. The impaction of a gallstone at the papilla Vateri causes obstruction not only of the common bile duct but also of the pancreatic duct. Behind the impacted stone a common channel is created which allows bile to enter the pancreatic duct. This hypothesis is simulated by retrograde injection of bile or bile salts into the pancreatic duct[3,47,48].

2. The impacted stone causes mechanical obstruction of the main pancreatic duct, which subsequently increases duct pressure, which in turn leads to blockage of secretion and damage to pancreatic acinar cells and ductal cells. In most animal models that make use of this hypothesis the main pancreatic duct is surgically ligated[48]. The pancreatic duct obstruction leads to mild acute pancreatitis, as recently shown by our group[49,50].

3. The third hypothesis predicts that the passage of a gallstone through the sphincter of Oddi leads to transient or permanent sphincter insufficiency and therefore retrograde influx of duodenal secretion into the pancreatic duct. Recent studies from our own group have excluded this mechanism as the underlying cause of human acute pancreatitis[50,51].

Duct infusion/injection modes

In 1856 Claude Bernard, the father of French physiology, injected olive oil and later bile into the pancreatic main duct of a dog, which resulted in an episode of acute necrotizing pancreatitis[52]. Since that time numerous combinations of bile and activated proteases have been tested for their ability to induce acute necrotizing pancreatitis after injection into the duct of Wirsung. Some evidence suggests that pancreatic lipase might be actively involved in the destruction of the pancreas in this model[53]. The major limitation of this model is that not only the toxic effect of the solutions injected affects the development of acute pancreatitis, but several other factors influence its severity, which limits its reproducibility. Even non-toxic substances such as saline can induce the disruption of cell junctions and damage of acinar cell membrane if injected at a sufficiently high pressure[54]. To prevent any pressure-related damage it is a prerequisite for any model to apply a constant low pressure and inject compounds over a predetermined time period. Moreover, there are differences in the composition of the bile salts injected which influence the severity of the animal model. Several studies show that non-conjugated bile salts display an 8 times higher toxicity compared to chenodeoxycholic acid and deoxycholic acid[55]. Combinations of bile salts with trypsin or pancreatic juice increases the severity of the disease[56]. The infusion of sodium taurocholate has been best standardized and characterized. Injection of 0.2 ml of a 3%, 4.5% or 5% sodium taurocholate solution into the duct of Wirsung leads to a mortality of 0%, 23.5% or 71% over the following 72 h. The development of acute necrotizing pancreatitis is associated with mild-oedema in the animals treated with saline, and involves severe pancreatic necrosis in the taurocholate groups. Most likely the toxic effect of sodium taurocholate on pancreatic acinar cells is mediated by its detergenic effect which dissolves the lipid bilayer membrane. Whether this effect mimics any pathophysiological conditions in humans is doubtful. We have reasons to believe that the pressure in the pancreatic duct is higher than that in the common bile duct and therefore reflux into the duct of Wirsung seems unlikely[57]. Furthermore, we were able to disprove Opie's second hypothesis which suggested that reflux of bile into the main pancreatic duct is responsible for the development of acute pancreatitis[51,58].

A different approach was established by Reber and his group, who used a prograde injection of toxic mediators such as ethanol or aspirin followed by activated pancreatic proteases into the main pancreatic duct[59]. In this animal model of oedematous pancreatitis in cats the toxic solutions were infused via a catheter placed into the main duct via the pancreatic tail. The advantage of this model is that the pressure applied on the pancreatic duct epithelium does not exceed a physiological range (20 cmH$_2$O). In addition the model can be converted into a model of haemorrhagic necrotizing pancreatitis by the application of prostaglandin E2[60]. The Reber model has not been adopted by many researchers to study acute pancreatitis, but has its place for the investigation of chronic pancreatitis.

Pancreatic duct ligation

Several clinical conditions such as gallstones, motility dysfunction of the sphincter of Oddii, inflammatory oedema or adenoma of the papilla Vateri, as well as parasites, can cause a complete or partial obstruction of the duct of Wirsung. Temporal obstruction of the pancreatic duct in rats and rabbits produces mild interstitial pancreatic oedema, while ligation of the common biliopancreatic duct in rats induces early pancreatitis, posthepatic obstructive jaundice and a clinical syndrome similar to multi-organ failure seen in humans[61]. The ultra-structural analysis of this model confirms the development of pancreatic oedema, inflammatory infiltrates, and considerable dilation of the small pancreatic duct, combined with structural damage to the acinar cell membrane[62]. This model mimics several early events of acute pancreatitis in humans. In the opossum, ligation of both ducts results in haemorrhagic necrotizing pancreatitis associated with a 14-day mortality rate of 100%[63]. Furthermore, as the pancreaticobiliary anatomy of the opossum is very similar to that in humans this model has been used to study the pathophysiology of acute biliary pancreatitis. It is therefore not surprising that the essential finding that pancreatitis begins in acinar cells and not, as previously proposed, in the periductular or perilobular space, was made in this model[3]. In addition we were able to demonstrate in this model that bile reflux into the pancreatic duct, via a common biliopancreatic channel, is not reqired for the development of pancreatitis due to gallstones[51,64,65]. Duct ligation models are easy to perform and avoid the addition of artificial agents. Nevertheless, while duct ligation models have demonstrated that impairment of pancreatic secretion, rather than a theoretical reflux of bile into the pancreatic duct, triggers gallstone pancreatitis, an unphysiological pressure in the pancreatic duct may still serve as a pathogenetic factor[65] (Figure 2).

Closed duodenal loop

As early as in 1910 Seidel and co-workers developed the closed duodenal loop technique as one of the first experimental models for acute necrotizing pancreatitis[66]. In this experimental setting in mongrel dogs the first 10 cm of the duodenum distal to the pylorus were mobilized and the common bile duct ligated. Therefore only the main pancreatic duct communicated with the blind loop. Subsequently a gastroduodenostomy was performed to bypass the blind duodenal loop. After 4 h oedematous swelling of the pancreatic head and body was observed, and haemorrhagic pancreatitis developed during the next 9–12 h. The pathophysiological hypothesis of this model was based on the idea that the duodenal loop is overdistended and that brush-border-activated proteases will reflux into the main pancreatic duct[67]. This model has been utilized in numerous studies on a number of animal species and has undergone a variety of modifications, such as additional ligation of the pancreatic duct, performing gastrojejunostomy and insertion of a bypass cannula (Herrera fistula); restoration of the continuity of the gastrointestinal tract with an intraduodenal tube before ligating the duodenal loop under pressure; and temporary occlusion of the duodenum and the common bile duct for 2 min with administration of

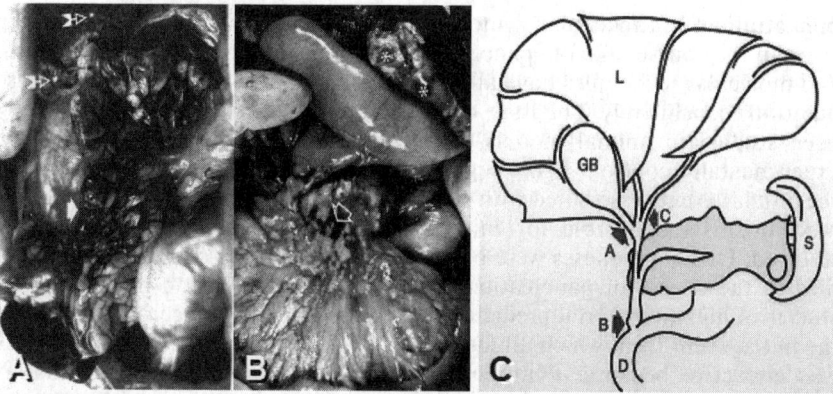

Figure 2 Experimental pancreatitis induced by pancreatic duct ligation in the American opossum. Early macroscopic changes can be observed after 24 h (**A**) and consist of haemorrhage (filled arrow) and extrapancreatic fat necrosis (winged arrows). After 7 days (**B**) pancreatic parenchymal necrosis is extensive (asterisks) and also involves the mesentery (open arrow). The advantages of the opossum model include its anatomy which permits testing of the various hypotheses that have been proposed to explain gallstone pancreatitis. These ducts can be ligated separately, such as the cystic duct (**A**), the common pancreatic–bile duct (**B**), and the bile duct without the pancreatic duct (**C**)

sodium taurocholate and trypsin intraluminally[68,69]. The closed duodenal loop model has mainly been used to clarify the aetiology of acute pancreatitis. Various degrees of severity of acute pancreatitis can be mimicked in this model, and it was therefore also used to test new treatment strategies. However, the main focus in investigating the model of the closed duodenal loop was to determine the pathophysiological role of duodenal reflux for the development of acute pancreatitis. Recent studies by our own group have shown that duodenal reflux is not an event required or associated with human gallstone-induced pancreatitis[51]. The disadvantages of this model are clear: the surgical intervention not only causes SIRS by itself but the pressure applied on the pancreatic duct far exceeds physiological conditions, and the model shares the problems of pancreatitis induction by sodium taurocholate.

FROM ANIMAL EXPERIMENTS TO CLINICAL USE – FROM BENCH TO BEDSIDE

Protective or dangerous proteases

About a century ago the pathologist Hans Chiari suggested that the pancreas of patients who had died during episodes of acute necrotizing pancreatitis 'had succumbed to its own digestive properties', and he postulated that pancreatic 'autodigestion' is the underlying pathophysiological mechanism of the disease[1]. Since then many attempts have been made to prove or disprove the role of premature and intracellular zymogen activation as an initial or an initiating event in the course of acute pancreatitis. Only recent advances in biochemical and molecular techniques have allowed investigators to address some of these questions conclusively. The issue of premature protease activation has mostly been studied in animal models of the disease[2,24,25]. These models can be experimentally controlled, are highly reproducible and recapitulate many of the cellular events associated with clinical disease. Issues relating to the site and mechanisms responsible for initiating pancreatitis have not been easily resolved. Early hypotheses were based on autopsy studies of patients who had died in the course of pancreatitis. An early theory based on morphological studies of human material predicted that peripancreatic fat necrosis represents the initial event from which all later alterations are derived[70]. This hypothesis was attractive because it implicated pancreatic lipase, an enzyme that is secreted from acinar cells in its active form and does not require activation by brush-border hydrolases, as the culprit for pancreatic necrosis. Another hypothesis suggested that periductular cells represent the site of initial damage, and that the extravasation of pancreatic juice from the ductal system was responsible for initiating the disease[4]. Subsequent controlled studies performed in animal models that simulate human disease have demonstrated that the acinar cell is the initial site of morphological damage[3]. This conclusion has been supported by genetic studies that linked the hereditary form of pancreatitis to mutations in the trypsinogen gene[71,72]. Trypsinogen and other pancreatic proteases are synthesized in the acinar cell as inactive proenzyme precursors (zymogens) and stored in membrane-bound zymogen granules. However, premature activation of large amounts of trypsinogen can overwhelm these protective mechanisms. This may lead to damage of zymogen-confining membrane and release of activated zymogens into the cytosol. Moreover, release of large amounts of calcium from the zymogen granule into the cytosol may activate calcium-dependent proteases such as calpains that contribute to cell injury. The suggestion that zymogen activation plays a central role in the pathogenesis of pancreatitis is based on the following observations: (a) pancreatic trypsin and elastase activities both increase early in the course of experimental pancreatitis[5,6]; (b) the activation peptides of trypsinogen and carboxypeptidase A_1 (PCA$_1$), which are cleaved from the respective proenzyme during the process of activation, are released into the serum early in the course of acute pancreatitis[73]; (c) serine protease inhibitors reduce injury in experimental pancreatitis[74,75]; and (d) forms of the hereditary variety of pancreatitis associated with mutations in the trypsinogen gene that could render trypsinogen more prone to premature activation or may render active trypsin more resistant to degradation by other proteases[76,77]. These observations, mostly derived from different animal models and investigations employing isolated pancreatic acini, provide compelling evidence that the premature and intracellular zymogen activation plays a critical role in initiating acute pancreatitis.

A number of recent studies involving patients have made therapeutic use of this concept and greatly contributed to understanding the role of zymogen activation in pancreatitis. A clinical trial in which a small molecular weight protease inhibitor (41.7 kDa) was administered to patients before they underwent ERCP reduced the incidence of ERCP-related pancreatitis[78]. Although protease inhibitors have been shown to be ineffective when used therapeutically in patients with clinically established pancreatitis[79], the result of the ERCP study suggests that the activation of pancreatic proteases is an inherent feature of the onset of the disease, and that its prevention can potentially lower the incidence of pancreatitis. In this multicentre double-blind placebo-controlled trial, conducted by Cavallini et al., gabexate was applicated for the prevention of post-ERCP pancreatitis in 418 patients. Gabexate (ethyl-guanidine-hexanol-oxy-dibenzoate-methyl-sodium-sulphonate) is a protease inhibitor with broad-spectrum inhibitor capacity with effects on trypsin, kallikrein, plasmin, α_2-macroglobulin, thrombin and antithrombin III, phospholipase A2 and C1-esterase. Sixteen patients in the placebo group and only five in the gabexate treatment group developed acute pancreatitis. This study gave evidence that prophylactic anti-proteatic treatment is effective in reducing pancreatic damage related to ERCP[78-80]. This report might function as one example in which a pathophysiological hypothesis was evaluated in several animal models and found its way from bench to bedside as a treatment option for the prevention of post-ERCP pancreatitis.

Immunomodulatory therapy

A change in the understanding of the pathophysiology of acute pancreatitis occurred with the suggestion that the initial phase of severe acute pancreatitis depends on neutrophil activation, accompanied by the systemic inflammatory response syndrome (SIRS)[81-83]. Platelet-activating factor (PAF) was implicated as playing an important role as a proinflammatory cytokine for the development of SIRS. PAF is involved not only via increasing the vascular permeability, by inducing leucocyte infiltration, oedema and tissue injury, but also has a negative inotropic effect. This made PAF a particularly promising target for the therapy of acute pancreatitis as its administration was shown to induce acute experimental pancreatitis, and PAF antagonist ameliorated the severity of acute pancreatitis in several models of the disease. Lexipafant is a potent PAF inhibitor for which therapeutic administration in a phase II trial enrolling 133 patients showed a significant improvement in organ failure scores[84,85]. Subsequently a multicentre, double-blind, placebo-controlled, randomized parallel-group phase III study was designed, and as primary objective the frequency of systemic or local complications in a patient cohort of 290 patients after lexipafant treatment during the first 72 h after the onset of pain due to acute pancreatitis was evaluated. To the authors' surprise the adequately powered study showed that the inhibition of PAF activity by itself was not sufficient to ameliorate SIRS in severe acute pancreatitis. As an explanation why the study failed to demonstrate its primary endpoint the investigators stated that patients admitted to the participating hospitals already suffered from established organ failure, which made this primary endpoint unemployable[86]. In contrast to the gabexate trial for the prevention of ERCP pancreatitis the lexipafant trial illustrates that even carefully conducted animal studies, as well as a promising concept, cannot necessarily predict a beneficial effect in a clinical trial.

CONCLUSION

No model is entirely appropriate to re-create all events causing and characterizing acute pancreatitis in humans. It is equally impossible to study either the initial subcellular events in a model of fulminant severity, or the pathogenesis of necrosis in a self-limiting mild model, or the validity of treatment in a model of irreversible pancreatic damage. However, when appropriate models are chosen to address specific cell biological, pathophysiological or clinical questions regarding pancreatitis they are an extremely useful and quite irreplaceable tools for pancreatic research. Whether a treatment modality found beneficial in an animal model of pancreatitis will find its way into clinical practice, even after the most careful selection of the appropriate model, will always have to be determined in controlled, preferably multicentre clinical trials.

References

1. Chiari H. Über die Selbstverdauung des menschlichen Pankreas. Z Heilk 17, 69–96, 1896
2. Gorelick FS, Adler G, Kern HF: Cerulein-induced pancreatitis. In: Go GVLW, Di Magno EP, Gardner JD, Lebenthal E, Reber HA, Scheele, GA, editors. The Pancreas: Biology, Pathobiology, and Disease. New York: Raven Press, 1993:501–26.
3. Lerch MM, Saluja AK, Runzi M, Dawra R, Saluja M, Steer ML. Acute necrotising pancreatitis in the opossum: earliest morphologic changes involve acinar cells. Gastroenterology. 1992;103:205–13.
4. Foulis AK. Histological evidence of initiating factors in acute necrotizing pancreatitis in man. J Clin Pathol. 1980;33:1125–31.
5. Bialek R, Willemer S, Arnold R, Adler G. Evidence of intracellular activation of serine proteases in acute cerulein-induced pancreatitis in rats. Scand J Gastroenterol. 1991;26: 190–6.
6. Luthen R, Niederau C, Grendell JH. Intrapancreatic zymogen activation and levels of ATP and glutathione during caerulein pancreatitis in rats. Am J Physiol. 1995;268:G592–604.
7. Rinderknecht H. Activation of pancreatic zymogens. Normal activation, premature intrapancreatic activation, protective mechanisms against inappropriate activation. Dig Dis Sci. 1986;31:314–21.
8. Mouret J. Contribution á l'etude des cellules glandulaires (pancreas). J Anat Physiol. 1895; 31:221-36.
9. Adler G, Gerhards G, Schick J, Rohr G, Kern HF. Effects of in vivo cholinergic stimulation of rat exocrine pancreas. Am J Physiol. 1983;244:G623–9.
10. Niederau C, Ferrell LD, Grendell JH. Caerulein-induced acute necrotizing pancreatitis in mice: protective effects of proglumide, benzotript, and secretin. Gastroenterology. 1985;88: 1192–204.
11. Saluja A, Saito I, Saluja M et al. In vivo rat pancreatic acinar cell function during supramaximal stimulation with caerulein. Am J Physiol. 1985;249:G702–10.
12. Watanabe O, Baccino FM, Steer ML, Meldolesi J. Supramaximal caerulein stimulation and ultrastructure of rat pancreatic acinar cell: early morphological changes during development of experimental pancreatitis. Am J Physiol. 1984;246:G457–67.
13. Pantoja JL, Renner IG, Abramson SB, Edmondson HA. Production of acute hemorrhagic pancreatitis in the dog using venom of the scorpion, Buthus quinquestriatus. Dig Dis Sci. 1983;28:429–39.
14. Ji B, Bi Y, Simenone D, Mortensen RM, Logsdon CD. Human pancreatic acinar cells do not respond to cholecystokinin. Pharmacol Toxicol. 2002;91:327–32.
15. Lampel M, Kern HF. Acute interstitial pancreatitis in the rat induced by excessive doses of a pancreatic secretagogue. Virchows Arch Pathol Anat Histol. 1977;373:97–117.
16. Scheele G, Palade G. Studies on the pancreas of the guinea pig – parallel discharge of exocrine enzyme activities. J Biol Chem. 1975;250:2660–70.

17. Lerch MM, Albrecht E, Ruthenburger M, Mayerle J, Halangk W, Kruger B. Pathophysiology of alcohol-induced pancreatitis. Pancreas. 2003;27:291–6.
18. Lerch MM, Lutz MP, Weidenbach H et al. Dissociation and reassembly of adherens junctions during experimental acute pancreatitis. Gastroenterology. 1997;113:1355–66.
19. Lerch MM, Saluja AK, Runzi M, Dawra R, Steer ML. Luminal endocytosis and intracellular targeting by acinar cells during early biliary pancreatitis in the opossum. J Clin Invest. 1995;95:2222–31.
20. Lerch MM, Saluja AK, Dawra R, Saluja M, Steer ML. The effect of chloroquine administration on two experimental models of acute pancreatitis. Gastroenterology. 1993; 104:1768–79.
21. Adler G, Rohr G, Kern HF. Alteration of membrane fusion as a cause of acute pancreatitis in the rat. Dig Dis Sci. 1982;27:993–1002.
22. Jungermann J, Lerch MM, Weidenbach H, Lutz MP, Kruger B, Adler G. Disassembly of rat pancreatic acinar cell cytoskeleton during supramaximal secretagogue stimulation. Am J Physiol. 1995;268:G328–38.
23. Halangk W, Lerch MM, Brandt-Nedelev B et al. Role of cathepsin B in intracellular trypsinogen activation and the onset of acute pancreatitis. J Clin Invest. 2000;106:773–81.
24. Lerch MM, Adler G. Experimental pancreatitis. Curr Opin Gastroenterol. 1993;9:752–9.
25. Lerch MM, Adler G. Experimental animal models of acute pancreatitis. Int J Pancreatol. 1994;15:159–70.
26. Lerch MM, Halangk W, Krüger B. The role of cysteine proteases in intracellular pancreatic serine protease activation. Adv Exp Med Biol. 2000;477:403–11.
27. Mooren F, Turi S, Günzel D et al. Calcium-magnesium interactions in pancreatic acinar cells. FASEB J. 2001;15:660–72.
28. Krüger B, Weber IA, Albrecht E, Mooren FC, Lerch MM. Effect of hyperthermia on premature intracellular trypsinogen activation in the exocrine pancreas. Biochem Biophys Res Comm. 2001;282:159–65.
29. Halangk W, Krüger B, Ruthenbürger M, Stürzebecher J, Lippert H, Lerch M. The role of trypsin in premature, intrapancreatic trypsinogen activation and inactivation of trypsin activity. Am J Physiol Gastrointest Liver Physiol. 2002;282:G367–74.
30. Lerch MM, Albrecht E, Ruthenburger M, Mayerle J, Halangk W, Kruger B. Pathophysiology of alcohol-induced pancreatitis. Pancreas. 2003;27:291–6.
31. Mayerle J, Simon P, Lerch MM. Medical management of acute pancreatitis. Gastroclin N Am. 2004 (In press).
32. Mizunuma T, Kawamura S, Kishino Y. Effects of injecting excess arginine on rat pancreas. J Nutr. 1984;114:467–71.
33. Tani S, Itoh H, Okabayashi Y et al. New model of acute necrotizing pancreatitis induced by excessive doses of arginine in rats. Dig Dis Sci. 1990;35:367–74.
34. Delaney CP, Mc Greeney KF, Dervan P, Fitzpatrick JM. Pancreatic atrophy: new model using serial intraperitoneal injections of L-arginine. Scand J Gastroenterol. 1993;28:1086–90.
35. Weaver C, Bishop AE, Polak JM. Pancreatic changes elicited by chronic administration of excess L-arginine. Exp Mol Pathol. 1994;84:147–56.
36. Hegyi P, Rakonczay Z, Sari R et al. L-Arginine-induced experimental pancreatitis. World J Gastroenterol. 2004;10:2003–9.
37. Griffith WH, Wade NJ. The occurrence and prevention of hemorrhagic degeneration in young rats on a low choline diet. J Biol Chem. 1938;131:567–77.
38. De Almeida AL, Grossman MI. Experimental production of pancreatitis with ethionine. Gastroenterology. 1952;20:554–77.
39. Lombardi B, Estes LW, Longecker DS. Acute hemorrhagic (massive necrosis) with fat necrosis induced in mice with DL-ethionine fed with a choline deficient diet. Am J Pathol. 1975;79:465–80.
40. Niederau C, Luthen R, Niederau MC, Grendell JH, Ferrell LD. Acute experimental hemorrhagic pancreatitis induced by feeding a choline-deficient, ethionine-supplemented diet. Methodology and standards. Eur Surg Res. 1992;24:40–54.
41. Gilliland L, Steer ML. Effects of ethionine on digestive enzyme synthesis and discharge by mouse pancreas. Am J Physiol. 1980;239:G418–26.
42. Rao KN, Eagon PK, Okamura K et al. Acute hemorrhagic pancreatic necrosis in mice. Induction in male mice treated with estradiol. Am J Pathol. 1982;109:8–14.

43. Leli U, Saluja A, Picard L, Zavertnik A, Steer ML. Effects of choline-deficient ethionine-supplemented diet on phospholipase activity in mouse pancreatic acinar cell membranes and electropermeabilized mouse pancreatic acini. J Pharmacol Exp Ther. 1990;253:847–50.
44. Thal A, Brackney E. Acute hemorrhagic pancreatic necrosis produced by local Shwartzman reaction. J Am Med Assoc. 1954;155:569–74.
45. Janigan DT, Nevalainen TJ, MacAulay MA, Vethmany VG. Foreign serum induced pancreatitis in mice. A new model of pancreatitis. Lab Invest. 1975;33:591–607.
46. Nevalainen TJ, Fowlie FE, Janigan DT. Foreign serum induced pancreatitis in mice. Secretory disturbances in acinar cells. Lab Invest. 1977;36:469–73.
47. Opie EL The etiology of acute hemorrhagic pancreatitis. Johns Hopkins Hosp Bull. 1901;12:182–8.
48. Opie EL, The relation of cholelithiasis to disease of the pancreas and to fat-necrosis. Johns Hopkins Hosp Bull. 1901;12:19–21.
49. Mooren FCh, Hlouschek V, Finkes T et al. Early changes in pancreatic acinar cell calcium signaling after pancreatic duct obstruction. J Biol Chem. 2003;278:9361–9.
50. Stone HH, Fabian TC, Dunlop WE. Gallstone pancreatitis: biliary tract pathology in relation to time of operation. Ann Surg. 1981;194:305–10.
51. Hernandez CA, Lerch MM. Sphincter stenosis and gallstone migration through the biliary tract. Lancet. 1993;341:1371–3.
52. Bernard C. Lecons de Physiologie Experimental. Paris: Baillière, 1856;2:278.
53. Nagai H, Heinrich H, Wünsch PH, Fischbach W, Mössner J. Role of pancreatic enymes and their substrates in autodigestion of the pancreas. Gastroenterology. 1989;96:838–47.
54. Arendt T. Bile induced acute pancreatitis in cats; roles of bile, bacteria and pancreatic duct pressure. Dig Dis Sci. 1993;38:39–44.
55. Hansson K. Experimental and clinical studies in the aetiological role of bile reflux in acute pancreatitis. Acta Chir Scand. 1967;375:1–102.
56. Schmidt J, Rattner DW, Lewandrowski K et al. A better model of acute pancreatitis for evaluating therapy. Ann Surg. 1992;215:44–56.
57. Carr-Locke D, Gregg JA. Endoscopic manometry of pancreatic and biliary sphincter zones in man. Dig Dis Sci. 1981;26:7–15.
58. Whitrock RM, Hine D, Crane J, McCorkel HJ. The effect of bile flow through the pancreas. Surgery. 1955;38:122–33.
59. Reber HA, Robert C, Way LW. The pancreatic duct mucosal barrier. Am J Surg. 1979; 137:128–34.
60. Wedgewood DR, Framer RC, Reber HA. A model of hemorrhagic pancreatitis in rats – the role of 16-dimethyl prostaglandin E2. Gastroenterology. 1986;90:32–9.
61. Oshio G, Saluja A, Steer ML. Effects of short-term pancreatic duct obstruction in rats. Gastroenterology. 1991;100:196–202.
62. Senninger N, Moody FG, Coelho JC, Van Buren DH. The role of biliary obstruction in the pathogenesis of acute pancreatitis in the opossum. Surgery. 1986;99:688–93.
63. Schiller WR, Suryapa C, Anderson MC. A review of experimental pancreatitis. J Surg Res. 1974;16:69–90.
64. Lerch MM, Weidenbach H, Hernandez CA, Preclik G, Adler G. Pancreatic outflow obstruction as the critical event for human gall stone induced pancreatitis. Gut. 1994;35: 1501–3.
65. Lerch MM, Hernandez CA, Adler G. Gallstones and acute pancreatitis–mechanisms and mechanics. Dig Dis. 1994;12:242–7.
66. Seidel H. Bemerkungen zu meiner Methode der experimentellen Erzeugung der akuten hämorhagischen Pankreatitis. Zentralbl Chir. 1910.
67. Pfeffer RB, Stasio O, Hinton JW. The clinical picture of the sequential development of hemorrhagic pancreatitis in the dog. Surg Forum. 1957;8:248–51.
68. Paulino-Netto A, Dreiling DA. Chronic duodenal obstruction: a mechanovascular aetiology of pancreatitis. Dig Dis Sci. 1983;28:429–39.
69. De Rai P, Franciosi C, Confalonieri GM et al. Effects of somatostatin on acute pancreatitis induced in rats by injection of taurocholate and trypsin into a temporarily closed duodenal loop. Int J Pancreatol. 1988;3:367–73.
70. Kloppel G, Dreyer T, Willemer S, Kern HF, Adler G. Human acute pancreatitis: its pathogenesis in the light of immunocytochemical and ultrastructural findings in acinar cells. Virchows Arch A. 1986;409:791–803.

71. Whitcomb DC, Gorry MC, Preston RA et al. Hereditary pancreatitis is caused by a mutation on the cationic trypsinogen gene. Nat Genet. 1996;14:141–5.
72. Whitcomb DC. Genes means pancreatitis. Gut. 1999;44:150.
73. Schmidt J, Fernandez-del Castillo C, Rattner DW, Lewandrowski K, Compton CC, Warshaw AL. Trypsinogen-activation peptides in experimental rat pancreatitis: prognostic implications and histopathologic correlates. Gastroenterology. 1992;103:1009–16.
74. Lasson A, Ohlsson K. Protease inhibitors in acute pancreatitis: correlation between biochemical changes and clinical course. Scand J Gastroenterol. 1984;19:779–86.
75. Niederau C, Grendell JH. Intracellular vacuoles in experimental acute pancreatitis in rats and mice are an acidified compartment. J Clin Invest. 1988;81:229–36.
76. Gorry MC, Gabbaizedeh D, Furey W et al. Mutations in the cationic trypsinogen gene are associated with recurrent acute and chronic pancreatitis. Gastroenterology. 1997;113:1063–8.
77. Varallyay E, Pal G, Patthy A, Szilagyi L, Graf L. Two mutations in rat trypsin confer resistance against autolysis. Biochem Biophys Res Commun. 1998;243:56–60.
78. Cavallini G, Tittobello A, Frulloni L, Masci E, Mariana A, Di Francesco V. Gabexate for the prevention of pancreatic damage related to endoscopic retrograde cholangiopancreatography. N Engl J Med. 1996;335:919–23.
79. Masci E, Cavallini G, Mariani A et al. Gabexate in Digestive Endoscopy–Italian Group II. Comparison of two dosing regimens of gabexate in the prophylaxis of post-ERCP pancreatitis. Am J Gastroenterol. 2003;98:2182–6.
80. Buchler M, Malfertheiner P, Uhl W et al. Gabexate mesilate in human acute pancreatitis. German Pancreatitis Study Group. Gastroenterology. 1993;104:1165–70.
81. Rinderknecht H. Fatal pancreatitis, a consequence of excessive leukocyte stimulation? Int J Pancreatol. 1988;3:105–12.
82. Gross V, Leser HG, Heinisch A. Inflammatory mediators and cytokines – new aspects of the pathophysiology and assessment of severity of acute pancreatitis? Hepatogastroenterology. 1993;40:522–33.
83. Tenner S, Hughues M, Sica G. Relationship of necrosis to organ failure in severe acute pancreatitis. Gastroenterology. 1997;113:899–903.
84. Kingsnorth AN, Galloway SW, Formela LJ. Randomized double-blind phase II trial of lexipafant, a platelet activating factor antagonist, in human pancreatitis. Br J Surg. 1995;82:1414–20.
85. McKay C, Curran FJM, Sharples CE. Prospective placebo controlled randomized trial of lexipafant in predicted severe acute pancreatitis. Br J Surg. 1997;84:1239–43.
86. Johnson CD, Kingsnorth AN, Imrie CW et al. Double blind, randomized, placebo controlled study of a platelet activating factor antagonist lexipafant, in the treatment and prevention of organ failure in predicted severe acute pancreatitis. Gut. 2001;48:62–9.

Acute pancreatitis I

Section II
Clinical presentation, diagnosis, staging

Chair: C.D. JOHNSON and M.V. SINGER

3
Acute pancreatitis: epidemiology and aetiology

P. G. LANKISCH, P. MAISONNEUVE and A. B. LOWENFELS

PRELIMINARY REMARKS: EPIDEMIOLOGY

Data on the epidemiology of acute pancreatitis vary considerably. This may be explained by several factors:

1. Data concerning the epidemiology of acute pancreatitis are limited and only available from eight countries, which are mainly European (Table 1); therefore, little is known about the epidemiology of the disease in most of the world.

2. The time periods (Table 1), vary considerably among the reports, as well as the availability and/or the use of imaging procedures such as ultrasound or computed tomography. This may lead to an underestimation of the disease.

3. The reports come from different types of centres. This may have an influence not only on the incidence rate but also on the aetiology. An urban hospital is more likely to report on alcohol-induced pancreatitis, whereas a rural hospital is more likely to report on biliary pancreatitis.

4. Death certificates, as a basis for epidemiological studies, are unreliable.

5. The post-mortem ratios differ considerably. There are a substantial number of diagnoses that are made at post-mortem and not during the patient's lifetime (Table 2)[2,10]. This may also lead to an underestimation of the disease.

6. Referral rates differ from country to country. This is due to the criteria laid down by general practitioners and/or health insurance companies. A study from the Netherlands[20] showed that only 2% of patients who definitely had acute pancreatitis were not referred to hospital; thus, in hospital-based studies, due to non-referral, the incidence of acute pancreatitis will not be

Table 1 Overall incidence of acute pancreatitis in various countries, ranked according to the first year of assessment

Reference	Localization	Period	Incidence (10^5) population/year
Trapnell and Duncan[1]	Bristol, England	1961–1967	5.4
Corfield et al.[2]	Bristol, England	1968–1979	7.3
Tran and Schilfgaarde[3]	Netherlands	1971	6.5
	Netherlands	1990	10.2
Thomson[4]	North and NE Scotland	1968–1980	9.4
Giggs et al.[5]	Nottingham, England	1977–1983	11.7
Lankisch et al.[6]	Lüneburg, Germany	1988–1995	19.7
Thomson et al.[7]	NE Scotland	1983–1985	24.2
Worning[8]	Denmark	1981	26.8
		1990	35.4
McKay et al.[9]	Scotland	1984–1995	31.8
Appelros and Borgström[10]	Malmö, Sweden	1985–1994	23.4
Eland et al.[11]	Netherlands	1985	12.4
		1995	15.9
Go[12]	United States of America	1987	49.5
			79.8
Jaakkola and Nordback[13]	Finland	1970	46.6
		1989	73.4
Halvorsen and Ritland[14]	Buskerud, Norway	1992	41.5
Floyd et al.[15]	North Jutland, Denmark	1981	17.1–18.0
	North Jutland, Denmark	1999	27.1–37.8
Goldacre and Roberts[16]	Southern England	1973–1974	4.9
	Southern England	1975–1986	7.7
	Southern England	1987–1998	9.8

Table 2 Undetected fatal acute pancreatitis in different countries

Reference	Time period	Deceased patients (n)	Percentage of deceased of whom the diagnosis was made post-mortem
Corfield et al.[2]	1968–1979	125	35
Wilson and Imrie[17]	1974–1984	126	42
Lankisch et al.[18]	1980–1985	43	30
Mann et al.[19]	1988–1992	50	12
Appelros and Borgström[10]	1985–1994	31	52

underestimated. However, the diagnosis of acute pancreatitis made by general practitioners was, when checked, not substantiated in 24%, probable in 24%, and definite only in 53%.

7. Different centres use different diagnostic criteria. The 'usual suspects' for the diagnosis of acute pancreatitis are abdominal pain and increased serum enzyme levels. However, it is unclear what the enzyme levels should be, in order to diagnose or evaluate the severity of the disease. The current use of > 3 times the upper limit of normal as a cut-off point for pancreatic enzymes in the diagnosis of acute pancreatitis, can be misleading. We found that patients with only mildly increased amylase/lipase levels can also have or develop acute pancreatitis[21]. When patients were divided into two groups according to the serum enzyme levels (group 1 ≤3n; group 2 >3n), 31% (amylase) and 18% (lipase) were in the first group. However, there were no significant differences between groups with regard to organ failure, fluid collections/pseudocysts, an indication for a necrosectomy and mortality.

8. Finally, prognostic scores and/or classification systems for imaging procedures are not widely used; thus information on the severity of the disease is often lacking.

INCIDENCE RATE

The incidence rates of acute pancreatitis per 100 000 inhabitants/year differ considerably. Remarkably, it is high in all Scandinavian countries. In the United Kingdom it is higher in Scotland than in England (Table 1).

The increased incidence of acute pancreatitis was significantly correlated with alcohol consumption in the Netherlands[3] and in Finland[13]. It was also associated with an increase in male, but not in female patients, in Finland[13], Scotland[22], and Denmark[8].

However, a recent study from Denmark has shown that, between 1981 and 2000, there was an increased incidence of acute pancreatitis. During this time the incidence in women surpassed that in men. This was between 1999 and 2000 (incidence in male patients 1981, 18.0, in 2000, 17.1; in female patients 27.1 and 37.1, respectively, per 100 000 persons/year)[15]. The reasons for this change are unknown.

In Lüneburg County, where we performed the first epidemiological study in a well-defined German population, the incidence rate of acute pancreatitis was 19.7 per 100 000 inhabitants/year during the period from 1988 to 1995. This was more than three times higher than the same incidence for chronic pancreatitis (6.4)[6]. When incidence rates were plotted against age groups it was shown that acute pancreatitis noticeably peaked in men aged 35–44 years, followed by a similar peak for chronic pancreatitis in those aged 45–54. Although distinctly lower, there was an incidence peak for acute pancreatitis in women aged between 25 and 34, which was followed by a small peak for chronic pancreatitis in those who were 10 years older (Figure 1)[6]. In England, age-standardized hospital admission rates for acute pancreatitis rose by 43%

Incidence - Men

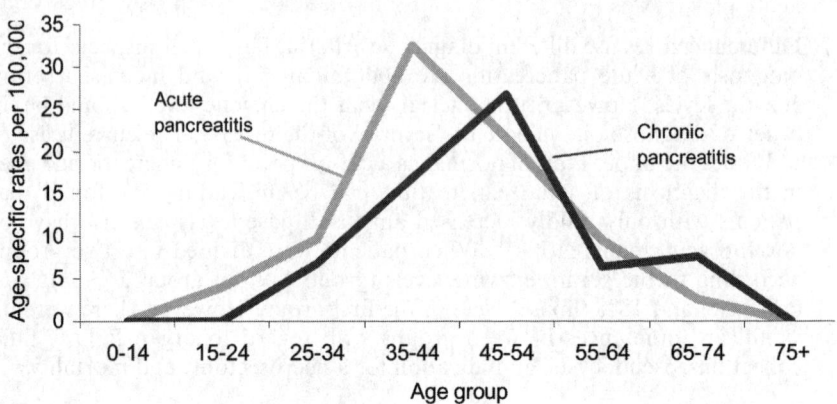

Incidence - Women

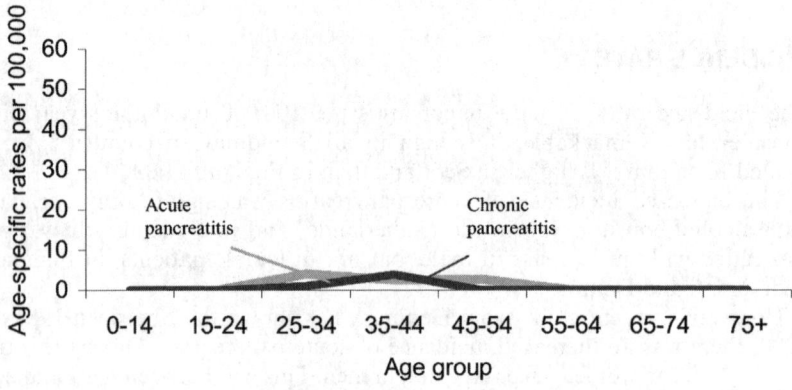

Figure 1 Age-specific incidence rates for acute pancreatitis by aetiology in Lüneburg County during 1988–1995[6]

between 1989/1990 and 1999/2000, whilst in the same period the incidence of chronic pancreatitis rose by 100%. Similarly, New York State reported a rise in the incidence of hospitalization for acute pancreatitis between 1991 and 2001[23]. This time interval may reflect either that chronic pancreatitis is the consequence of a necrosis–fibrosis sequence[24], or the development of pancreatic fibrosis without intermittent pancreatic necrosis. In each case it will probably take some time, and several attacks of acute pancreatitis, before chronic pancreatitis develops[25].

PRELIMINARY REMARKS: AETIOLOGY

Worldwide, biliary disease and alcohol abuse are the main aetiological factors for acute pancreatitis (Table 3)[1,2,4,6,7,10], but there are certain issues regarding these factors. It is unknown how much alcohol is needed to induce alcoholic pancreatitis, and the studies designed to assess the aetiology of the disease vary considerably. Some believe that >80 g alcohol/day for more than 5 years, or social or weekend abuse[44], is likely to induce acute pancreatitis. We consider alcohol abuse to be the cause of acute pancreatitis when the patient or the relatives report regular alcohol consumption of at least 60 g per day of pure alcohol in the form of beer, wine or schnapps, or when an excessive amount of alcohol has been consumed immediately before the attack. However, there are many other definitions.

In a study from Lüneburg County the crude incidence rates for alcoholic pancreatitis for men and women in the general population, between 1988 and 1995, were 10.1 and 1.3 per 100 000 inhabitants/year, respectively. However, the risk of developing acute pancreatitis, in heavy drinkers ($\geqslant$60 g alcohol/day) was almost the same for men and women: 91.5 versus 81.9 patients per 100 000 heavy drinkers/year. Over a 20- or 30-year period the risk of developing alcoholic pancreatitis in this group is unlikely to be more than 2–3%[45]. For the same period the crude incidence rates for biliary pancreatitis in the general population were 5.7 for men and 9.7 for women. However, the rate of biliary pancreatitis in male patients with gallstones was distinctly higher than that for female patients: 75.0 versus 58.1 per 100 000 inhabitants/year. These gender-related differences were especially apparent in the older individuals (Figure 2)[46]. Again, over a 20- or 30-year period, the risk of developing biliary pancreatitis in patients with asymptomatic gallstones is unlikely to be greater than 2%[46]. Therefore, the low frequency of pancreatitis among heavy drinkers and patients with gallstones implies that other as-yet-undetected environmental or genetic factors are important. In this context a study by Ramstedt[47], which examined alcohol and pancreatitis mortality in 14 countries, is interesting. Higher alcohol consumption was associated with a rise in pancreatitis mortality, whereas a decline was followed by lower pancreatitis death rates. Although not statistically significant, the effect of the same increase in alcohol consumption tended to be larger in northern Europe (not Finland) than in other parts of Europe and Canada, and increased by 25% per extra litre, compared with 9% in central Europe, 6% in southern Europe and 5% in Canada. Thus, there may be national differences regarding the importance of alcohol.

In another study Kratzer et al.[48] investigated the prevalence of gallstones in sonographic surveys worldwide. Astonishingly, the prevalence of gallstones in some countries, for example Sweden, is high, but in that country alcohol abuse has become the dominating aetiology of acute pancreatitis in recent years.

About 23 studies, each including more than 100 patients, have been published during the past three decades, with detailed data concerning gender distribution and the aetiology of acute pancreatitis (first attack) (Table 3). In 16 of these biliary disease was the dominating aetiology and in the remaining seven alcohol abuse. Based on these data, a map of Europe showing the

Table 3 Studies, each involving more than 100 patients, published during the past 3 decades, with detailed data concerning gender distribution and the aetiology of acute pancreatitis (first attack). Data from the incidence of idiopathic pancreatitis or pancreatitis due to other causes are not given as the definitions for these aetiological factors varied considerably between the studies

Reference and place of investigation	Period	Patients (n)	Men (%)	Women (%)	Aetiology (%) Biliary	Alcoholism
Renner et al.[26] Los Angeles	1949–1978	405	62.7	37.3	27.9	67.7
Trapnell and Duncan[1] Bristol	1950–1969	590	38.3	61.7	53.6	4.4
Edlund et al.[27] Göteborg	1956–1960	460	52.2	47.8	68.0	13.0
Imrie[28] Glasgow	1960–1970	140	47.8	52.2	50.0	12.2
Madsen and Schmidt[29] Copenhagen	1960–1970	122	68.8	31.2	14.0	40.0
Jacobs et al.[30] Boston	1963–1969	519	54.9	45.1	47.0	31.0
Satiani and Stone[31] Atlanta	1966–1975	389	59.9	40.1	3.1	91.8
Lukash[32] Bethesda	Not mentioned	100	82.0	18.0	23.0	66.0
Ong et al.[33] Hong Kong	1967–1976	311	39.5	60.5	52.4	15.1
Svensson et al.[34] Göteborg	1968–1969 1974–1975	105 204	83.0 77.0	17.0 23.0	20.0 26.0	68.0 66.0
Corfield et al.[2] Bristol	1968–1979	638	48.7	51.3	50.0	8.0
Thomson[4] Aberdeen	1968–1980	632	47.8	52.2	44.0	19.0
Ranson and Spencer[35] New York	1971–1977	450	78.0	22.0	16.0	70.0
Thomson et al.[7] Aberdeen	1983–1985	359	52.6	47.4	40.9	15.3
Fan et al.[36] Hong Kong	1983–1986	268	42.9	57.1	50.0	12.3
Fan et al.[37] Hong Kong	1988–1991	176	39.2	60.8	57.4	12.5
De Beaux et al.[38] Edinburgh	1989–1993	279	61.6	38.4	41.6	34.8
Lankisch et al.[39] Göttingen-Lüneburg	1980–1994	602	55.6	44.4	37.7	29.4
Appelros and Borgström[10] Malmö	1985–1994	547	58.1	41.9	38.4	31.8
Lankisch et al.[6] Lüneburg	1988–1995	228	59.6	40.4	40.0	32.0

Table 3   (continued)

Reference and place of investigation	Period	Patients (n)	Men (%)	Women (%)	Aetiology (%)	
					Biliary	Alcoholism
Chang et al.[40] Taiwan	1998–2000	1193	71.4	28.6	34.1	33.6
Uhl et al.[41] Bern/Ulm	Not mentioned	190	66.8	33.2	31.6	49.5
Pezzilli et al.[42] Bologna	1991–1995	158	58.2	41.8	70.9	16.5
Lindkvist et al.[43] Malmö	1985–1995	929	53.1	46.9	42.2	24.5
Total	1949–1995	7097	55.0	45.0	41.0	31.7

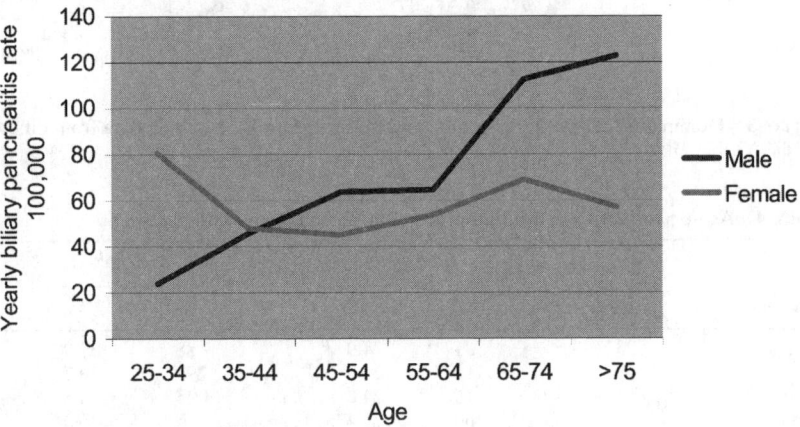

Figure 2   Estimated frequency of biliary acute pancreatitis in Lüneburg County during 1988–1995[46]

dominating aetiologies of acute pancreatitis in different countries reveals that alcohol is the prevailing cause in Sweden, Finland, northern France, and Hungary, whereas in the remaining countries biliary aetiology prevails (Figure 3).

However, these data should be viewed with caution. Five reports are from the United States. In four of them alcohol was the main cause, but in one it was biliary disease[26,35]. Three reports are from Sweden, one covering two different periods[34]. In the paper from Edlund et al.[27], and the more recent one from Lindkvist et al.[43], biliary disease was the dominating factor, whereas in the study from Svensson et al.[34], covering the periods from 1968–1969 and 1974–1975, alcohol was certainly the main aetiology. The study from Taiwan[40] shows

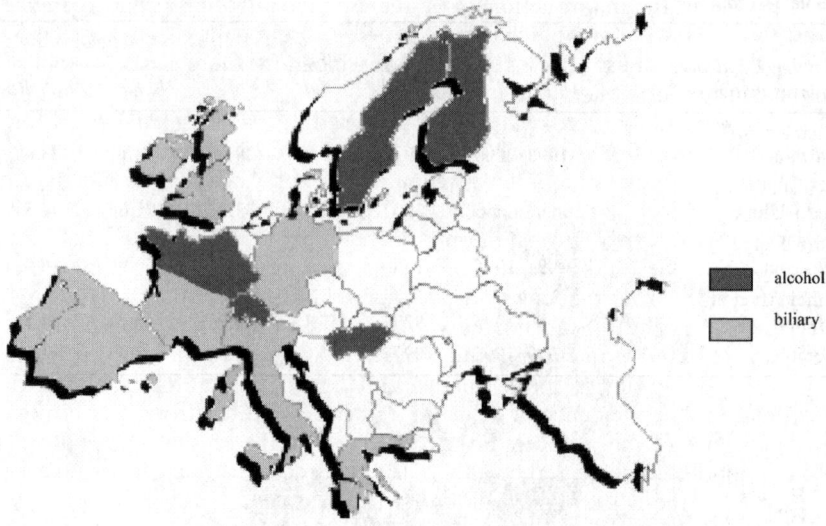

Figure 3 Dominating aetiologies of acute pancreatitis in Europe, based on data from different studies (Table 3)[1,2,4,6,7,10]

Table 4 Acute pancreatitis in five European countries: aetiology in 1068 patients[44]

Country	No. of patients	Gallstones		Alcohol	
		No.	(%)	No.	(%)
Germany	232	81	34.9	88	37.9
Hungary	483	116	24.0	293	60.7
France	65	16	24.6	25	38.5
Greece	84	60	71.4*	5	6.0*
Italy	204	123	60.3*	27	13.2*
Total	1068	396	37.1	438	41.0

*$p < 0.01$ versus the corresponding values of Germany, Hungary and France.

how difficult it is to define the aetiology of acute pancreatitis for one country. In this multi-centre study Taiwan was divided into the northern, middle, southern and eastern regions: in the northern region alcohol was the dominating factor, whereas in the other areas, gallstones were the main contributing factor.

More recently, Gullo et al.[44] designed a multi-centre study of 1068 patients from five European countries, who were admitted to hospital because of acute pancreatitis between January 1990 and December 1994. The aetiological factors varied considerably (Table 4)[44]. Gallstone disease was much more frequent in Greece and Italy compared to the corresponding values of Germany, Hungary and France[44]. The percentage dominance of one aetiological factor for acute pancreatitis may vary over the years.

A change in the major aetiology of acute pancreatitis has been reported at least twice. Mero[49] found a change of aetiology from gallstone disease (1967–1968) to alcohol abuse (1977–1978), during which time there was a 2.5-fold rise in the consumption of alcohol in Finland.

In a recent study, Lindkvist et al.[43] reported on 929 first attacks of acute pancreatitis in Malmö, the third largest city in Sweden. Similar to Lüneburg, Malmö is in a unique situation in Sweden. It is the only hospital serving the city, and there are no referrals of patients to or from this hospital; thus the risk of selection bias is low. During the period between 1985 and 1999 this group reported that the total incidence of acute pancreatitis increased by 3.9% per year. However, the incidence of gallstone-related pancreatitis increased by 6.6% per year, and this correlated with an increase in the incidence of other gallstone-related conditions and obesity. Alcohol-induced pancreatitis decreased during this period by minus 5.1% per year, and this correlated with a decrease in the incidence of delirium tremens, mortality from liver cirrhosis and incidence of lung cancer. From 1980 to 1996 the amount of legally sold alcohol in Malmö decreased by about 36%. This decrease was due to a marked reduction in the sales of hard liquor, whereas sales of wine and beer were stable[43]. Interestingly, a specific correlation of acute pancreatitis with hard liquor, but not wine and beer, had been reported in Sweden earlier[50].

In the 24 studies on the aetiology of acute pancreatitis 17 presented more men than women, whereas in the remaining six studies more women were presented (three of them were from the same centre in Hong Kong, two from the same centre in Bristol, one from Glasgow and one from Aberdeen). In all seven centres biliary disease was the dominating aetiological factor; that may, in part, explain the gender difference.

It has frequently been questioned whether the aetiology of acute pancreatitis has any effect on the severity of the prognosis of the disease.

Two large studies, one[41] comprising 190 patients, the other[51] comprising 602 patients with a first attack of acute pancreatitis, showed that the aetiology had no influence on the mortality of the disease.

As our prospective study on the diagnosis and prognosis of acute pancreatitis continues in Lüneburg, first results have been reported earlier[52], and data from 1987 to 2004 are now available; they show no significant differences among the aetiological subgroups concerning the prognostic parameters of Ranson and Imrie (Table 5). The higher incidence of patients with severe acute pancreatitis, according to the APACHE II score in biliary disease, is explained by the significantly higher mean age of patients with biliary as opposed to alcohol-induced pancreatitis ($x \pm$ SD: 63.4 ± 17.1 and 44.6 ± 12.3; $p < 0.001$), since the APACHE II score, in contrast to the two other scores, is heavily age-weighted. Patients with alcohol-induced pancreatitis had significantly more pancreatic necrosis (Table 6), more fluid collections/pseudocysts (Table 7) and usually needed more artificial ventilation (Table 8). However, the indication for a necrosectomy and the mortality rate did not differ. As previously stated[52], patients with alcohol-induced acute pancreatitis should be monitored intensely, in order to prevent respiratory insufficiency and other complications, as the need for artificial ventilation in alcoholics is high. Whether this is due to a higher incidence of smokers in this group, who presumably have some lung

Table 5 Aetiology of acute pancreatitis and prognostic parameters in Lüneburg County from 1987 to 2004

Aetiology	Ranson >3 points (n, %)	Imrie >3 points (n, %)	Apache II ≥8 points (n, %)	p-Value
Alcohol	5 (3)	6 (4)	28 (18) ⎫	<0.0001
Biliary	4 (2)	11 (5)	95 (43) ⎬	
Other			8 (16) ⎭	
Unknown	3 (3)	4 (4)	40 (35)	
Total	12 (2)*	21 (4)*	171 (32)	

*Not significant.

Table 6 Aetiology of acute pancreatitis and CT score (Balthazar) in Lüneburg County from 1987 to 2004

Aetiology	CT score >4 (n, %)		
Alcohol		26 (20) ⎫	
Biliary	11 (7) ⎫		p = 0.0002
Other	2 (6) ⎬	21 (8) ⎬	
Unknown	8 (10) ⎭		
Total		47 (12)	

Table 7 Aetiology of acute pancreatitis and fluid collections/pseudocysts in Lüneburg County from 1987 to 2004

Aetiology	Fluid collections/pseudocysts (n, %)		
Alcohol		27 (23) ⎫	
Biliary	14 (19) ⎫		p = 0.0002
Other	3 (9) ⎬	22 (9) ⎬	
Unknown	5 (7) ⎭		
Total		49 (13)	

Table 8 Aetiology of acute pancreatitis and artificial ventilation in Lüneburg County from 1987 to 2004

Aetiology	Artificial ventilation (n, %)		
Alcohol		13 (9) ⎫	
Biliary	4 (2) ⎫		p = 0.01
Other	2 (4) ⎬	13 (3) ⎬	
Unknown	7 (6) ⎭		
Total		26 (5)	

damage prior to acute pancreatitis, is unknown, but it should be a subject for future prospective studies. Some investigations have shown that alcohol abuse *per se* has a negative effect on the lung[53,54].

Several groups have investigated the development of pancreatic pseudocysts in acute pancreatitis of different aetiologies. In two of these studies the incidence of pancreatic pseudocysts was the same in all aetiological subgroups[55,56]. In contrast, Thomson et al.[7] found that patients with alcohol-induced pancreatitis were more likely to develop pancreatic pseudocysts than those patients with biliary acute pancreatitis. In these studies a differentiation between fluid collections and pancreatic pseudocysts was not clarified. Whether a higher incidence of fluid collections/pseudocysts in patients with alcohol-induced acute pancreatitis indicates a later progression from acute to chronic pancreatitis remains an open question[25].

Finally, we could indicate earlier that the aetiology of acute pancreatitis and the absence or presence of initial organ failure have an impact on the later course of the disease. Patients with alcohol abuse and initial organ failure (arterial $pO_2 \leqslant 60$ mmHg and/or serum creatinine > 2 mg/dl after rehydration) deteriorated more significantly than other subgroups, requiring artificial ventilation and/or dialysis treatment. If, on admission, there was no initial organ failure, there were no differences within the aetiological subgroups. Thus, patients with alcohol-induced acute pancreatitis, plus initial organ failure, represent a major risk group, requiring special attention and intensive care. If necessary they should be transferred to a specialized centre. Secondly, patients with no initial organ failure are at lower risk of organ failure and usually do not need intensive care[57].

OUTLOOK

To conclude, we need multicentre studies from different countries in a defined population taken from comparable settings, to evaluate the true incidence of acute pancreatitis, the severity and outcome. These data could meet the new restrictions of the various health insurance schemes throughout the world, and could generate diagnosis-related groups and payment. We need clearer, internationally accepted definitions for alcohol abuse and biliary disease as the aetiological factors of acute pancreatitis, in order to evaluate and compare the data from different centres. We should pay special attention to patients with a first attack of alcohol-induced acute pancreatitis, because they tend to have a higher incidence of necrotizing pancreatitis and respiratory organ failure and represent an 'at risk' group. Probably the higher incidence of fluid collections and/or pseudocysts in this group is indicative of a later progression to chronic pancreatitis. These and other open questions concerning the diagnosis, prognosis and outcome of acute pancreatitis could be answered by groups of pancreatologists or clubs and associations such as the International Association of Pancreatology, the European Pancreatic Club, and the American Pancreatic Association.

Acknowledgements

Supported by the Italian Association for Cancer Research (Associazione Italiana per la Ricerca sul Cancro, AIRC); A.B.L. was supported in part by the CD Smithers Foundation

References

1. Trapnell JE, Duncan EHL. Patterns of incidence in acute pancreatitis. Br Med J. 1975;2: 179–83.
2. Corfield AP, Cooper MJ, Williamson RCN. Acute pancreatitis: a lethal disease of increasing incidence. Gut. 1985;26:724–9.
3. Tran DD, Van Schilfgaarde R. Prevalence and mortality from acute pancreatitis in the Netherlands during 1971–1990. Digestion. 1994;55:342–3 (abstract).
4. Thomson HJ. Acute pancreatitis in North and North-East Scotland. J R Coll Surg Edinb. 1985;30:104–10.
5. Giggs JA, Bourke JB, Katschinski B. The epidemiology of primary acute pancreatitis in Greater Nottingham: 1969–1983. Soc Sci Med. 1988;26:79–89.
6. Lankisch PG, Assmus C, Maisonneuve P, Lowenfels AB. Epidemiology of pancreatic diseases in Lüneburg County – a study in a defined German population. Pancreatology. 2002;2:469–77.
7. Thomson SR, Hendry WS, McFarlane GA, Davidson AI. Epidemiology and outcome of acute pancreatitis. Br J Surg. 1987;74:398–401.
8. Worning H. Acute interstitial (edematous) pancreatitis in Denmark. In: Bradley III EL, editor. Acute Pancreatitis: Diagnosis and Therapy. New York: Raven Press, 1994:265–9.
9. McKay CJ, Evans S, Sinclair M, Carter CR, Imrie CW. High early mortality rate from acute pancreatitis in Scotland, 1984–1995. Br J Surg. 1999;86:1302–5.
10. Appelros S, Borgström A. Incidence, aetiology and mortality rate of acute pancreatitis over 10 years in a defined urban population in Sweden. Br J Surg. 1999;86:465–70.
11. Eland IA, Sturkenboom MJCM, Wilson JHP, Stricker BHC. Incidence and mortality of acute pancreatitis between 1985 and 1995. Scand J Gastroenterol. 2000;35:1110–16.
12. Go VLW. Etiology and epidemiology of pancreatitis in the United States. In: Bradley III EL, editor. Acute Pancreatitis: Diagnosis and Therapy. New York: Raven Press, 1994:235–9.
13. Jaakkola M, Nordback I. Pancreatitis in Finland between 1970 and 1989. Gut. 1993;34: 1255–60.
14. Halvorsen F-A, Ritland S. Acute pancreatitis in Buskerud County, Norway. Incidence and etiology. Scand J Gastroenterol. 1996;31:411–14.
15. Floyd A, Pedersen L, Lauge Nielsen G, Thorlacius-Ussing O, Sorensen HT. Secular trends in incidence and 30-day case fatality of acute pancreatitis in North Jutland County, Denmark. A register-based study from 1981–2000. Scand J Gastroenterol. 2002;37:1461–5.
16. Goldacre MJ, Roberts SE. Hospital admission for acute pancreatitis in an English population, 1963–98: database study of incidence and mortality. Br Med J. 2004;328: 1466–9.
17. Wilson C, Imrie CW. Deaths from acute pancreatitis: why do we miss the diagnosis so frequently? Int J Pancreatol. 1988;3:273–82.
18. Lankisch PG, Schirren CA, Kunze E. Undetected fatal acute pancreatitis: why is the disease so frequently overlooked? Am J Gastroenterol. 1991;86:322–6.
19. Mann DV, Hershman MJ, Hittinger R, Glazer G. Multicentre audit of death from acute pancreatitis. Br J Surg. 1994;81:890–3.
20. Eland IA, Sturkenboom MJCM, van der Lei J, Wilson JHP, Stricker BHC. Incidence of acute pancreatitis. Scand J Gastroenterol. 2002;37:124.
21. Lankisch PG, Burchard-Reckert S, Lehnick D. Underestimation of acute pancreatitis: patients with only a small increase in amylase/lipase levels can also have or develop severe acute pancreatitis. Gut. 1999;44:542–4.
22. Wilson C, Imrie CW. Changing patterns of incidence and mortality from acute pancreatitis in Scotland, 1961–1985. Br J Surg. 1990;77:731–4.

23. Fiorianti J, Sullivan T, Lowenfels AB. Rising incidence of hospitalization for acute pancreatitis in New York State from 1991 to 2001. Pancreas. 2003;27:381–2.
24. Klöppel G, Maillet B. Chronic pancreatitis: evolution of the disease. Hepatogastroenterology. 1991;38:408–12.
25. Lankisch PG. Progression from acute to chronic pancreatitis. A physician's view. Surg Clin N Am. 1999;79:815–27.
26. Renner IG, Savage III WT, Pantoja JL, Renner VJ. Death due to acute pancreatitis. A retrospective analysis of 405 autopsy cases. Dig Dis Sci. 1985;30:1005–18.
27. Edlund Y, Norbäck B, Risholm L. Acute pancreatitis, etiology and prevention of recurrence. Follow-up study of 188 patients. Rev Surg. 1968;25:153–7.
28. Imrie CW. Observations on acute pancreatitis. Br J Surg. 1974;61:539–44.
29. Madsen OG, Schmidt A. Acute pancreatitis. A study of 122 patients with acute pancreatitis observed for 5–15 years. World J Surg. 1979;3:345–52.
30. Jacobs ML, Daggett WM, Civetta JM et al. Acute pancreatitis: analysis of factors influencing survival. Ann Surg. 1977;185:43–51.
31. Satiani B, Stone HH. Predictability of present outcome and future recurrence in acute pancreatitis. Arch Surg. 1979;114:711–16.
32. Lukash WM. Complications of acute pancreatitis. Unusual sequelae in 100 cases. Arch Surg. 1967;94:848–52.
33. Ong GB, Lam KH, Lam SK, Lim TK, Wong J. Acute pancreatitis in Hong Kong. Br J Surg. 1979;66:398–403.
34. Svensson J-O, Norbäck B, Bokey EL, Edlund Y. Changing pattern in aetiology of pancreatitis in an urban Swedish area. Br J Surg. 1979;66:159–61.
35. Ranson JHC, Spencer FC. The role of peritoneal lavage in severe acute pancreatitis. Ann Surg. 1978;187:565–75.
36. Fan ST, Choi TK, Lai CS, Wong J. Influence of age on the mortality from acute pancreatitis. Br J Surg. 1988;75:463–6.
37. Fan S-T, Lai ECS, Mok FPT, Lo C-M, Zheng S-S, Wong J. Prediction of the severity of acute pancreatitis. Am J Surg. 1993;166:262–9.
38. De Beaux AC, Palmer KR, Carter DC. Factors influencing morbidity and mortality in acute pancreatitis; an analysis of 279 cases. Gut. 1995;37:121–6.
39. Lankisch PG, Burchard-Reckert S, Petersen M et al. Morbidity and mortality in 602 patients with acute pancreatitis seen between the years 1980–1994. Z Gastroenterol. 1996; 34:371–7.
40. Chang M-C, Su C-H, Sun M-S et al. Etiology of acute pancreatitis – a multicenter study in Taiwan. Hepatogastroenterology. 2003;50:1655–7.
41. Uhl W, Isenmann R, Curti G, Vogel R, Beger HG, Büchler MW. Influence of etiology on the course and outcome of acute pancreatitis. Pancreas. 1996;13:335–43.
42. Pezzilli R, Billi P, Morselli-Labate AM. Severity of acute pancreatitis: relationship with etiology, sex and age. Hepatogastroenterology. 1998;45:1859–64.
43. Lindkvist B, Appelros S, Manjer J, Borgström A. Trends in incidence of acute pancreatitis in a Swedish population: is there really an increase? Clin Gastroenterol Hepatol. 2004;2: 831–7.
44. Gullo L, Migliori M, Oláh A et al. Acute pancreatitis in five European countries: etiology and mortality. Pancreas. 2002;24:223–7.
45. Lankisch PG, Lowenfels AB, Maisonneuve P. What is the risk of alcoholic pancreatitis in heavy drinkers? Pancreas. 2002;25:411–12.
46. Lowenfels AB, Lankisch PG, Maisonneuve P. What is the risk of biliary pancreatitis in patients with gallstones? Gastroenterology. 2000;119:879–80.
47. Ramstedt M. Alcohol and pancreatitis mortality at the population level: experiences from 14 western countries. Addiction. 2004;99:1255–61.
48. Kratzer W, Mason RA, Kächele V. Prevalence of gallstones in sonographic surveys worldwide. J Clin Ultrasound. 1999;27:1–7.
49. Mero M. Changing aetiology of acute pancreatitis. Ann Chir Gynaecol. 1982;71:126–9.
50. Schmidt DN. Apparent risk factors for chronic and acute pancreatitis in Stockholm county. Int J Pancreatol. 1991;8:45–50.
51. Lankisch PG, Burchard-Reckert S, Petersen M et al. Etiology and age have only a limited influence on the course of acute pancreatitis. Pancreas. 1996;13:344–9.

52. Lankisch PG, Assmus C, Pflichthofer D, Struckmann K, Lehnick D. Which etiology causes the most severe acute pancreatitis? Int J Pancreatol. 1999;26:55–7.
53. Lange P, Groth S, Mortensen J et al. Pulmonary function is influenced by heavy alcohol consumption. Am Rev Respir Dis. 1988;137:1119–23.
54. Garshick E, Segal MR, Worobec TG, Salekin CMS, Miller MJ. Alcohol consumption and chronic obstructive pulmonary disease. Am Rev Respir Dis. 1989;140:373–8.
55. Schulze S, Baden H, Brandenhoff P, Larsen T, Burcharth F. Pancreatic pseudocysts during first attack of acute pancreatitis. Scand J Gastroenterol. 1986;21:1221–3.
56. Nguyen B-LT, Thompson JS, Edney JA, Bragg LE, Rikkers LF. Influence of the etiology of pancreatitis on the natural history of pancreatic pseudocysts. Am J Surg. 1991;162:527–31.
57. Lankisch PG, Pflichthofer D, Lehnick D. Acute pancreatitis: which patient is most at risk? Pancreas. 1999;19:321–4.

4
Acute pancreatitis: diagnostic gold standard – new perspectives?

L. GULLO

INTRODUCTION

There are several laboratory tests and imaging procedures which are very useful for the diagnosis of acute pancreatitis and its complications[1,2]. However, despite this, an important point remains unsolved; i.e. early diagnosis of the severe forms. Early recognition of severe forms of acute pancreatitis is important for rapid admission of patients to appropriate wards, for appropriate therapy and for improving prognosis. Therefore I believe that, among the possible diagnostic gold standards in acute pancreatitis, an important one could be the diagnostic mean able to recognize the severe forms of acute pancreatitis as soon as possible. The diagnostic means for early recognition of severe acute pancreatitis could be the following three: (1) the clinician's assessment, (2) laboratory tests, and (3) imaging procedures.

Concerning the first, several British investigators[3–8] have compared the clinician's assessment of severity, soon after admission of patients, with other more objective parameters, and showed that this assessment has a poor sensitivity but good specificity (Table 1). According to these results, experienced physicians can correctly predict severe attacks in only 37% of patients on admission, a percentage that is too low to be taken into consideration.

Concerning point 3, i.e. imaging procedures, at present none of these procedures is able to recognize the severe forms of acute pancreatitis during the first hours of the development of an attack.

Table 1 Clinician's assessment in predicting severity of acute pancreatitis

No. of patients	Sensitivity	Specificity	+ PV	– PV
1253	37% (113/308)	94% (878/937)	64%	81%

+ PV, positive predictive value; – PV, negative predictive value.

From references 1, 3–8.

The only remaining possibility, therefore, is the search for a laboratory test. To be a diagnostic gold standard this must be simple, quick to perform and inexpensive, and able to confirm diagnosis and predict severity of acute pancreatitis as early as possible (the first 8–12 h from clinical onset), guide therapy and positively influence prognosis. The sensitivity and specificity must also be 100% or so.

In the past 15 years several markers have been studied for the diagnosis of acute pancreatitis and some of them seem to be useful for early diagnosis of the more severe forms of acute pancreatitis[1,2]. Most of these markers are an expression of the early pathogenetic events of acute pancreatitis and their levels in serum or urine increase early, especially in the more severe forms of the disease. These markers can be divided into two groups: (1) markers of trypsinogen activation, and (2) markers of inflammation. There are many of these markers, but I will mention only the ones that have been most studied to date.

MARKERS OF TRYPSINOGEN ACTIVATION

The main markers of this group are listed in Table 2.

Table 2 Markers of trypsinogen activation

Trypsinogen activation peptide (TAP)
Carboxypeptidase B activation peptide (CAPAP)
Trypsinogen-2–α_1-antitrypsin complex (trypsin-2-AAT)

Trypsinogen activation peptide (TAP)

Among the markers of trypsinogen activation, trypsinogen activation peptide (TAP) in the urine is one of the most studied[9–13]. TAP is a small peptide (eight amino acids, molecular weight approximately 900 daltons) that is cleaved from the amino-terminal end of trypsinogen during its activation to trypsin. Since trypsin activation is the first event in the pathogenesis of acute pancreatitis, TAP appears very early in the course of the disease, especially in the more severe forms.

One of the first studies on TAP is the one by Gudgeon et al.[9] published 15 years ago, on 55 patients with acute pancreatitis – 40 mild and 15 severe. This study concluded that, in predicting disease severity, the urine TAP concentration is as good as or better than multifactorial scoring at 48 h, and is much better than the C-reactive protein (CRP) assay.

In a subsequent study on a larger series of patients (139 acute pancreatitis – 99 mild and 40 severe), Tenner et al.[10] concluded that urinary TAP obtained within the first 48 h of the onset of symptoms can distinguish patients with severe acute pancreatitis.

More recently, Neoptolemos et al.[11] studied the diagnostic value of urinary TAP in 172 patients with acute pancreatitis – 137 mild and 35 severe. The results were compared with those of CRP and of three clinicobiochemical scoring systems (APACHE II, Ranson and Imrie systems). They showed that the sensitivity of TAP (> 35 mmol/L) in early prediction of severity (24 h after clinical onset) was about 60%, while that of CRP (> 150 mg/L) was 0%. The negative predictive value for severe disease was high (86%) and this is important because a high proportion of patients with mild acute pancreatitis can be managed in low-cost wards. The early sensitivity of TAP was even better than that of the Ranson, Imrie and APACHE II systems, which are complex scoring systems. The authors concluded that urinary TAP provides accurate severity prediction 24 h after onset of symptoms, and that this simple marker of severity in acute pancreatitis deserves routine clinical application. It should nevertheless be pointed out that TAP sensitivity during the first 24 h of severe acute pancreatitis was only 58%; an improvement of this percentage could be possible, perhaps by selecting patients with the more severe forms of acute pancreatitis.

A study published in 2004 seems to support this hypothesis. In this paper Johnson et al.[12] studied urinary TAP in 190 cases of acute pancreatitis – 164 mild and 26 severe; they used a stringent definition of severity, and patients with transient organ failure were excluded from this study. The conclusion was that TAP is a useful predictor of severe acute pancreatitis, particularly in the early phase of the disease, in patients admitted to hospital within 24 h of onset of symptoms. In this study urinary TAP estimation was as accurate as the APACHE II system.

On the basis of the results of the above four studies on TAP, obtained on a total of 556 cases of acute pancreatitis – 440 mild and 116 severe, I believe it can be concluded that this test could be very useful in clinical practice for the early diagnosis of the severity of acute pancreatitis.

Unfortunately, the only TAP dosage method currently available was a radioimmunoassay method, and we must hope that a simple and fast dosage method, to test in clinical practice, will soon be available.

Carboxypeptidase B activation peptide (CAPAP)

Carboxypeptidase B is a protease synthesized by acinar cells as an inactive proenzyme, procarboxypeptidase B. In acute pancreatitis this proenzyme is activated very rapidly within the pancreatic cells by trypsin, with consequent release of carboxypeptidase B activation peptide (CAPAP). This peptide is considerably larger (95 amino acids) than TAP, making its measurement more reliable. Moreover, it is stable in both serum and urine, which is an advantage over TAP.

Several studies have been carried out on the diagnostic value of this peptide, and the results have been promising. Appelros et al.[14] studied urine and serum samples obtained within 48 h of admission from 40 patients with acute pancreatitis, and found that levels of CAPAP correlated with the severity of the attack. They concluded that CAPAP could be a valuable tool in the diagnosis and early determination of severity in acute pancreatitis.

Three other studies have recently been published with similar results. In the first study[15], 60 patients with acute pancreatitis – 48 mild and 12 severe – were studied and the conclusion was that measurement of CAPAP in urine and serum is an accurate way to predict the severity of acute pancreatitis. In the second study, by Muller et al.[16], 85 patients with acute pancreatitis were studied, and the results were similar to those of the previous study. In the third study, carried out in 2004 by Saez et al.[17], 52 patients – 35 with mild acute pancreatitis and 17 with severe acute pancreatitis – were studied; the conclusion was that serum and urine CAPAP levels and urinary TAP are accurate in the early assessment of severity in acute pancreatitis. Urine CAPAP levels were the most accurate marker 24 h after onset of symptoms.

On the basis of these results it seems that measurement of CAPAP is a very useful test for early recognition of the severity of acute pancreatitis. Further studies are, however, necessary to confirm whether this is real progress or just another marker.

Trypsin-2–α_1-antitrypsin complex (trypsin-2-AAT)

This is a complex which is formed in blood between trypsin and α_1-antitrypsin.

It has been shown that serum concentrations of trypsin-2–α_1-antitrypsin complex (trypsin-2-AAT) correlate to the severity of acute pancreatitis. Hedstrom et al.[18] studied 110 patients with acute pancreatitis, which was mild in 82 and severe in 28, and 66 patients with acute abdominal diseases of extrapancreatic origin, and concluded that trypsin-2-AAT was very accurate in differentiating between acute pancreatitis and extrapancreatic disease, and in predicting a severe course for acute pancreatitis. During the first 12 h after admission this complex was more accurate than CRP.

In a subsequent study Hedstrom et al.[19] compared the diagnostic value of serum levels of trypsinogen-2 and trypsin-2-AAT with serum lipase and amylase in 64 patients with acute pancreatitis – 43 mild and 21 severe. They concluded that these two markers displayed the best accuracy for predicting severe acute pancreatitis on admission, which makes these markers superior for clinical purposes.

On the basis of the results of these studies trypsin-2-AAT also appears to be a good marker for the rapid recognition of severe acute pancreatitis, although further studies are necessary to be able to draw a definite conclusion. It should be noted that high serum levels of this complex have also been reported in patients with perforated duodenal ulcer and other acute gastrointestinal disorders[20].

MARKERS OF INFLAMMATION

The second group of tests proposed in the last 15 years for the diagnosis of severe acute pancreatitis includes markers that are in relation to the inflammatory reaction that accompanies acute pancreatitis. High levels of these markers are also observed in other conditions of severe inflammation. The main markers in this group are listed in Table 3.

Table 3 Markers of inflammation

Interleukin-6 (IL-6)
Granulocyte elastase
Serum amyloid A (SAA)

Interleukin-6 (IL-6)

Interleukin-6 (IL-6) is an important marker of inflammation. Numerous studies have been performed on its diagnostic value in acute pancreatitis, and they all concluded in its favour. For this marker, too, these studies began about 15 years ago and, despite the favourable results, its dosage has not yet become part of clinical practice. This is essentially due to the fact that a simple and rapid method for its determination has not yet been developed.

In 1991, in one of the first studies on the diagnostic value of IL-6, performed in 50 patients with acute pancreatitis – 25 mild and 25 severe – Leser et al.[21] concluded that elevated serum concentrations of IL-6 followed by increased levels of CRP reflect the severity of acute pancreatitis.

Many other studies[22–32] have since been carried out on the value of IL-6 in the early diagnosis of severe acute pancreatitis, and all concluded that IL-6 is a good marker of severity during the first 24 h of the disease. In particular, a survey of 13 papers[21–32] published between 1991 and 2004, in which a total of 481 patients with acute pancreatitis were studied, showed that the conclusion in all these studies was that IL-6 is able to predict severity of acute pancreatitis during the first 24 h of the disease.

On the basis of these results I believe we can say that IL-6 has been widely studied to date, and that a simple, rapid and inexpensive test is now needed so that it can be included and tested in clinical practice.

Granulocyte elastase

Another marker of inflammation is granulocyte elastase. One of the first studies on this marker is the one by Gross et al.[33] who studied 75 patients with acute pancreatitis – 34 mild and 41 severe. They concluded that granulocyte elastase is a good early marker for the severity of acute pancreatitis. Moreover, it has been shown that, compared with elevated levels of CRP and α_1-antitrypsin, release of granulocyte elastase reflects an event that precedes acute-phase protein induction.

Dominguez-Munoz et al.[34] published the results of a multicentre study on the clinical usefulness of this marker, which comprised 182 patients with acute pancreatitis – 154 with a mild disease and 28 with a severe form – and concluded that it is a very early and reliable marker in the diagnosis of the severity of acute pancreatitis. The highest values of granulocyte elastase were found in patients who developed local and/or systemic complications.

These two studies[33,34] concluded that granulocyte elastase is an early and reliable marker of severity in acute pancreatitis, and it should be taken into consideration. Here again we need a simple and rapid method to test this promising marker on a large scale.

Serum amyloid A (SAA)

Serum amyloid A (SAA) is an acute-phase protein which has been reported to be a very early marker of inflammation and tissue injury in a variety of conditions; generally, changes in this protein mirror those of CRP[35–37]. Studies of its value in acute pancreatitis have shown that it may be a useful early marker of severity of this disease[38–40]. In particular, Mayer et al.[40], in a study of 137 patients with mild and 35 with severe acute pancreatitis, found that SAA concentrations were significantly higher in patients with severe acute pancreatitis than in those with mild disease, on admission, at 24 h or less after symptom onset, and subsequently. SAA levels predicted severity significantly better than CRP on admission and at 24 h following symptom onset. Further studies of SAA on large series of patients with acute pancreatitis are warranted.

All the markers described so far are dosed with radioimmunoassay and cannot therefore be used as a rapid test in clinical practice. At present the only rapid test available is the dosage of trypsinogen 2 in the urine. Some authors have reported that urinary trypsinogen is a simple and rapid method useful in the early prediction of the severity of acute pancreatitis[41], while others did not find similar results[42,43].

CONCLUSIONS

Several other markers, in addition to those presented here, have been described, but I have limited my discussion to those that have to date been studied the most. Among these, those which seem to be the best candidates for clinical use as early predictors of severity of acute pancreatitis are TAP and IL-6. Whether they can be considered as a diagnostic gold standard is difficult to say at the moment; we must at least wait for the results of their use on a large scale in clinical practice. However, as to the question in the title of this chapter, i.e. 'are there new perspectives regarding the diagnostic gold standard in acute pancreatitis'? I believe that the answer could be yes.

References

1. Steinberg WM. Predictors of severity of acute pancreatitis. Gastroenterol Clin N Am. 1990; 19:849–61.
2. Sandberg AA, Borgstrom A. Early prediction of severity in acute pancreatitis. Is this possible? J Pancreas. (Online). 2002;3:116–25.
3. Corfield AP, Cooper MJ, Williamson RCN et al. Prediction of severity in acute pancreatitis: prospective comparison of three prognostic indices. Lancet. 1985;2:403–7.
4. Larvin M, McMahon MJ. APACHE-II score for assessment and monitoring of acute pancreatitis. Lancet. 1989;2:201–5.
5. Mayer AD, McMahon MJ, Bowen M et al. C reactive protein: an aid to assessment and monitoring of acute pancreatitis. J Clin Pathol. 1984;37:207–11.
6. Mayer AD, McMahon MJ. The diagnostic and prognostic value of peritoneal lavage in patients with acute pancreatitis. Surg Gynecol Obstet. 1985;160:507–12.

7. McMahon MJ, Playforth MJ, Pickford IR. A comparative study of methods for the prediction of severity of attacks of acute pancreatitis. Br J Surg. 1980;67:22–5.
8. Wilson C, Heads A, Shenkin A et al. C reactive protein, antiproteases and complement factors as objective markers of severity in acute pancreatitis. Br J Surg. 1989;76:177–81.
9. Gudgeon AM, Heath DI, Hurley P et al. Trypsinogen activation peptides assay in the early prediction of severity of acute pancreatitis. Lancet. 1990;335:4–8.
10. Tenner S, Fernandez-del Castillo C, Warshaw A et al. Urinary trypsinogen activation peptide (TAP) predicts severity in patients with acute pancreatitis. Int J Pancreatol. 1997; 21:105–10.
11. Neoptolemos JP, Kemppainen EA, Mayer JM et al. Early prediction of severity in acute pancreatitis by urinary trypsinogen activation peptide: a multicentre study. Lancet. 2000; 355:1955–60.
12. Johnson CD, Lempinen M, Imrie CW et al. Urinary trypsinogen activation peptide as a marker of severe acute pancreatitis. Br J Surg. 2004;91:1027–33.
13. Kemppainen E, Mayer J, Puolakkainen P, Raraty M, Slavin J, Neoptolemos JP. Plasma trypsinogen activation peptide in patients with acute pancreatitis. Br J Surg. 2001;88:679–80.
14. Appelros S, Thim L, Borgstrom A. Activation peptide of carboxypeptidase B in serum and urine in acute pancreatitis. Gut. 1998;42:97–102.
15. Appelros S, Petersson U, Toh S, Johnson C, Borgstrom A. Activation peptide of carboxypeptidase B and anionic trypsinogen as early predictors of the severity of acute pancreatitis. Br J Surg. 2001;88:216–21.
16. Muller CA, Appelros S, Uhl W, Buchler MW, Borgstrom A. Serum levels of procarboxy-peptidase B and its activation peptide in patients with acute pancreatitis and non-pancreatic diseases. Gut. 2002;51:229–35.
17. Saez J, Martinez J, Trigo C et al. A comparative study of the activation peptide of carboxypeptidase B and trypsinogen as early predictors of the severity of acute pancreatitis. Pancreas. 2004;29:e9 (abstract).
18. Hedstrom J, Sainio V, Kemppainen E et al. Serum complex of trypsin 2 and α1 antitrypsin as diagnostic and prognostic marker of acute pancreatitis: clinical study in consecutive patients. Br Med J. 1996;313:333–7.
19. Hedstrom J, Kemppainen E, Andersen J, Jokela H, Puolakkainen P, Stenman UH. A comparison of serum trypsinogen-2 and trypsin-2–α1 antitrypsin complex with lipase and amylase in the diagnosis and assessment of severity in the early phase of acute pancreatitis. Am J Gastroenterol. 2001;96:424–30.
20. Borgstrom A, Lasson A, Ohlsson K. Patterns of immunoreactive trypsin in serum from patients with acute abdominal disorders. Scand J Clin Lab Invest. 1989;49:757–62.
21. Leser HG, Gross V, Scheibenbogen C et al. Elevation of serum interleukin-6 concentrations precedes acute-phase response and reflects severity in acute pancreatitis. Gastroenterology. 1991;101:782–5.
22. Viedma JA, Perez-Mateo M, Dominguez JE, Carballo F. Role of interleukin-6 in acute pancreatitis. Comparison with C-reactive protein and phosholipase A. Gut. 1992;33:1264–7.
23. Curley PJ, McMahon MJ, Lancaster F et al. Reduction in circulating levels of CD4-positive lymphocytes in acute pancreatitis: relationship to endotoxin, interleukin 6 and disease severity. Br J Surg. 1993;80:1312–15.
24. Pezzilli R, Billi P, Miniero R et al. Serum interleukin-6, interleukin-8, and β2-micro-globulin in early assessment of severity of acute pancreatitis. Comparison with serum C-reactive protein. Dig Dig Sci. 1995;40:2341–8.
25. Stoelben E, Nagel M, Ockert D, Quintel M, Scheibenbogen C, Klein B. Clinical significance of cytokines IL-6, IL-8 and C-reactive protein in serum of patients with acute pancreatitis. Chirurg. 1996;67:1231–6.
26. Inagaki T, Hoshino M, Hayakawa T et al. Interleukin-6 is a useful marker for early prediction of the severity of acute pancreatitis. Pancreas. 1997;14:1–8.
27. Ikei S, Ogawa M, Yamaguchi Y. Blood concentrations of polymorphonuclear leucocyte elastase and interleukin-6 are indicators for the occurrence of multiple organ failures at the early stage of acute pancreatitis. J Gastroenterol Hepatol. 1998;13:1274–83.
28. Berney T, Gasche Y, Robert J et al. Serum profiles of interleukin-6, interleukin-8, and interleukin-1 in patients with severe and mild acute pancreatitis. Pancreas. 1999;18:371–7.

29. Brivet FG, Emilie D, Galanaud P. Pro- and anti-inflammatory cytokines during acute severe pancreatitis: an early and sustained response, although unpredictable of death. Parisian Study Group on Acute Pancreatitis. Crit Care Med. 1999;27:749–55.
30. Naskalski JW, Kusnierz-Cabala B, Panek J, Kedra B. Poly-C specific ribonuclease activity correlates with increased concentrations of IL-6, IL-8 and sTNFR55/sTNFR75 in plasma of patients with acute pancreatitis. J Physiol Pharmacol. 2003;54:439–48.
31. Pooran N, Indaram A, Singh P, Bank S. Cytokines (IL-6, IL-8, TNF): early and reliable predictors of severity in acute pancreatitis. J Clin Gastroenterol. 2003;37:263–6.
32. Mentula P, Kylanpaa ML, Kemppainen E et al. Plasma anti-inflammatory cytokines and monocyte human leucocyte antigen-DR expression in patients with acute pancreatitis. Scand J Gastroenterol. 2004;39:178–87.
33. Gross V, Scholmerich J, Leser HG et al. Granulocyte elastase in assessment of severity of acute pancreatitis. Comparison with acute-phase proteins C-reactive protein, α_1-antitrypsin, and protease inhibitor α_2-macroglobulin. Dig Dis Sci. 1990;35:97–105.
34. Dominguez-Munoz JE, Carballo F, Garcia MJ et al. Clinical usefulness of polymorphonuclear elastase in predicting the severity of acute pancreatitis: results of a multicentre study. Br J Surg. 1991;78:1230–4.
35. Maury CPJ. Comparative study of serum amyloid A protein and C-reactive protein in disease. Clin Sci. 1985;68:233–8.
36. Mozes G, Friedman N, Shainkin-Kestenbaum R. Serum amyloid A: an extremely sensitive marker for intensity of tissue damage in trauma patients and indicator of acute response in various disease. J Trauma. 1989;29:71–4.
37. Malle E, De Beer FC. Human serum amyloid A (SAA) protein: a prominent acute-phase reactant for clinical practice. Eur J Clin Invest. 1996;26:427–35.
38. Rau B, Steinbach G, Baumgart K, Gansauge F, Grunert A, Beger HG. Serum amyloid A versus C-reactive protein in acute pancreatitis: clinical value of an alternative acute-phase reactant. Crit Care Med. 2000;28:736–42.
39. Pezzilli R, Melzi d'Eril GV, Morselli-Labate AM, Merlini G, Barakat B, Bosoni T. Serum amyloid A, procalcitonin, and C-reactive protein in early assessment of severity of acute pancreatitis. Dig Dis Sci. 2000;45:1072–8.
40. Mayer JM, Raraty M, Slavin J. et al. Serum amyloid A is a better early predictor of severity than C-reactive protein in acute pancreatitis. Br J Surg. 2002;89:163–7141.
    Lempinen M, Kylanpaa-Back ML, Stenman UH et al. Predicting the severity of acute pancreatitis by rapid measurement of trypsinogen-2 in urine. Clin Chem. 2001;47:2103–7.
42. Hedstrom J, Korvuo A, Kenkimaki P et al. Urinary trypsinogen-2 test strip for acute pancreatitis. Lancet. 1996;347:729–31.
43. Pezzilli R, Morselli-Labate AM, D'Alessandro A, Barakat B. Time-course and clinical value of the urine trypsinogen-2 dipstick test in acute pancreatitis. Eur J Gastroenterol Hepatol. 2001;13:269–74.

5
Acute pancreatitis: when to perform computed tomography

P. C. FREENY

INTRODUCTION

Acute pancreatitis is characterized by a spectrum of inflammatory disease ranging from *mild* (interstitial or oedematous pancreatitis) to *severe* (pancreatitis with associated parenchymal and/or peripancreatic fat necrosis, pancreatic abscess, pseudocyst, or other local or systemic complications). As the severity of the inflammatory process increases, the associated morbidity and mortality also increase. Thus, early diagnosis, differentiation of acute oedematous from acute necrotizing pancreatitis, and detection of complications is important for appropriate patient management.

Dynamic contrast-enhanced computed tomography (DCT) is the imaging modality of choice for diagnosis and detection of complications of acute pancreatitis. Other techniques, such as sonography, ERCP, and angiography are useful for problem solving, for specific evaluation of the pancreatic and biliary ducts and vascular system when involvement is known to be present, for obtaining more precise anatomical information when required, and for follow-up evaluation of a known fluid collection or pseudocyst.

The following guidelines for the use of CT in patients with acute pancreatitis are suggested:

INITIAL DCT SCAN

1. Patients presenting initially with clinically severe acute (based on Ranson criteria, APACHE II score, or other classification systems).

2. Patients who do not show significant clinical improvement within 72 h of conservative medical treatment.

53

3. Patients with clinically mild acute pancreatitis who demonstrate clinical improvement during initial medical therapy but then manifest an acute change in clinical status suggesting a developing complication (e.g. fever, pain, inability to tolerate oral intake, hypotension, falling haematocrit, etc.).

FOLLOW-UP DCT SCAN

1. A follow-up DCT scan is recommended if there is a change in the patient's clinical status which suggests a developing complication, or if the patient does not continue to respond to appropriate medical or surgical therapy.

2. A follow-up scan is recommended at 7–10 days if the initial scan shows severe pancreatitis or gland necrosis. The resolution of the CT manifestations of pancreatic and peripancreatic inflammation virtually always lags behind the improving clinical status of the patient. Thus, if the patient's clinical status is improving, additional follow-up scans during hospitalization are recommended only if the clinical status deteriorates or fails to show continued improvement. However, because some important complications can develop prior to becoming clinically evident, e.g. evolution of a fluid collection into a pseudocyst or development of an arterial pseudoaneurysm, DCT may be obtained at the time of hospital discharge or during subsequent follow-up to confirm resolution and lack of sequelae of known complications.

CT DETECTION OF COMPLICATIONS

Multiple studies have shown that CT should be performed early in the course of acute pancreatitis to accurately identify patients with necrotizing pancreatitis and existing or potential complications[1–3].

Necrosis

Necrotizing pancreatitis (Figure 1) can be differentiated from interstitial/oedematous pancreatitis (Figure 2) by DCT by demonstrating focal or diffuse areas of diminished pancreatic parenchymal contrast enhancement[4–6]. The accuracy of CT detection of parenchymal necrosis was investigated by Maier and colleagues in a large series of patients who underwent both DCT and surgery. The overall accuracy for CT was 87%. The false negative rate was 21% in patients with minor necrosis, but in cases of major or extended necrosis (>50%), the false negative rate was only 11%. There were no false positive CT scans, giving a specificity of 100%[7]. Bradley and co-workers subsequently confirmed these results and indicated that CT detection of gland necrosis had important prognostic implications[4].

It should be noted that most patients with acute pancreatitis who develop necrotizing pancreatitis do so within the first 24 h, and virtually all within the

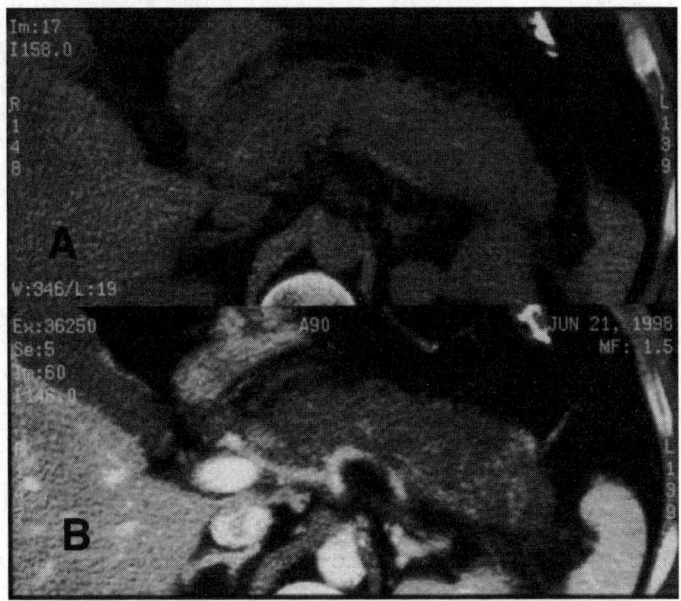

Figure 1 Acute necrotizing pancreatitis. **A**: CT without intravenous contrast shows homogeneous pancreatic parenchyma and only minimal peripancreatic inflammatory changes. **B**: CT with intravenous contrast shows virtually total lack of parenchymal enhancement indicating necrosis

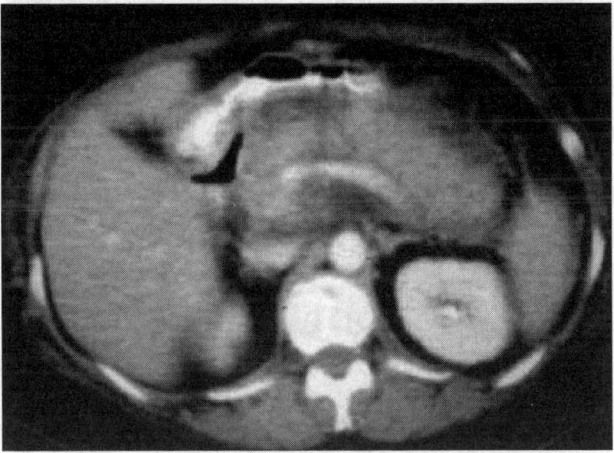

Figure 2 Acute interstitial (oedematous) pancreatitis. CT with intravenous contrast shows homogeneous enhancement of pancreatic parenchyma, moderate gland enlargement, and mild peripancreatic inflammatory changes

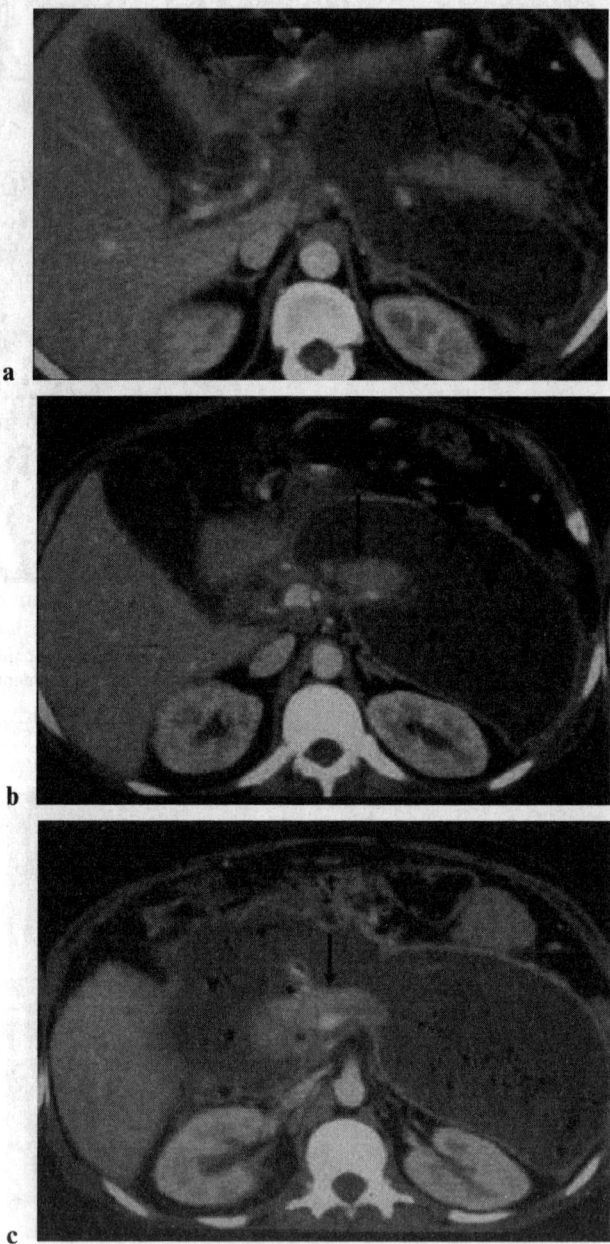

Figure 3 Acute interstitial pancreatitis and peripancreatic fluid collection. CT with intravenous contrast shows homogeneous enhancement of the pancreas (arrows). The gland is surrounded by a large fluid collection containing gas bubbles. Needle aspiration confirmed bacterial infection of the collection

first 72 h following the onset of clinical symptoms. Because the CT findings of necrosis may be equivocal during the first 24–48 h, the initial CT scan obtained in patients with clinically severe acute pancreatitis should be postponed until 72 h unless the patient is critically ill and potentially in need of emergent surgery.

The presence of infection within necrotic pancreatic tissue has a significant effect on patient morbidity and mortality. In Beger's series of 114 patients with pancreatic necrosis, intestinal microorganisms were cultured from the necrotic tissue in 39.4% of cases[8]. Patients with less than 50% gland necrosis showed an increase in mortality from 12.9% to 38.9% if the necrotic tissue was infected, and patients with subtotal necrosis (>50%), showed an increase in mortality from 14.3% to 66.7% in the presence of infection.

Many patients with necrotizing pancreatitis manifest SIRS (systemic inflammatory response syndrome) manifested by fever and elevated white blood cell count. Thus, because a clinical diagnosis of sepsis may not be possible, patients with necrosis who manifest clinical signs of sepsis should undergo fine-needle aspiration with CT or ultrasound guidance to determine the presence of bacterial contamination[9,10].

Fluid collections

Fluid collections (Figures 3 and 4) develop in or around the pancreas in as many as 50% or more of patients with acute pancreatitis[11,12]. Because the presence or absence of secondary infection within these collections often cannot be determined accurately by DCT, guided fine-needle aspiration should be performed. If percutaneous drainage is planned, DCT should always be

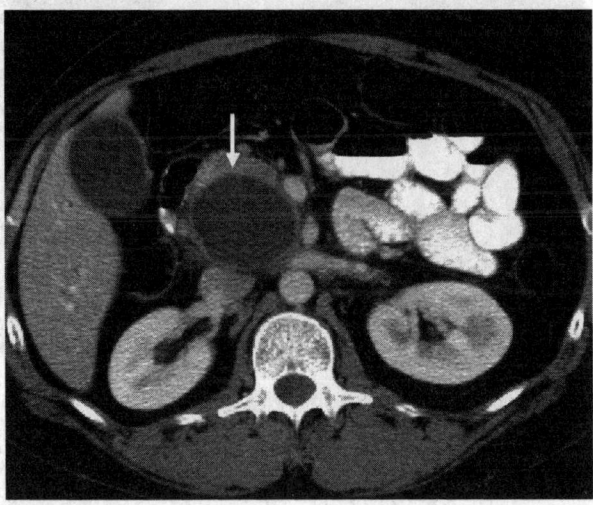

Figure 4 Acute pancreatitis and pseudocyst. CT with intravenous contrast performed 6 weeks following an episode of acute pancreatitis with associated fluid collection now shows a round fluid collection with a slightly enhancing wall typical of pseudocyst

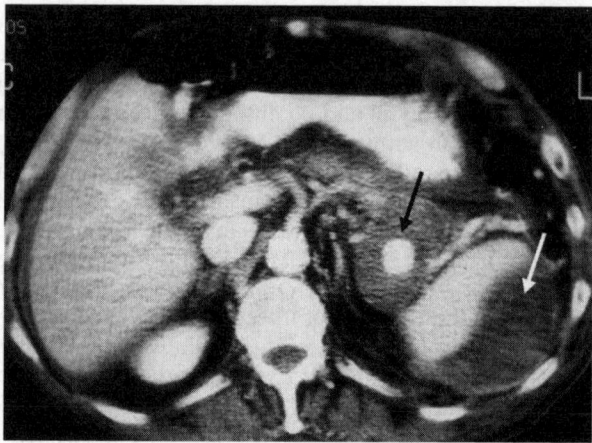

Figure 5 Arterial pseudoaneurysm within pseudocyst. CT with intravenous contrast shows a pseudocyst in the tail of the pancreas also involving the spleen (white arrow). In the centre of the pseudocyst an arterial pseudoaneurysm (black arrow) shows contrast enhancement equal to the aorta. Subsequent arteriogram showed the aneurysm to fill from the splenic artery and successful embolotherapy was performed

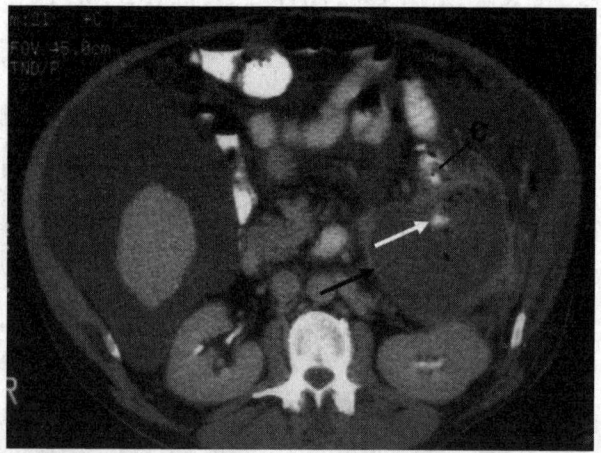

Figure 6 Pseudocyst eroding into colon following episode of acute pancreatitis. CT with intravenous contrast shows a pseudocyst in the tail of the pancreas (black arrow). Orally administered bowel contrast material opacifies the splenic flexure of the left colon (C) and has entered the pseudocyst (white arrow) indicating direct erosion. Gas bubbles are also present within the pseudocyst. The cyst was drained percutaneously and the fistula closed spontaneously without surgical intervention

obtained to define the precise anatomical relationship of the collection to surrounding structures and vessels, so that the catheter can be placed safely in the appropriate location[13,14].

Vascular complications

Involvement of the peripancreatic arteries and veins by the inflammatory process associated with acute pancreatitis is common, and can be detected accurately by DCT. Complications include erosion of intrapancreatic or peripancreatic arteries with acute haemorrhage, formation of arterial pseudoaneurysms (Figure 5), and thrombosis of branches of the portal venous system with formation of varices or acute mesenteric infarction[15].

Biliary tract involvement

The most common biliary tract abnormality associated with acute pancreatitis is cholelithiasis and/or choledocholithiasis. Biliary tract involvement by the inflammatory process associated with acute pancreatitis can be manifested by transient obstruction of the intrapancreatic segment of the common bile duct owing to periductal inflammation, or to compression by an adjacent pseudocyst or fluid collection, or chronic obstruction owing to a ductal stricture caused by the surrounding inflammatory process. Pancreatic pseudocysts can also involve the common bile duct directly, or they can invade into the liver, resulting in an intrahepatic biliary fistula[16].

Gastrointestinal tract involvement

While conventional contrast studies can detect abnormalities of the gastrointestinal tract caused by acute pancreatitis, DCT provides important information concerning the extent of the inflammatory process extrinsic to or surrounding the involved segment of the gastrointestinal tract[17]. The aetiology of the involvement can usually be elucidated (e.g. fluid collection, pseudocyst, or direct extension of the inflammatory process), and the appropriate surgical or interventional treatment can be planned (Figure 6).

Solid organ involvement

The inflammatory process of acute pancreatitis can extend to involve the contiguous solid organs, particularly the spleen, left kidney, and liver [18].

References

1. Balthazar E, Robinson D, Megibow A et al. Acute pancreatitis: value of CT in establishing prognosis. Radiology. 1990;174:331–6.
2. Balthazar E, Ranson J, Naidich D et al. Acute pancreatitis: prognostic value of CT. Radiology. 1985;156:767–72.
3. Beger H, Büchler M. Outcome of necrotizing pancreatitis in relation to morphological parameters. In: Malfertheiner P, Ditchuneit H, editors. Diagnostic Procedures in Pancreatic Disease. Springer-Verlag: Berlin, 1986:130–2.

4. Bradley E, Murphy F III, Ferguson C. Prediction of pancreatic necrosis by dynamic pancreatography. Ann Surg. 1989;210:495–504.
5. Johnson C, Stephens D, Sarr M. CT of acute pancreatitis: correlation between lack of contrast enhancement and pancreatic necrosis. Am J Roentgenol. 1991;156:93–5.
6. Larvin M, Chalmers A, McMahon M. Dynamic contrast enhanced computed tomography: a precise technique for identifying and localising pancreatic necrosis. Br Med J. 1990;300: 1425–8.
7. Maier W. Early objective diagnosis and staging of acute pancreatitis by contrast enhanced CT. In: Beger H, Büchler M, editors. Acute Pancreatitis. Springer-Verlag: Berlin, 1987:132–40.
8. Beger H, Bittner R, Block S et al. Bacterial contamination of pancreatic necrosis. A prospective study. Gastroenterology. 1986;91:433–8.
9. Banks P. Infected necrosis: morbidity and therapeutic consequences. Hepatogastroenterology. 1991;38:116–19.
10. Banks P. The role of needle-aspiration bacteriology in the management of necrotizing pancreatitis. In: Bradley E III, editor. Acute Pancreatitis: Diagnosis and Therapy. Raven Press: New York, 1994:99–103.
11. Kourtesis G, Wilson S, Williams R. The clinical significance of fluid collections in acute pancreatitis. Am Surg. 1990;56:796–99.
12. Yeo C, Bastidas J, Lynch-Nyhan A et al. The natural history of pancreatic pseudocysts documented by computed tomography. Surg Gynecol Obstet. 1990;170:411–17.
13. Freeny P, Lewis G, Traverso L et al. Infected pancreatic fluid collections: percutaneous catheter drainage. Radiology. 1988;167:435–41.
14. vanSonnenberg E, Casola G, Varney R et al. Imaging and interventional radiology for pancreatitis and complications. Radiol Clin N Am. 1989;27:65–72.
15. Vujic I. Vascular complications of pancreatitis. Radiol Clin N Am. 1989;27:81–91.
16. Rohrmann C, Baron R. Biliary complications of pancreatitis. Radiol Clin N Am. 1989; 27:93–104.
17. Safrit H, Rice R. Gastrointestinal complications of pancreatitis. Radiol Clin N Am. 1989; 27:73–9.
18. Freeny P, Lawson T. Radiology of the Pancreas. New York: Springer-Verlag, 1982.

Acute pancreatitis II

Section III
Controversial issues of therapy

Chair: M.W. BÜCHLER and U.R. FÖLSCH

6
Controversies in the treatment of acute pancreatitis: antibiotic therapy – when and why?

J. WERNER and M. W. BÜCHLER

INTRODUCTION

There has been great improvement in knowledge of the natural course and pathophysiology of acute pancreatitis over the past 20 years[1–5]. The clinical course of acute pancreatitis varies from a mild transitory form to a severe necrotizing disease. Most episodes of acute pancreatitis (80%) are mild and self-limiting, subsiding spontaneously within 3–5 days. Patients with mild pancreatitis respond well to medical treatment and generally do not need intensive-care treatment or pancreatic surgery. Thus, morbidity and mortality rates are below 1%[6–10]. In contrast, severe pancreatitis is associated with organ failure and/or local complications such as necrosis, abscess formation, or pseudocysts[11]. Severe pancreatitis can be observed in 15–20% of all cases.

PATHOPHYSIOLOGY OF SEVERE ACUTE PANCREATITIS

Severe pancreatitis develops in two phases. The first 2 weeks after onset of symptoms are characterized by the systemic inflammatory response syndrome (SIRS). The release of proinflammatory mediators is thought to contribute to the pathogenesis of SIRS-associated pulmonary, cardiovascular, and renal insufficiency. Mediators include pancreatic proteases, cytokines, reactive oxygen species, and many more[3,12–14]. In parallel, pancreatic necrosis develops within the first 4 days after the onset of symptoms to its full extent[15]. However, it is important that SIRS in the early phase of severe pancreatitis may be found in the absence of significant pancreatic necrosis and is frequently found in the absence of pancreatic infection[16,17]. In contrast, infection of pancreatic necrosis is still the major risk factor of sepsis-related multiple organ failure and the main life-threatening complication in the later phase of severe acute pancreatitis[6,18]. Infection of pancreatic necrosis develops most frequently in the second and third weeks after the onset of symptoms. Naturally pancreatic infection corelates with the duration of the disease, and up to 70% of all patients with necrotizing disease present with infected pancreatic necrosis 4 weeks after the onset of the disease[15,19,20]. Moreover, the risk of infection increases with the extent of intra- and extra-pancreatic necrosis[15,18].

DIAGNOSIS AND STAGING OF ACUTE PANCREATITIS

Although the majority of patients will have mild disease that resolves spontaneously, it is difficult to detect patients at risk of complications early on admission to hospital. The main problem has been the lack of accurate predictors of disease severity indicating development of necrosis and organ failure in the early stages, and infected necrosis, multi-organ failure, and sepsis in the later phase.

Contrast enhanced computed tomography (CE-CT) is the 'gold standard' for the diagnosis of pancreatic necrosis[4,21] (Figure 1). However, it will not reveal the complete extent of pancreatic necrosis before the fourth day after the onset of the disease[15]. The presence of more than 50% of pancreatic necrosis on CT scanning is predictive for severe disease, and helps to identify patients who might develop septic complications[22]. In most cases CE-CT is not capable of revealing the presence of superinfected necrosis in the later course of the disease[21,23], and the diagnosis of pancreatic necrosis does not predict the development of remote organ complications[16,17]. Several scoring systems for the assessment of severity of acute pancreatitis exist, including the Ranson, Glasgow, and APACHE II score[24,25]. However, they are only moderately accurate in assessing the disease severity of an individual patient. Although multiple single markers have been proposed as predictors of disease severity, C-

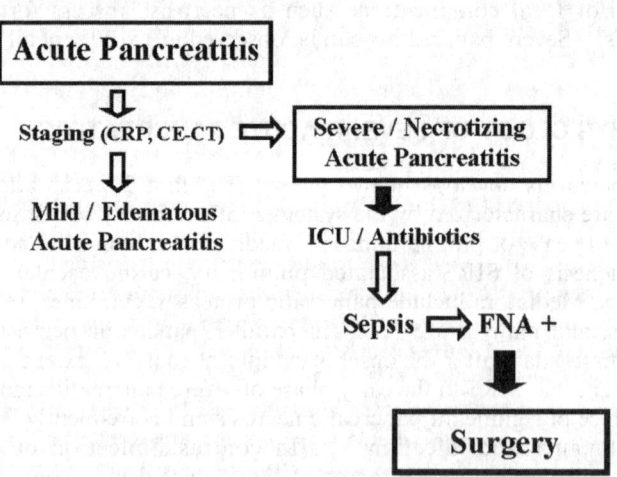

Figure 1 Therapeutical algorhithm of acute pancreatitis

reactive protein (CRP) is still the reference parameter of all single indicators[26]. CRP predicts severe pancreatitis and pancreatic necrosis accurately from the third day after onset of symptoms onwards[26–28]. Moreover, measurement of CRP is readily available almost everywhere. In contrast, no single parameter has been developed which is suitable for early prediction of infected pancreatic necrosis. Consequently, it is wise to treat every patient aggressively until disease severity has been established[6–10].

When pancreatic necrosis has developed, the differentiation between sterile and infected necrosis is essential for the management of patients, since infected pancreatic necrosis is an indication for surgical intervention[6,8] (Figure 1). Infection of necrotic pancreatic tissue is usually suspected in patients who develop clinical signs of sepsis[8]. These patients should undergo CT- or ultrasonography-guided fine-needle aspiration (FNA) of pancreatic or peri-pancreatic necrosis[6,8]. FNA is an accurate, safe, and reliable approach to differentiate between sterile and infected necrosis 19, 29. It is important to note that only those patients who present clinical signs of sepsis should undergo FNA, since FNA bears a potential risk of secondary infection. SIRS in the early phase of acute pancreatitis is no indication for FNA at our institution.

MANAGEMENT OF ACUTE PANCREATITIS

There are two primary objectives in the early treatment of patients with acute pancreatitis, The first is to provide supportive therapy and the second to prevent specific complications, especially superinfection of pancreatic necrosis.

Supportive treatment

All patients with signs of moderate to severe acute pancreatitis should be admitted to an intensive-care unit and referred to specialized centres for maximum supportive care[7,9,10]. Since complications may develop at any time, frequent reassessment and continuous monitoring is necessary. The most important supportive therapy is an adequate and prompt fluid resuscitation with intravenous fluids and supplemental oxygen with a liberal indication for assisted or controlled ventilation to guarantee optimal oxygen transport[30–32]. Cardioinotropic drugs, haemofiltration or dialysis may also be needed to allow optimal fluid therapy despite acute renal failure or hypoperfusion. Due to the popular belief that the pancreas should be put to 'rest' during acute pancreatitis, the parenteral route of administering nutrition is still predominantly used in acute pancreatitis[9,10,33]. However, there has been increasing concern regarding the gut being the main source of microorganisms causing infectious pancreatic complications and multiple organ failure[34]. In patients with severe pancreatitis, oral intake is inhibited by nausea and subileus. Whereas some reports have demonstrated that enteral feeding is possible in acute pancreatitis and associated with fewer septic complications[35,36], others did not show any beneficial effects[37]. Although the evidence is not conclusive to support enteral nutrition in all patients with severe acute pancreatitis, the enteral route may be used if that can be tolerated.

The supportive therapy also includes an adequate analgesia[30,31]. Several treatment regimens including opioids, or epidural blockade, have been widely advocated. However, these strategies of pain management are based on empirical experience rather than on results of controlled, prospective trials[38]. Treatment of acute pancreatitis is still symptomatic, with no specific medication being available today (Figure 1).

Antibiotic treatment

The development of infection of pancreatic necrosis is the main determinant of morbidity and mortality in the second phase of necrotizing pancreatitis. Unlike the use of antibiotics in the treatment of proven infection, the rationale for the use of prophylactic antibiotics in severe pancreatitis is to prevent infection from affecting areas of pancreatic necrosis, and consequently reducing the need for surgery and mortality. Evidence for the effectiveness of prophylactic antibiotics in the treatment of necrotizing pancreatitis has been given by various randomized controlled trials[39–45] (Table 1) and also by several meta-analyses[46,47]. Two meta-analyses have shown a positive benefit for prophylactic antibiotics in reducing mortality in acute pancreatitis[46,47]. However, the advantage was limited to patients with severe pancreatitis who received broad-spectrum antibiotics that achieved therapeutic pancreatic tissue levels. A more recent meta-analysis of the Cochrane Library[48] concluded that 'there was strong evidence that intravenous antibiotic prophylactic therapy for 10 to 14 days decreased the risk of superinfection of necrotic tissue and mortality in patients with severe acute pancreatitis with proven pancreatic necrosis at CT'. Therefore prophylactic antibiotic therapy is the only treatment in acute necrotizing pancreatitis in which significant benefit has been demonstrated by several meta-analyses which represent the highest level of evidence available.

The choice of the antibiotic agent is critical, since it must penetrate the pancreas and must have the right spectrum of activity against the microorganisms commonly found in infected necrosis. Büchler et al.[49,50] and Bassi et al.[51] have identified imipenem as the antibiotic agent of first choice because it reached higher pancreatic tissue levels and provided higher bactericidal activity against most of the bacteria present in pancreatic infection compared to other types of antibiotics. This finding may be reflected by a significantly lower infection rate of pancreatic necrosis with imipenem compared to pefloxacin[44]. No significant differences have been shown between imipenem and meropenem, a new carbapenem antibiotic[45]. An alternative antibiotic regimen is either ciprofloxacin or ofloxacin in combination with metronidazole. However, a recently published double-blind, placebo-controlled multicentre trial evaluating ciprofloxacin in combination with metronidazole compared to a placebo group detected no benefit of antibiotic prophylaxis with respect to the risk of developing infected pancreatic necrosis[43]. Importantly, in that study almost 50% of patients in the placebo group were started on antibiotic therapy because of septic complications that emerged during the course of the trial. The severity of the disease may also have been low in many of these patients, since mortality and infection rates of the control group were just 7% and 9%, respectively.

Table 1 Prospective randomized trials of prophylactic antibiotic therapy in severe acute pancreatitis

Reference	Drug	No. of patients		Rate of pancreatic infection (%)		Rate of MOF/major organ complications		Mortality (%)	
		Control	Case	Control	Case	Control	Case	Control	Case
Pederzoli et al.[39]	Imipenem	33	41	30	12[a]	39	29	12	7
Sainio et al.[40]	Cefuroxime	30	30	40	30			23	3[b]
Schwarz et al.[41]	Ofloxacin/metronidazole	13	13	53	61			15	0
Nordback et al.[42]	Imipenem	33	25			25	7[c]	5	2
Isenmann et al.[43]	Ciprofloxacin/metronidazole	56	58	9	12			5	7
Bassi et al.[44]	Pefloxacin vs. imipenem	Pefloxacin 30	Imipenem 30	Pefloxacin 34	Imipenem 10[d]	Pefloxacin	Imipenem	Pefloxacin 24	Imipenem 10
Manes et al.[45]	Meronem vs. imepenem	Meronem 88	Imepenem 88	Meronem 11	Imipenem 14	Meronem 7/34	Imipenem 9/38	Meronem 14	Imipenem 11

MOF: multiple organ failure.
[a] $p < 0.01$; [b] $p = 0.028$; [c] $p < 0.001$; [d] $p \leq 0.05$.

CONCLUSIONS

The most significant change in the clinical course of acute pancreatitis over the past decade has undoubtedly been the decrease in mortality. Overall mortality is now about 5%, and for severe cases in the range of 10–20%[6,16,52–54]. The major improvements include intensive-care medicine, the accurate diagnosis of necrosis by CE-CT, the reliable diagnosis of infected necrosis by FNA, the ERCP concept in gallstone pancreatitis, and the administration of prophylactic antibiotics in severe necrotizing pancreatitis[54].

Today there is no doubt that pancreatic infection is the major risk factor in necrotizing pancreatitis with regard to morbidity and mortality in the later phase of the disease[6,15,55]. The infection is usually due to gut-derived aerobic organisms. Although many antibiotics could be used, several groups of antibiotics do not reach therapeutically relevant levels in the pancreas and thus cannot be effective. Imipenem has been identified as the antibiotic agent of first choice because it showed higher pancreatic tissue levels and provided higher bactericidal activity against most of the bacteria present in pancreatic infection. An alternative regimen is either ciprofloxacin or ofloxacin in combination with[50].

Several randomized controlled trials have demonstrated that prophylactic administration of antibiotics prevents superinfection of pancreatic necrosis, decreases septic complications, and mortality (Table 1). So far only one multicentre trial using ciprofloxacin and metronidazole has reached the conclusion that there is no benefit of antibiotic prophylaxis with respect to the risk of developing infected necrosis.

Despite variations in drug agent, case mix, duration of treatment and methodological quality, there is the strongest evidence possible (evidence level Ia) that intravenous antibiotic prophylactic therapy for 10–14 days decreases the risk of superinfection of necrotic tissue, septic complications, and mortality in patients with severe acute pancreatitis[56]. Further studies are required to confirm all of the benefits suggested, to provide more adequate data on adverse effects and germ shift, and to address the choice of antibacterial agents and effects of varying duration of therapy.

References

1. Buter A, Imrie C, Carter C et al. Dynamic nature of early organ dysfunction determines outcome in acute pancreatitis. Br J Surg. 2002;89:298–302.
2. Isenmann R, Beger H. Natural history of acute pancreatitis and the role of infection. Baillieres Best Pract Res Clin Gastroenterol. 1999;13:291–301.
3. Johnson C, Kingsnorth A, Imrie C et al. Double blind, randomised, placebo controlled study of a platelet activating factor antagonist, lexipafant, in the treatment and prevention of organ failure in predicted severe acute pancreatitis. Gut. 2001;48:62–9.
4. Uhl W, Roggo A, Kirschstein T et al. Influence of contrast-enhanced computed tomography on course and outcome in patients with acute pancreatitis. Pancreas. 2002;24:191–7.
5. Klar E, Werner J. New pathophysiological findings in acute pancreatitis. Chirurg. 2000;71: 253–64.
6. Buchler MW, Gloor B, Müller CA et al. Acute necrotizing pancreatitis: treatment strategy according to the status of infection. Ann Surg. 2000;232:619–26.

7. Rünzi M, Layer P, Büchler M. The therapy of acute pancreatitis. General guidelines. Working Group of the Society for Scientific–Medical Specialities. Z Gastroenterol. 2000; 38:571–81.
8. Uhl W, Warshaw A, Imrie C et al. IAP guidelines for the surgical management of acute pancreatitis. Pancreatology. 2002;175.
9. United Kingdom guidelines for the management of acute pancreatitis. Gut. 1998;42:S1–13.
10. Dervenis C, Johnson CD, Bassi C et al. Diagnosis, objective assessment of severity, and management of acute pancreatitis. Int J Pancreatol. 1999;25:195–200.
11. Bradley ELD. A clinically based classification system for acute pancreatitis. Summary of the International Symposium on Acute Pancreatitis, Atlanta, GA, September 11–13, 1992. Arch Surg. 1993;128:586–90.
12. Steer ML, Meldolesi J. The cell biology of experimental pancreatitis. N Engl J Med. 1987; 316:144–50.
13. Werner J, Z'Graggen K, Fernandez-del Castillo C et al. Specific therapy for local and systemic complications of acute pancreatitis with monoclonal antibodies against ICAM-1. Ann Surg. 1999;229:834–40.
14. Norman J. The role of cytokines in the pathogenesis of acute pancreatitis. Am J Surg. 1998; 175:76–83.
15. Beger HG, Bittner R, Block S, Büchler M. Bacterial contamination of pancreatic necrosis – a prospective clinical study. Gastroenterology. 1986;91:433–41.
16. Tenner S, Sica G, Hughes M et al. Relationship of necrosis to organ failure in severe acute pancreatitis. Gastroenterology. 1997; 113:899–903.
17. Lankisch P, Pflichthofer D, Lehnick D. No strict correlation between necrosis and organ failure in acute pancreatitis. Pancreas. 2000;20:319–22.
18. Isenmann R, Rau B, Beger H. Bacterial infection and extent of necrosis are determinants of organ failure in patients with acute necrotizing pancreatitis. Br J Surg. 1999;86:1020–4.
19. Gerzof SG, Banks PA, Robbins AH et al. Early diagnosis of pancreatic infection by computed tomography-guided aspiration. Gastroenterology. 1987;93:1315–20.
20. Bassi C, Falconi M, Girelli F. Microbiological findings in severe pancreatitis. Surg Res Commun. 1989;5:1–4.
21. Balthazar E, Robinson D, Megibow A, Ranson J. Acute pancreatitis: value of CT in establishing prognosis. Radiology. 1990;174:331–6.
22. Isenmann R, Buchler M, Uhl W et al. Pancreatic necrosis: an early finding in severe acute pancreatitis. Pancreas. 1993;8:358–61.
23. Kemppainen E, Sainio V, Haapiainen R et al. Early localization of necrosis by contrast-enhanced computed tomography can predict outcome in severe acute pancreatitis. Br J Surg. 1996;83:924–9.
24. Ranson J, Rifkind K, Roses D et al. Prognostic signs and the role of operative management in acute pancreatitis. Surg Gynecol Obstet. 1974;139:69–81.
25. Wilson C, Heath DI, Imrie CW. Prediction of outcome in acute pancreatitis: a comparative study of APACHE II, clinical assessment and multiple factor scoring systems. Br J Surg. 1990;77:1260–4.
26. Werner J, Hartwig W, Uhl W et al. Useful markers for predicting severity and monitoring progression of acute pancreatitis. Pancreatology. 2003;3:115–27.
27. Wilson C, Heads A, Shenkin A, Imrie CW. C-reactive protein, antiproteases and complement factors as objective markers of severity in acute pancreatitis [see comments]. Br J Surg. 1989;76:177–81.
28. Buchler MW, Malfertheiner P, Schoetensack C et al. Sensitivity of antiproteases, complement factors and C-reactive protein in detecting pancreatic necrosis: results of a prospective clinical trial study. Int J Pancreatol. 1986;1:227–35.
29. Banks P, Gerzof S, Langevin R et al. CT-guided aspiration of suspected pancreatic infection: bacteriology and clinical outcome. Int J Pancreatol. 1995;18:265–70.
30. Niederau C, Schulz H. Current conservative treatment of acute pancreatitis: evidence from animal and human studies. Hepatogastroenterology. 1993;40:538–49.
31. Sigurdson G. Acute pancreatitis: therapeutic options in multiple organ failure. In: Büchler M, Uhl W, Friess H, Malfertheiner P, editors. Acute Pancreatitis: Novel Concepts in Biology and Therapy. Oxford: Blackwell Science, 1999:395–410.
32. Werner J, Klar E. Effective treatment regimens in the management of acute pancreatitis. Chir Gastroenterol. 1999;15:328–33.

33. Grant J, James S, Grabowski V, Trexler K. Total parenteral nutrition in pancreatic disease. Ann Surg. 1984;200:627–31.
34. Runkel N, Rodriguez L, Moody F. Mechanisms of sepsis in acute pancreatitis in oppossums. Am J Surg. 1995;169:227–32.
35. Kalfarentzos F, Kehagias J, Mead N et al. Enteral nutrition is superior to parenteral nutrition in severe acute pancreatitis: results of a randomized prospective trial. Br J Surg. 1997;84:1665–9.
36. Windsor A, Kanwar S, Li A et al. Compared with parenteral nutrition, enteral feeding attenuates the acute phase response and improves severity in acute pancreatitis. Gut. 1998; 42:431–5.
37. Powell J, Murchison J, Fearon K et al. Randomized controlled trial of the effect of early enteral nutrition on markers of the inflammatory response in predicted severe acute pancreatitis. Br J Surg. 2000;87:1375–81.
38. Mössner J. Current standards for the management of acute pancreatitis and pain. In: Büchler M, Uhl W, Friess H, Malfertheiner P, editors. Acute Pancreatitis: Novel Concepts in Biology and Therapy. Oxford: Blackwell Science, 1999:293–7.
39. Pederzoli P, Bassi C, Vesentini S, Campedelli A. A randomized multicenter clinical trial of antibiotic prophylaxis of septic complications in acute necrotizing pancreatitis with imipenem. Surg Gynecol Obstet. 1993;176:480–7.
40. Sainio V, Kemppainen E, Puolakkainen P. Early antibiotic treatment of severe acute alcoholic pancreatitis. Lancet. 1995;346:663–7.
41. Schwarz M, Isenmann R, Meyer H, Beger H. Antibiotics in necrotizing pancreatitis. Results of a controlled study. Dtsch Med Wochenschr. 1997;122:356–61.
42. Nordback I, Sand J, Saaristo R, Paajanen H. Early treatment with antibiotics reduces the need for surgery in acute necrotizing pancreatitis – a single-center randomized study. J Gastrointestinal Surg. 2001;5:113–20.
43. Isenmann R, Runzi M, Kron M et al. Prophylactic antibiotic treatment in patients with predicted severe acute pancreatitis: a placebo-controlled, double-blind trial. Gastroenterology. 2004;126:997–1004.
44. Bassi C, Falconi M, Talamini G. Controlled clinical trial of pefloxacin versus imipenem in severe acute pancreatitis. Gastroenterology. 1998;115:1513–17.
45. Manes G, Rabitti P, Menchise A et al. Prophylaxis with meropenem of septic complications in acute pancreatitis: a randomized, controlled trial versus imipenem. Pancreas. 2003;27: 79–83.
46. Golub R, Siddiqi F, Pohl D. Role of antibiotics in acute pancreatitis: a meta-analysis. J. Gastrointest Surg. 1998;2:496–503.
47. Sharma VK, Howden CW. Prophylactic antibiotic sepsis and mortality in acute necrotizing pancreatitis: a meta-analysis. Pancreas. 2001;22:28–31.
48. Villatoro E, Larvin M, Bassi C. Antibiotic therapy for prophylaxis against infection of pancreatic necrosis in acute pancreatitis. Cochrane Database of Systematic Reviews. 2003; 4:CD002941.
49. Buchler M, Malfertheiner P, Friess H et al. The penetration of antibiotics into human pancreas. Infection. 1989;17:20–5.
50. Buchler M, Malfertheiner P, Friess H et al. Human pancreatic tissue concentration of bactericidal antibiotics. Gastroenterology. 1992;103:1902–8.
51. Bassi C, Pederzoli P, Vesentini S. Behaviour of antibiotics during human necrotizing pancreatitis. Antimicrob Agents Chemother. 1994;38:830–6.
52. Bradley A, Allen K. A prospective longitudinal study of observation versus surgical intervention in the management of necrotizing pancreatitis. Am J Surg. 1991;161:19–24.
53. Sarr MG, Nagorney DM, Mucha P Jr et al. Acute necrotizing pancreatitis: management by planned, staged pancreatic necrosectomy/debridement and delayed primary wound closure over drains. Br J Surg. 1991;78:576–81.
54. Bank S. Clinical course of acute pancreatitis: what has changed in recent years? In: Büchler MW, Friess H, Uhl W, Malfertheiner P, editors. Acute Pancreatitis: Novel Concepts in Biology and Therapy. Berlin, Vienna: Blackwell Science, 1999:164–9.
55. Widdison AL, Karanjia ND. Pancreatic infection complicating acute pancreatitis. Br J Surg. 1993;80:148–54.
56. Uhl W, Warshaw A, Imrie C et al. IAP guidelines for the surgical management of acute pancreatitis. Pancreatology. 2002;175.

7
Acute pancreatitis: benefit of early enteral feeding?

D. BIMMLER

INTRODUCTION

A mere decade ago, to treat a patient with acute pancreatitis seemed rather straightforward for just about every resident: it meant intravenous fluids, adequate painkillers and a strict nil-by-mouth regimen for at least a couple of days. Nutritional support was given, if at all, via the parenteral route.

The rationale behind this regimen was the concept that any stimulation of the inflamed gland must be avoided as it would aggravate the disease.

However, things have changed. In a recent publication[1], Flint and colleagues describe the nutritional support of patients treated for severe acute pancreatitis in their intensive-care unit: over a 10-year period a predominantly parenteral nutrition has been replaced by mostly enteral feeding.

Mitchell et al. state in their review paper on acute pancreatitis[2]: 'Enteral feeding by nasojejunal tube ... has largely replaced total parenteral nutrition in the management of patients with severely catabolic acute pancreatitis'.

At the University Hospital of Zurich we had followed the same path in the late 1990s. When preparing this chapter, I was curious to learn about the present policy in other parts of Switzerland. I thus sent out a very short questionnaire to the major hospitals in every Canton of Switzerland. The return rate was 79% (49 of 62), with an equal distribution of medical and surgical units. The answers are therefore representative for the whole country.

The first question asked the recipients to choose the correct or best description of their therapeutic approach in a freshly diagnosed case of acute pancreatitis: The patient

(a) shall be kept on a nil-by-mouth regimen until the inflammation subsides clinically and chemically (i.e. possibly for more than 48 h),

(b) shall in case of a mild course of the disease start eating within 48 h at the most, independent of clinical or chemical signs of inflammation.

Only one out of four opted for a strict nil-by-mouth regimen, while 75% start refeeding their patients early.

The second question dealt with severe cases and patients who could not tolerate eating due to nausea or vomiting. Regarding these patients a choice of three was given: The patient receives

(a) total parenteral nutrition,

(b) enteral nutrition via a nasojejunal tube,

(c) enteral nutrition via a nasogastric tube.

A distinct majority (55%) of medical and surgical units in major Swiss hospitals apply enteral nutrition via nasojejunal tube to give nutritional support to their patients with severe acute pancreatitis. Only a few feed by way of a nasogastric tube. Roughly 40% prefer total parenteral nutrition.

What are the advantages of early enteral nutrition that seem to have convinced the majority of our colleagues to take such a U-turn in their therapeutic strategy?

In trying to answer this question I shall start by listing some of the more recent guidelines for the management of acute pancreatitis, then proceed to the evidence basis regarding pancreas and gut pathophysiology, and last, but not least comment on the prospective randomized controlled trials comparing enteral nutrition, total parenteral nutrition or no nutritional support.

GUIDELINES

In the late 1990s, according to the American College of Gastroenterologists[3], nutritional support was indicated only for patients who had been without oral nutrition for at least a week, and parenteral nutrition was recommended in such cases. The British guidelines[4] that were issued shortly afterwards did not even mention nutritional support. Some five years later the situation had changed: the World Congress of Gastroenterology[5] recommended enteral nutrition, as did the Japanese Society of Emergency Abdominal Medicine[6]. The European Society of Parenteral and Enteral Nutrition (ESPEN), on the other hand, remained cautious in their consensus statement[7]: 'Thus far, there is no generally accepted or standardized approach for handling nutrition in patients with acute pancreatitis'.

PANCREAS PATHOPHYSIOLOGY

Pancreatic secretion underlies a complex neurohumoral control. We distinguish a cephalic, a gastric and an intestinal phase of stimulation. Synthesis and secretion of enzymes are controlled by cholecystokinin and the vagal nerve, while bicarbonate secretion is stimulated by secretin and the vasoactive intestinal polypeptide.

With respect to enteral nutrition, it seems important that lipids or proteins delivered into the duodenum represent a powerful stimulus for the pancreas, while the same nutrients delivered into the jejunum exert only a minor stimulation. The latter can be reduced further by replacing these nutrients with an elemental diet.

Bodoky and colleagues[8] reported that enteral nutrition administered via catheter feeding jejunostomy does not stimulate pancreatic secretion more than parenteral nutrition. Regarding acute pancreatitis, our traditional belief was that oral feeding would cause a cholecystokinin release and thereby stimulate pancreatic enzyme synthesis and secretion. This in turn would aggravate the inflammatory process that had been initiated by premature trypsin activation. This belief had led to the concept of 'pancreatic rest', a concept based mainly on studies performed in healthy human individuals. However, things are different in acute pancreatitis. Thanks to experimental data from animals we know that secretion is suppressed during acute pancreatitis[9]. This secretory block also seems to occur in humans[10].

When Qin and co-authors[11] investigated nutritional support in severe acute pancreatitis provoked in dogs, they found no relevant stimulation of enzyme release or pancreatic juice secretion, nor a deterioration of acute pancreatitis in animals fed intrajejunally.

Another observation in line with these findings refers to the effects of somatostatin. Somatostatin and its analogues strongly inhibit pancreatic secretion. However, it had no effect on the course of acute pancreatitis in two multicentre studies[12,13]. With the secretory block during acute pancreatitis in mind this does not come as a surprise.

Severe acute pancreatitis can be described as a state of catabolic stress, characterized by a systemic inflammatory response, often leading to multiple organ failure, associated with nutritional deterioration.

The questions to answer are:

1. Is nutritional support important with regard to recovery?

2. Should we apply total parenteral nutrition or enteral nutrition?

It seems that acute pancreatitis is associated with a significant delay in small-intestinal transit time and with a reduced intestinal oxygen and nutrient delivery due to impaired blood supply. Such a state will favour bacterial overgrowth and may lead to increased bacterial translocation.

It is well known that infection of pancreatic necrosis is the main cause of a late death from severe acute pancreatitis. The most important sources of bacterial infection are indwelling catheters and the gut. One of the primary goals in our therapeutic strategy must therefore be the prevention of bacterial translocation. Thus the patient needs an intact mucosal barrier function and, to ensure the latter, an adequate delivery of oxygen and nutrients to the gut. We therefore have to guarantee an adequate blood supply to the gut and, as some of us believe, provide for enteral feeding.

Foitzik has demonstrated, in a rat model of severe acute pancreatitis, that enterally supplied nutrients stabilize the intestinal mucosal barrier[14].

GUT PATHOPHYSIOLOGY

The intestinal tract has several distinct tasks: it is meant to digest nutrients and absorb them. It is an important source of cytokines, and it represents an immunological barrier. Any condition of intestinal ischaemia, e.g. severe acute pancreatitis, can cause an overactivation of gut macrophages and of the gut-associated lymphoid tissue (GALT), leading to a release of cytokines and other mediators and thus to a systemic inflammatory response.

The purpose of the gut barrier is to prevent bacteria and endotoxins from entering the systemic circulation. Several factors add up to the gut barrier function; i.e. peristalsis, the mucus, the indigenous gastrointestinal microflora, an intact epithelial layer, secretory immunoglobulins, and the GALT. In order to reliably assess the correct functioning of the gut barrier, a microbiological examination of the normally sterile extraintestinal tissue must be performed.

In animals, fasting leads to mucosal atrophy; this probably weakens the gut barrier. However, epithelial cell turnover differs from species to species. The cell migration time from the base of the crypt to the villus tips where exfoliation occurs takes 6–7 days in humans, but only 1–2 days in rodents[15]. While bowel rest in rats is associated with mucosal atrophy within days, no dramatic changes occur in human mucosal architecture after periods of bowel rest that last up to 1 month. MacFie could not find any difference in mucosal architecture comparing patients who had been supplied with total parenteral nutrition for 10 days preoperatively to patients who had eaten normally before the operation[15].

It is furthermore interesting that in patients with severe acute pancreatitis no association was found between the early increase in intestinal permeability or systemic endotoxin exposure and systemic bacterial translocation[16]. This was investigated by assessment of microbial DNA in the blood of such patients.

There are three possible pathways by which gut bacteria may get into the pancreas: the lymphatic, the haematogenous, and the transmural way. Under normal conditions, however, bacteria that migrate from the gut lumen are entrapped and killed by immunocompetent cells[17].

Concluding from animal studies, there are several risk factors for bacterial translocation: reduced splanchnic blood flow, impaired host immune defence (GALT), and alterations of the gut microflora (due to antibiotics or nutritional changes). Only the last one has also been shown to be a risk factor in humans[15].

ADVANTAGES OF ENTERAL NUTRITION

Advantages of enteral nutrition primarily seem to consist in the lack of disadvantages associated with total parenteral nutrition.

In a randomized controlled trial comparing early total parenteral nutrition (TPN) to no nutritional support, Sax and colleagues[18] found no benefit of TPN regarding hospital stay or complications, but a high rate of catheter-related infections. Heyland and co-authors, in 1998, made a rather pronounced and provocative statement[19]: They equalled TPN with 'Total poisonous nutrition'. In their meta-analysis of trials comparing TPN and no nutritional support they found a 1.78-fold increased risk of dying during critical illness in the parenterally fed group. For others, e.g. MacFie, it seems to be less clear. Studies comparing TPN with enteral nutrition were not always isocaloric. Enteral nutrition often achieved only some 50% of the target intake. The negative effects of TPN, therefore, may be due to overfeeding with consecutive hyperglycaemia and impaired complement fixation, not due to TPN in general[15].

On the other hand, studies from trauma surgery have demonstrated earlier that in severely injured patients enteral nutrition favourably alters the outcome[20].

Feasibility studies applying enteral nutrition to patients suffering from acute pancreatitis were reported in the late 1990s. Nasojejunal feeding did not reactivate the inflammatory process in moderate or severe acute pancreatitis, and was successfully installed in 20 out of 21 patients[21].

To the surprise of many among us, nasogastric delivery of a low-fat semi-elemental diet was equally successful in 22 of 26 patients with severe acute pancreatitis, without evidence of disease exacerbation[22].

PROSPECTIVE RANDOMIZED CONTROLLED TRIALS

In the meantime, several prospective randomized controlled trials have compared TPN and enteral nutrition. The first one, published in 1997 by McClave and co-authors[23], included patients with mild acute pancreatitis only, and its conclusions may thus not be relevant.

The study reported by Windsor and colleagues[24] did involve patients with mild and with severe acute pancreatitis. It showed a trend in favour of enteral nutrition, but only 13 of 34 patients had severe acute pancreatitis.

The hitherto most important trial comes from the Kalfarentzos group[25]. Following 38 patients with severe acute pancreatitis they found similar morbidity, hospital stay and mortality, but more catheter sepsis and hyperglycaemia in the TPN group.

Two prospective randomized controlled studies have been published more recently, one by Abou-Assi, the second by Gupta and co-authors. Abou-Assi and co-workers[10] studied 53 patients, 26 of whom displayed moderate or severe acute pancreatitis with a Ranson score of more than 3. Severe complications such as acute respiratory distress syndrome (ARDS) or multiple organ failure (MOF) and death occurred with similar incidence in both groups. However, nutritional support was necessary for a significantly shorter time with enteral nutrition than with TPN (6.7 vs 10.8 days, $p < 0.001$). Hyperglycaemia was significantly more frequent in the TPN group (more than 3-fold), catheter-related infections 9 times more frequent. While some 85% of the target calories were achieved with TPN, only 49% were reached with enteral nutrition. Total hospitalization costs and daily costs for feeding were significantly lower with enteral nutrition.

The study published by Gupta and colleagues[26] again reported only a very small number of patients ($n = 17$), albeit all of them with severe acute pancreatitis. Hospital stay was significantly shorter with enteral nutrition, organ failure occurred with TPN only. No new aspects evolved from this trial.

So far only one prospective randomized controlled trial has compared enteral nutrition to no nutritional support[27]. Powell and colleagues found only little benefit from enteral feeding and no amelioration with regard to acute-phase proteins such as IL-6, TNF-RI and CRP. They did, however, achieve only 21% of the target daily intake during the first 5 days, mainly due to ileus problems. Their results are thus rather questionable, primarily telling us that it may not always be easy to install enteral nutrition.

The prospective randomized controlled trial studying nasogastric versus nasojejunal delivery of enteral nutrition has so far been published in abstract form only[28]; it found no significant difference in mortality or morbidity.

Up to now, two meta-analyses with respect to our topic have been published, and these came to fairly similar conclusions[29,30]. In the more recent meta-analysis, Marik and co-workers looked at six prospective randomized controlled trials comparing enteral and total parenteral nutrition, involving 263 participants. The combined data resulted in a significantly lower incidence of infections in the enteral nutrition group, with a relative risk of 0.45. Surgical interventions were significantly less frequent (relative risk 0.48), and hospital stays shorter (mean reduction of 2.9 days) with enteral nutrition.

The authors of this meta-analysis pointed out various limitations, e.g. the different selection of patients and the different study designs. They made clear that the individual studies were underpowered and of relatively poor quality. They pointed out that conclusions from these studies can only be drawn thanks to the fact that their results are supported by experimental data and by clinical studies on parenteral or enteral nutrition in other critically ill patients[30].

The ESPEN consensus statement published in 2002 summarizes the evidence as follows[7]:

'Several prospective randomized controlled trials provide evidence that jejunal feeding is possible and safe, but the evidence that it is effective or beneficial remains tenuous. [In clinical practice] there is no evidence to support the thesis that prolonged TPN suppresses the immune system and promotes gastrointestinal leakage with the potential risk of subsequent bacterial translocation'.

As we have frequently seen in modern medicine, it seems rather difficult to provide a conclusive study showing which therapeutic approach is best for our patients. Looking at all the papers published on the topic of nutritional support in acute pancreatitis we cannot but realize that papers putting forward the authors' opinion by far outrange the papers presenting randomized trials.

Astonishingly, at least a part of the medical world seems to have changed its opinion on TPN or enteral nutrition in acute pancreatitis even before this scarce evidence was published.

The ESPEN, though, have remained cautious on the issue. Their consensus statement recommends that the route of nutrient delivery should be determined by patient tolerance. Nutritional therapy in patients with severe acute pancreatitis may be started with an enteral jejunal approach. Parenteral nutrition remains an alternative method when enteral nutrition is inadequate.

There is nothing to be added to this well-balanced statement, apart from maybe this: in order to carry out evidence-based medicine we would need larger trials on the matter, if possible including immuno-enhancing feeds.

References

1. Flint R, Windsor J, Bonham M. Trends in the management of severe acute pancreatitis: interventions and outcome. ANZ J Surg. 2004;74:335-42.
2. Mitchell R, Byrne MF, Baillie J. Pancreatitis. Lancet. 2003;361:1447-55.
3. Banks PA. Practice guidelines in acute pancreatitis. Am J Gastroenterol. 1997;92:377-86.
4. Anonymous. United Kingdom guidelines for the management of acute pancreatitis. British Society of Gastroenterology [see comment]. Gut. 1998;42(Suppl. 2):S1-13.
5. Toouli J, Brooke-Smith M, Bassi C et al. Guidelines for the management of acute pancreatitis. J Gastroenterol Hepatol. 2002;17:S15.
6. Mayumi T, Ura H, Arata S et al. Evidence-based clinical practice guidelines for acute pancreatitis: proposals. J Hepatobiliary Pancreat Surg. 2002;9:413-22.
7. Meier R, Beglinger C, Layer P et al. ESPEN guidelines on nutrition in acute pancreatitis. European Society of Parenteral and Enteral Nutrition. Clin Nutr. 2002;21:173-83.
8. Bodoky G, Harsanyi L, Tihanyi T, Flautner L, Pap A. Effect of enteral nutrition on exocrine pancreatic function. Am J Surg. 1991;161:144-8.
9. Niederau C, Niederau M, Luthen R, Strohmeyer G, Ferrell LD, Grendell JH. Pancreatic exocrine secretion in acute experimental pancreatitis [see comment]. Gastroenterology. 1990;99:1120-7.
10. Abou-Assi S, Craig K, O'Keefe SJD. Hypocaloric jejunal feeding is better than total parenteral nutrition in acute pancreatitis: results of a randomized comparative study. Am J Gastroenterol. 2002;97:2255-62.
11. Qin HL, Su ZD, Hu LG, Ding ZX, Lin QT. Parenteral versus early intrajejunal nutrition: effect on pancreatitic natural course, entero-hormones release and its efficacy on dogs with acute pancreatitis. World J Gastroenterol. 2003;9:2270-3.
12. D'Amico D, Favia G, Biasiato R et al. The use of somatostatin in acute pancreatitis – results of a multicenter trial. Hepatotgastroenterology. 1990;37:92-8.
13. Gjorup I, Roikjaer O, Andersen B et al. A double-blinded multicenter trial of somatostatin in the treatment of acute pancreatitis. Surg Gynecol Obstet. 1992;175:397-400.
14. Foitzik T. [Pancreatitis and nutrition. Significance of the gastrointestinal tract and nutrition for septic complications]. Z Chirurg. 2001;126:4-9.
15. MacFie J. Enteral versus parenteral nutrition: the significance of bacterial translocation and gut-barrier function. Nutrition. 2000;16:606-11.
16. Ammori B, Fitzgerald P, Hawkey P, McMahon M. The early increase in intestinal permeability and systemic endotoxin exposure in patients with severe acute pancreatitis is not associated with systemic bacterial translocation: molecular investigation of microbial DNA in the blood. Pancreas. 2003;26:18-22.
17. Deitch EA. Bacterial translocation of the gut flora. J Trauma Inj Inf Crit Care. 1990;30(12 Suppl.):S184-9.
18. Sax HC, Warner BW, Talamini MA et al. Early total parenteral nutrition in acute pancreatitis: lack of beneficial effects. Am J Surg. 1987;153:117-24.
19. Heyland DK, MacDonald S, Keefe L, Drover JW. Total parenteral nutrition in the critically ill patient: a meta-analysis [see comment]. J Am Med Assoc. 1998;280:2013-9.
20. Moore FA, Moore EE, Kudsk KA et al. Clinical benefits of an immune-enhancing diet for early postinjury enteral feeding. J Trauma Inj Inf Crit Care. 1994;37:607-15.
21. Nakad A, Piessevaux H, Marot J et al. Is early enteral nutrition in acute pancreatitis dangerous? About 20 patients fed by an endoscopically placed naso-gastro-jejunal tube. Pancreas. 1998;17:187-93.
22. Eatock F, Brombacher G, Steven A, Imrie C, McKay C, Carter R. Nasogastric feeding in severe acute pancreatitis may be practical and safe. Int J Pancreatol. 2000;28:23-9.
23. McClave S, Greene L, Snider H et al. Comparison of the safety of early enteral vs. parenteral nutrition in mild acute pancreatitis. J Parent Ent Nutr. 1997;21:14-20.
24. Windsor ACJ, Kanwar S, Li AGK et al. Compared with parenteral nutrition, enteral feeding attenuates the acute phase response and improves disease severity in acute pancreatitis. Gut. 1998;42:431-5.
25. Kalfarentzos F, Kehagias J, Mead N, Kokkinis K, Gogos C. Enteral nutrition is superior to parenteral nutrition in severe acute pancreatitis: results of a randomized prospective trial. Br J Surg. 1997;84:1665-9.

26. Gupta R, Patel K, Calder PC, Yaqoob P, Primrose JN, Johnson CD. A randomised clinical trial to assess the effect of total enteral and total parenteral nutritional support on metabolic, inflammatory and oxidative markers in patients with predicted severe acute pancreatitis (APACHE II > or = 6). Pancreatology. 2003;3:406–13.
27. Powell J, Murchison J, Fearon K, Ross J, Siriwardena A. Randomized controlled trial of the effect of early enteral nutrition on markers of the inflammatory response in predicted severe acute pancreatitis. Br J Surg. 2000;87:1375–81.
28. Eatock F. Abstract. Pancreatology. 2001;1:149a.
29. Al-Omran M, Groof A, Wilke D. Enteral versus parenteral nutrition for acute pancreatitis [update of Cochrane Database Syst Rev. 2001;(2):CD002837; PMID: 11406048]. Cochrane Database of Systematic Reviews, 2003;1.
30. Marik PE, Zaloga GP. Meta-analysis of parenteral nutrition versus enteral nutrition in patients with acute pancreatitis. Br Med J. 2004;328:1407.

8
Sterile necrosis and/or pseudocyst – endoscopic intervention, surgery, or wait and see?

P. A. BANKS

INTRODUCTION

According to the Atlanta Symposium of 1992, pancreatic necrosis was defined as local or diffuse areas of non-viable or dead pancreatic parenchyma often associated with peripancreatic fat necrosis. A pseudocyst was defined as a collection of pancreatic juice enclosed by a wall of fibrous or granulation tissue[1]. A third term that has come into use since the Atlanta symposium is organized necrosis[2]. This term characterizes the somewhat ovoid configuration of pancreatic necrosis once there has been resolution of the peripancreatic and pancreatic inflammatory components of necrotizing pancreatitis. Some investigators prefer to call this entity a pancreatic pseudocyst, whereas others prefer to restrict the use of the term pseudocyst to collections that persist mostly or completely in the peripancreatic area.

Most reports throughout the world indicate that approximately 65–70% of patients with necrotizing pancreatitis have sterile necrosis. In studies dating back more than 20 years, the mortality of sterile necrosis was thought to be approximately 10%, whereas that of infected necrosis was approximately 30%[3,4]. More recently a number of reports have indicated that the mortality of sterile necrosis may be reasonably close to that of infected necrosis[5,6]. In our recent experience the mortality of sterile necrosis was 11% whereas that of infected necrosis was 19%[6]. The most important correlation was the presence of multiple organ failure, which carried a mortality of approximately 50% in both infected necrosis and sterile necrosis[6]. We[4,6] and others[7,8] have also found that patients who experience organ failure at admission are much more likely to have a fatal outcome than those who do not have organ failure at admission. Furthermore, an important distinction has been made between transient organ failure (with a very low mortality of 1%) versus persistent organ failure (with a mortality of 35%)[9]. In summary, organ failure at or shortly after admission and the development of multi-system organ failure strongly correlated with mortality in necrotizing pancreatitis. These correlations appear to be as true for sterile necrosis as they are for infected necrosis. In the absence of organ failure the mortality of sterile necrosis is generally considered to be 0–2%; with single organ failure it is approximately 5–10%; and in the presence of multisystem organ failure it is 35–50%[6,9,10].

It should be kept in mind that various criteria are utilized in the name of the Atlanta Symposium pertaining to organ failure. Table 1 shows the criteria most often utilized. In many publications, including our own, only the first four criteria are utilized for organ failure.

Table 1   Criteria for organ failure

Systemic blood pressure $\leqslant$ 90 mmHg
$pO_2 \leqslant 60$ mmHg
Creatinine > 2 mg/dl
Gastrointestinal bleeding > 500 ml/24 h
Glasgow coma score < 13
Platelet count $\leqslant$ 80 000

THE ROLE OF INTERVENTION

In the absence of organ failure there is generally no need for intervention, and certainly no need for early intervention. In the presence of organ failure, intervention might serve one of the following goals:

1. Improve organ failure.

2. Prevent infected necrosis.

3. Reduce systemic toxicity (that is, elevated white blood count and temperature and possibly also tachycardia).

4. Treat abdominal pain.

STERILE NECROSIS – EARLY INTERVENTION (< 14 DAYS)

Surgical debridement

Whereas surgical debridement was generally considered the treatment of choice in patients with sterile necrosis and persistent organ failure until approximately 10–15 years ago, a variety of more recent reports have strongly suggested that surgical debridement within the first 14 days should be avoided[11–19]. In one randomized prospective study the patients who underwent necrosectomy within 3 days had a 56% mortality, whereas those who were operated on in a time interval greater than 12 days had a 27% mortality[19]. Although this difference was not statistically significant in a small sample size of 36, the study was discontinued because of the high mortality. In another more recent retrospective study among 62 patients, those who underwent early surgical debridement within 3 days had a 53% mortality compared to 22% who underwent necrosectomy in greater than 3 days[12]. Concerns regarding early surgery include the high mortality noted above, conversion of sterile necrosis into infected necrosis, and an increasing belief that the majority of patients who survive initial organ failure associated with sterile necrosis enter a later phase that would be more amenable to surgical treatment, if needed. In summary, early surgical necrosectomy was not shown to prevent or improve organ failure, prevent infection, reduce systemic toxicity, or ameliorate abdominal pain. Early surgery within 14 days is generally not recommended in patients with necrotizing pancreatitis[15].

Percutaneous debridement using multiple catheters

There is very little information regarding the efficacy of percutaneous debridement using multiple catheters that can be upsized with the goal of eliminating as much necrotic material and associated fluid as possible. Potential benefits would be to eliminate organ failure, prevent the later development of infected necrosis, reduce systemic toxicity such as leucocytosis and fever, and treat agonizing abdominal pain usually due to the accumulation of fluid under pressure in the lesser sac. In our experience we have seen some benefit in percutaneous drainage of peripancreatic fluid to ameliorate abdominal pain and possibly to reduce systemic toxicity (Figure 1). We have not been convinced that this prevents infected necrosis, and the use of indwelling catheters, even when properly managed, carries with it the potential not only of colonization but also possibly the development of a secondary infection. Furthermore, we do not have evidence that this prevents or eliminates organ failure. In our recent experience with 23 patients who underwent percutaneous drainage for these various indications, six (26%) died, one of whom had single organ failure and five had multiple organ failure; 50% of the patients with multiple organ failure died, a percentage that has been shown previously in our experience to take place among patients with sterile pancreatic necrosis who do not undergo percutaneous drainage techniques. As such, the role of percutaneous debridement with catheters remains unproven. It is possible that, when the duration of percutaneous drainage is only a few days, abdominal pain may be relieved and the catheter withdrawn before secondary infection develops.

Endoscopic stenting

Early stenting of the pancreatic duct in an effort to prevent extravasation of noxious pancreatic fluid into the retroperitoneum has been considered as a technique that might be helpful in improving organ failure, reducing systemic toxicity, and treating abdominal pain. This technique has not been subjected to prospective trials. A concern would be that the presence of a foreign body in the pancreatic duct would encourage infection of the surrounding necrotic tissue.

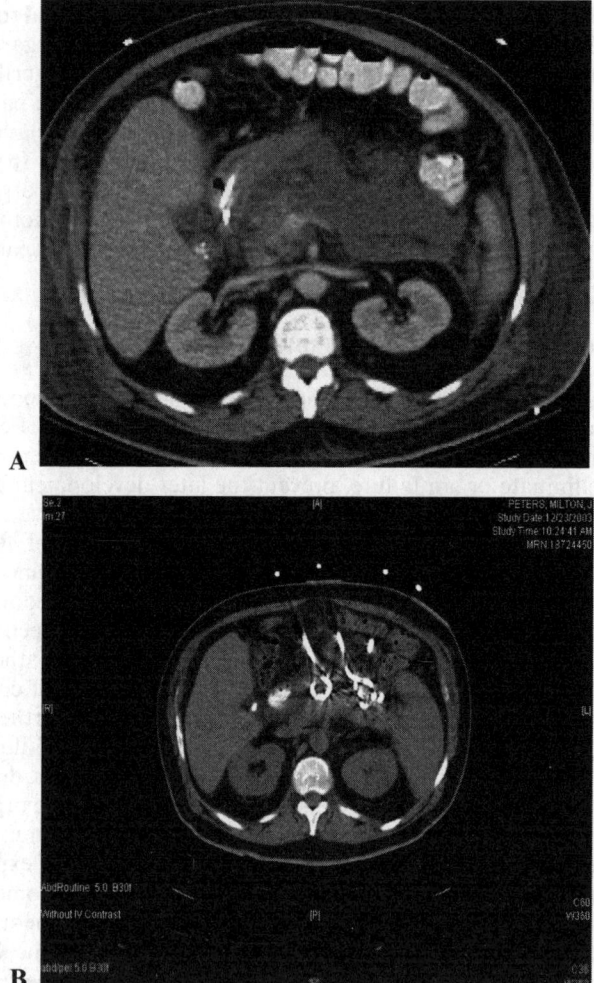

Figure 1 **A**: Axial contrast-enhanced CT scan image showing almost total necrosis of the pancreas. There is little, if any, viable pancreatic tissue. Small calcified gallstones are visible in gallbladder. There is a nasogastric tube in the descending duodenum. The patient was experiencing multi-system organ failure with hypoxaemia requiring assisted ventilation and renal failure. He was febrile to 102.8°F and had an elevated white blood count of greater than 25 000. **B**: Axial non-enhanced CT scan image showing multiple percutaneously placed catheters that have successfully debrided most of the pancreatic necrosis. A total of four pigtail catheters were utilized. The patient recovered completely without need for surgery and has resumed a normal life. Despite this apparent success of catheter drainage, the role of percutaneous catheter drainage in sterile pancreatic necrosis remains unclear

Summary

There are insufficient data to recommend early intervention by surgical debridement, percutaneous debridement, or endoscopic stenting in sterile necrosis.

STERILE NECROSIS – LATE INTERVENTION (> 21 DAYS)

The goals of intervening late (after 21 days) are, as follows:

1. Eliminate organ failure.

2. Treat abdominal pain.

The concept that lingering organ failure such as respiratory failure requiring prolonged intubation might be caused by persistence of inflammatory exudate below the diaphragm that compromises pulmonary function has never been subjected to a randomized prospective trial. It remains unproven that elimination of necrotic debris will facilitate improvement of respiratory function. The most important reason for late intervention is intractable abdominal pain preventing oral intake. Techniques that have been applied include surgical debridement, percutaneous debridement, endoscopic debridement, and endoscopic stenting.

Surgical debridement

Surgical debridement is generally indicated after 21 days among patients who are continuing to exhibit severe abdominal pain such that they cannot take sufficient oral intake. By this time the active inflammatory process in and around the pancreas has generally subsided, and the configuration of the organized inflammation resembles that of a pseudocyst. Another term that is frequently used is 'organized necrosis'. The value of this term is to call attention to the fact that there is a considerable amount of necrosis that must also be eliminated, and that simple drainage of fluid without removal of the necrotic debris frequently results in infection. There are many surgical techniques that have been utilized in this setting.

Percutaneous debridement

It is particularly difficult to evacuate semi-solid necrotic material even with relatively large-sized percutaneously placed catheters. Inability to evacuate semi-solid material frequently leads to infection. For this reason percutaneous debridement is generally not performed in this setting[20].

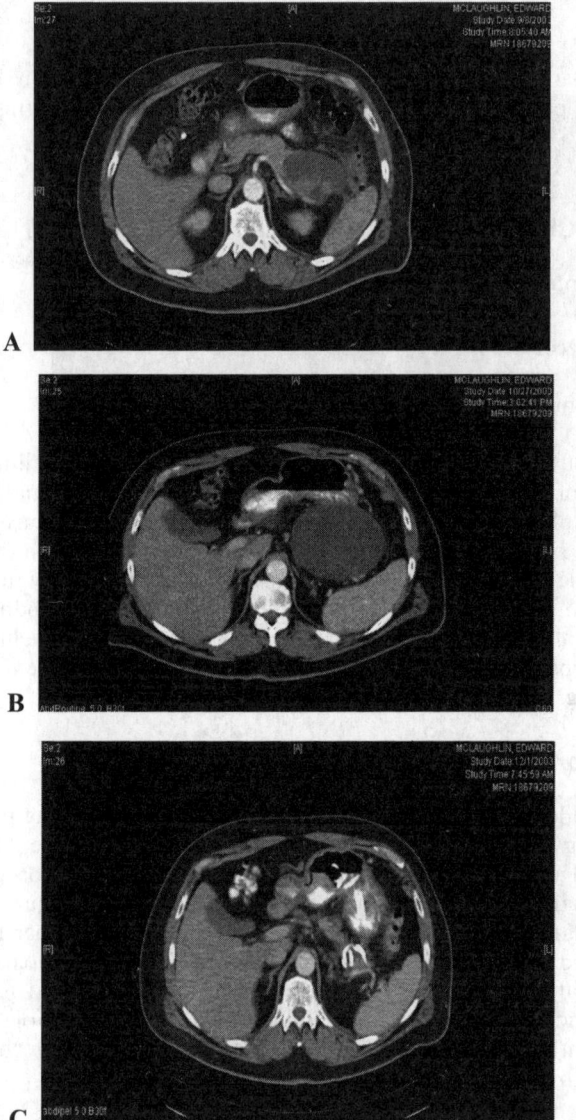

Figure 2 **A**: Axial contrast-enhanced CT scan image shows an area of organized pancreatic necrosis involving the tail of the pancreas. The patient was experiencing intractable abdominal pain. **B**: Axial contrast-enhanced CT scan image shows that the organized necrosis extends to the posterior wall of the stomach. Some might utilize the term pseudocyst to describe this entity. **C**: Axial contrast-enhanced CT scan image shows resolution of the organized necrosis following endoscopic debridement and placement of pigtail catheters between the stomach and the organized necrosis. The catheters were removed one month later, and the patient has remained well clinically. A follow-up CT scan several months later showed no recurrence of the organized necrosis

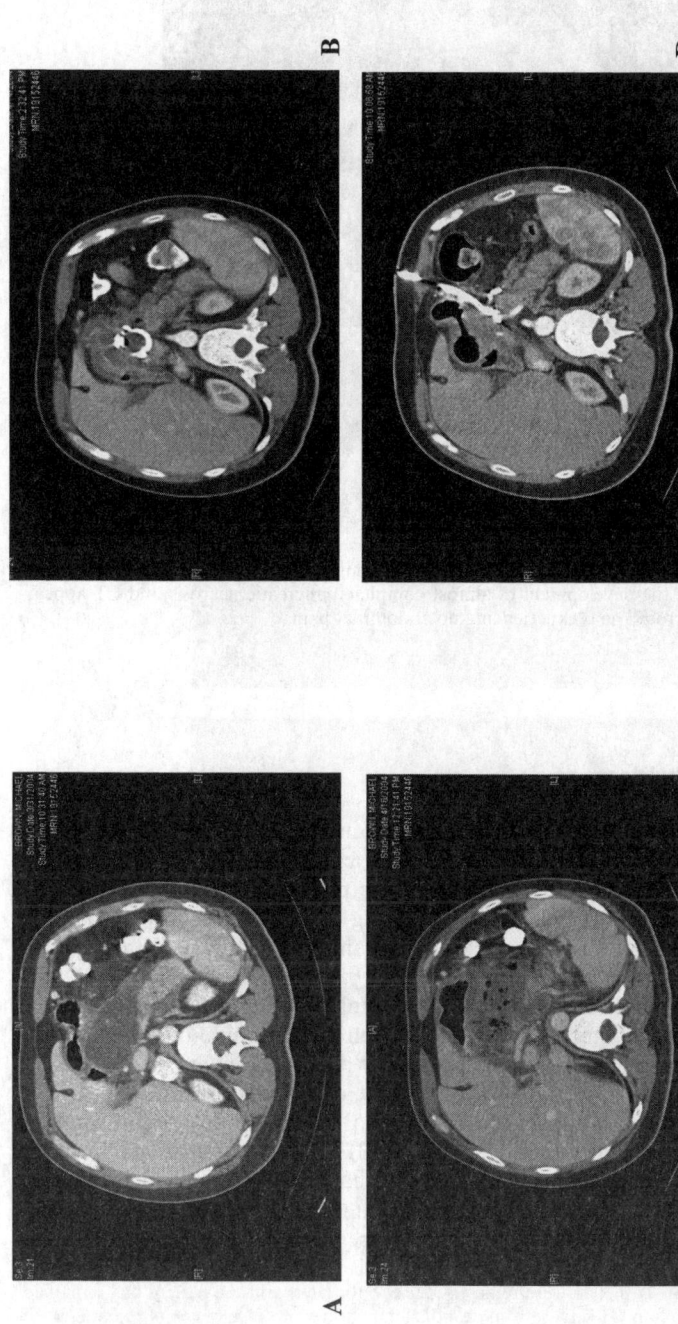

Figure 3 A: Axial contrast-enhanced CT scan image shows an area of organized necrosis in the body and tail of the pancreas with persistence of viable pancreatic parenchyma in the tail. The patient was experiencing intractable abdominal pain such that he was unable to eat. B: Axial contrast-enhanced CT scan image shows resolution of organized necrosis following endoscopic debridement and placement of two pigtail catheters between the stomach and the organized necrosis. C: Axial contrast-enhanced CT scan image shows the development of a pancreatic abscess in the lesser sac following the removal of the pigtail catheters. D: Axial contrast-enhanced CT scan image shows a percutaneously placed pigtail catheter with successful drainage of the pancreatic abscess. The catheter was later removed. The patient has remained clinically well. Follow-up CT scan showed no reaccumulation of fluid

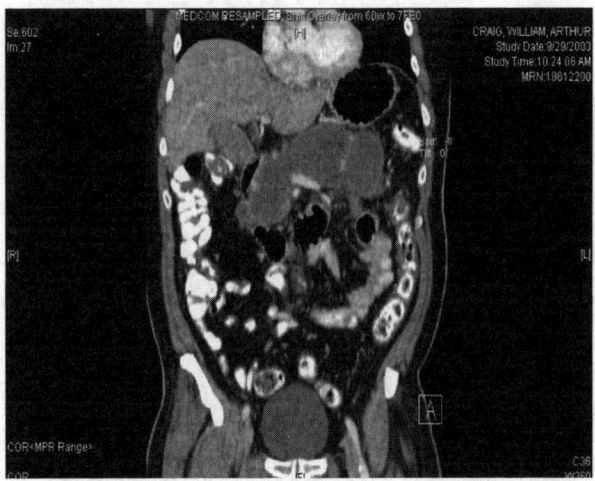

Figure 4 Contrast-enhanced coronal reformated CT scan image shows total pancreatic necrosis. The patient developed multi-system organ failure, was treated for several weeks in our intensive-care unit, and later made a complete recovery without need for intervention. He has resumed his normal life, and requires insulin for diabetes and pancreatic enzymes for steatorrhoea. Despite the development of almost complete pancreatic necrosis and CT appearance of organized necrosis, he is experiencing no abdominal pain

Endoscopic debridement

An endoscopic technique has developed to eliminate fluid and necrotic debris when organized necrosis is firmly attached to the posterior wall of the stomach. The first step is creation of an opening in the posterior wall of the stomach. Once this has occurred, the size of the opening can be increased with balloon dilation to facilitate the evacuation of the fluid and to allow the endoscope itself to be advanced into the cavity for removal of necrotic debris (Figure 2). The disadvantage of this technique is that the opening between the stomach and the cavity of the organized necrosis may close even when double-pigtail catheters are placed between the stomach and the cavity of the organized necrosis. With closure of the opening there is stasis within the cavity, and infection may then ensue which would require surgical, radiological treatment or possibly another attempt at endoscopic drainage[20–23] (Figure 3). Thus far there have been no randomized prospective trials comparing surgical and endoscopic debridement in this setting. In one study of 43 patients treated by endoscopic debridement, 37% developed complications, 29% had recurrences, and infectious complications were common[22].

Endoscopic stenting

When there is minimal pancreatic necrosis and persistence of abdominal pain and systemic toxicity associated with a ductal disruption, endoscopic stenting can be attempted to bridge the disruption and thereby prevent further extravasation of fluid[21,24]. After several weeks the stent can be removed. If the catheter cannot be advanced to a position that bridges the disruption, the disruption may not close. In general, the success of this technique is more favorable when pancreatic ductal disruption occurs in the context of chronic pancreatitis than with acute pancreatitis[24].

Summary

Surgical debridement remains the treatment of choice for intractable abdominal pain associated with organized necrosis. The threat of infection is particularly significant following attempts at percutaneous debridement. Endoscopic debridement requires further evaluation and possibly improvements in technique before it can be generally applied. Endoscopic stenting for a ductal disruption may be helpful in closing a ductal disruption in selected instances. When organized necrosis develops in the absence of abdominal pain or evidence of pancreatic infection, there is no need for intervention (Figure 4).

References

1. Bradley EL III. A clinically-based classification system for acute pancreatitis. Arch Surg. 1993;128:586–90.
2. Baron TH, Thaggard WG, Morgan DE, Stanley RJ. Endoscopic therapy for organized pancreatic necrosis. Gastroenterology. 1996;111:755–64.
3. Beger HG, Krautzberger W, Bittner R, Block S, Buchler M. Results of surgical treatment of necrotizing pancreatitis. World J Surg. 1985;9:972–9.
4. Tenner S, Sica G, Hughes M et al. Relationship of necrosis to organ failure in severe acute pancreatitis. Gastroenterology. 1997;113:899–903.
5. Rattner DW, Legermate DA, Lee MJ, Mueller PR, Warshaw AL. Early surgical debridement of symptomatic pancreatic necrosis is beneficial irrespective of infection. Am J Surg. 1992;163:105–10.
6. Perez A, Whang EE, Brooks DC et al. Is severity of necrotizing pancreatitis increased in extended necrosis and infected necrosis? Pancreas. 2002;3:229–33.
7. Beger HG, Rau B, Isenmann R. Natural history of necrotizing pancreatitis. Pancreatology. 2003;3:93–101.
8. Isenmann R, Rau B, Beger HG. Early severe acute pancreatitis: characteristics of a new subgroup. Pancreas. 2001;3:274–8.
9. Johnson CD, Abu-Hilal M. Persistent organ failure during the first week as a marker of fatal outcome in acute pancreatitis. Gut. 2004;53:1340–4.
10. Karimgani I, Porter KA, Langevin RE, Banks PA. Prognostic factors in sterile pancreatic necrosis. Gastroenterology. 1992;103:1636–40.
11. Ashley SW, Perez A, Pierce EA et al. Necrotizing pancreatitis: contemporary analysis of 99 consecutive cases. Ann Surg. 2001;4:572–80.
12. Hartwig W, Maksan S, Foitzik T, Schmidt J, Herfarth C, Klar E. Reduction in mortality with delayed surgical therapy of severe pancreatitis. J Gastrointest Surg. 2002;3:481–7.
13. Hartwig W, Werner J, Muller CA, Uhl W, Buchler MW. Surgical management of severe pancreatitis including sterile necrosis. J Hepatobil Pancreat Surg. 2002;9:429–35.
14. Steinberg WM, Barkin J, Bradley EL, Dimagno E, Layer P. Controversies in clinical pancreatology. Pancreas. 1996;3:219–25.

15. Uhl W, Warshaw A, Imrie C et al. IAP guidelines for the surgical management of acute pancreatitis. Pancreatology. 2002;2:565–73.
16. Yousaf M, McCallion K, Diamond T. Management of severe acute pancreatitis. Br J Surg. 2003;90:407–20.
17. Andersson R, Andersson B, Haraldsen P, Drewsen G, Eckerwall G. Incidence, management and recurrence rate of acute pancreatitis. Scand J Gastroenterol. 2004;9:891–4.
18. Buchler MW, Gloor B, Muller CA, Friess H, Seiler CA, Uhl W. Acute necrotizing pancreatitis: treatment strategy according to the status of infection. Ann Surg. 2000;5: 619–26.
19. Mier J, Luque-de Leon E, Castillo A, Robledo F, Blanco R. Early versus late necrosectomy in severe necrotizing pancreatitis. Am J Surg. 1997;173:71–5.
20. Hariri M, Silvka A, Carr-Locke DL, Banks PA. Pseudocyst drainage predisposes to infection when pancreatic necrosis is unrecognized. Am J Gastroenterol. 1994;89:1781–4.
21. Baillie J. Pancreatic pseudocysts. Gastrointest Endoscop. 2004;1:105–16.
22. Baron TH, Harewood GC, Morgan DE, Yates M. Outcome difference after endoscopic drainage of pancreatic necrosis, acute pancreatic pseudocyst, and chronic pancreatic pseudocyst. Gastrointest Endoscop. 2002;56:7–17.
23. Harewood GC, Wright CA, Baron TH. Impact on patient outcomes of experience in the performance of endoscopic pancreatic fluid collection drainage. Gastrointest Endoscop. 2003;2:230–5.
24. Telford JJ, Farrell JJ, Saltzman JR et al. Pancreatic stent placement for duct disruption. Gastrointest Endoscop. 2002;56:18–24.

9
Acute pancreatitis: evidence-based indications for surgery – the current concept*

M. SCHÄFER, S. HEINRICH and P.-A. CLAVIEN

INTRODUCTION

In most Western countries acute pancreatitis (AP) is caused either by symptomatic gallstone disease or excessive alcohol intake[1,2]. Due to improvements in management, disease-related mortality has declined during the past two decades despite an increase in the overall incidence of AP in many countries[3–5]. The vast majority of AP episodes do not require any intervention, since they are mild and self-limiting. Only 15% of all patients develop a severe form of AP, which is still associated with an increased mortality rate up to 30%[1,6,7]. Severe AP is characterized by necrosis formation of the pancreas and the surrounding tissue (necrotizing AP) that is best assessed by contrast-enhanced computed tomography[8,9]. According to the Atlanta classification, AP is predicted as severe if it is accompanied by organ failure, local complications, three or more Ranson criteria[10], or an APACHE II score of eight points or more[11].

The role of surgery has changed during the past 25 years from extensive pancreatic resections to a more conservative treatment aiming at preservation of the gland. The optimal timing and type of surgery for AP are still under debate. Some authors prefer re-explorations in 2-days intervals, while others perform a single necrosectomy followed by continuous postoperative lavage of the lesser sac. Following the actual trend to less invasive procedures, the feasibility of retroperitoneal necrosectomy as well as laparoscopic[12] and endoscopic[13] interventions has been demonstrated, but not yet prospectively evaluated.

In the past the main indications for surgery were pancreatic necrosis and deterioration of the patient's general status. With the development of the

*This chapter represents a part of a current study submitted to *Annals of Surgery* for publication.

concept of sterile and infected pancreatic necrosis, evidence showed that patients with sterile necrosis might recover without surgical intervention[6]. Thus, surgical interventions are increasingly restricted to patients who cannot successfully be treated using a conservative approach.

The aim of this analysis was to assess the clinical value of surgery for AP by reviewing the current literature on the treatment of AP. To secure the highest level of objectivity we used the evidence-based approach of Sackett to analyse the literature[14].

METHODS

An electronic search of the Medline database was performed using different keywords that covered selected topics of AP. In addition, we screened the Cochrane Library for publications on these topics. All publications which fulfilled the inclusion criteria and addressed the clinical questions of this analysis were further assessed. Review articles and abstracts publications were excluded. Only articles published in the English language from 1990 to 2004 were included.

The level of evidence of each publication was ranked in accordance with a modified Sackett's classification (Table 1)[14]. As a general rule only studies of the two highest available levels of evidence were used for the final data analysis. The grade of recommendation based on the available literature for each clinical question was also determined as proposed by Sackett (Table 1)[14].

Table 1 Modified classification of the level of evidence according to Sackett[14]

Level of evidence	Type of trial	Criteria for classification	Grade of recommendation
I	Large randomized trials with clear-cut results (and low risk for error)	Sample size calculation provided and fulfilled, study end-point provided, could be used in meta-analysis	A
II	Small randomized trials (and moderate to high risk for errors) Study end-point not provided, convincing comparative studies	Matched analysis, sample size calculation not given or not fulfilled	B
III	Non-randomized, contemporaneous controls	Non-comparative, prospective	C
IV	Non-randomized, historical controls	Retrospective analysis, cohort studies	–
V	No control, case series only, opinion of experts	Small series, review articles	–

RESULTS

Surgical versus endoscopic treatment of mild acute pancreatitis

One level I trial[15], but no level II or III trials have compared endoscopic retrograde cholangiography (ERC) and endoscopic sphincterotomy (+ ES) with primary cholecystectomy in patients with mild biliary AP. Chang et al. randomized patients to either ERC + ES followed by laparoscopic chole-cystectomy or to laparoscopic cholecystectomy followed by ERC + ES[15]. If laparoscopic cholecystectomy was performed first, ERC was performed only if common bile duct (CBD) stones were detected by intraoperative cholangio-graphy. The study end-point was hospital cost. Hospital stay and overall cost were significantly lower if laparoscopic cholecystectomy was performed first[15]; but costs for anaesthesia were not included in this analysis, and laparoscopic bile duct clearance was never attempted, so that the need for postoperative ERC could probably be further reduced.

Another three level I trials[16–18] and one level II[19] trial compared ERC + ES with cholecystectomy in patients with symptomatic CBD stones (not exclu-sively biliary AP). In three trials[16,17,19], patients with symptomatic CBD stones were randomized to open cholecystectomy or ERC + ES. Two of these trials demonstrated significantly less recurrent biliary symptoms in the cholecystect-omy group[16,17]; the late mortality was increased in the ERC group in one trial[19] and equal in two trials[16,17].

Cuschieri et al. compared laparoscopic cholecystectomy and CBD clearance with ERC + ES followed by laparoscopic cholecystectomy during the same hospitalization[18], but do not provide long-term results. However, ductal stone clearance, morbidity and mortality were not significantly different between the two groups[18].

Recommendations

1. Patients with mild biliary AP are best treated by primary laparoscopic cholecystectomy with intraoperative cholangiography (level B).

2. ERC should be performed postoperatively, if intraoperative cholangiogra-phy reveals CBD stones and laparoscopic bile duct clearance has failed (level B).

Indication for cholecystectomy after ERC + ES

Whereas emergency ERC is not indicated for mild biliary AP, it has been shown that emergency ERC + ES should be strongly considered in patients with severe biliary AP as well as in patients with cholangitis.

The indication for cholecystectomy after ERC + ES for biliary AP has been assessed in only three level III studies[20–22], whereas no level I or II trials have been performed. Therefore, the current literature does not support a well-based statement. For this reason we also analysed studies evaluating the indication of cholecystectomy after ES for CBD stones. One level I trial compared ERC + ES vs ERC + ES followed by laparoscopic cholecystectomy in patients with ASA scores I–III[23]. If laparoscopic cholecystectomy was performed within 6 weeks after ES, recurrent biliary symptoms occurred less often within 2 years (47% vs 2%, $p < 0.0001$)[23]. These results are supported by two prospective non-randomized trials in patients with biliary AP, in which recurrent biliary symptoms occurred in 15–52%, if cholecystectomy was omitted[21,22].

Similarly, recurrent biliary symptoms occurred in 16% of patients who did not undergo laparoscopic cholecystectomy compared to 7.6% of patients who underwent laparoscopic cholecystectomy after ERC + ES in a prospective cohort study (level III).

Recommendations

1. Cholecystectomy is indicated after ES for any event of symptomatic CBD stones or biliary AP in patients with ASA scores I–III, since biliary AP represents one major complication of CBD stones (level A).

2. Current literature does not support a well-based statement on laparoscopic cholecystectomy in patients with ASA scores IV and V, but a 'wait-and-see' policy after ERC + ES appears to be reasonable in these patients deemed too sick for cholecystectomy (level C).

Timing for cholecystectomy after ERC + ES

ERC + ES should be performed in patients with severe AP, cholangitis, and persistent cholestasis, and might be performed in selected cases with mild AP. If ES has been performed, laparoscopic cholecystectomy should be performed within 6 weeks[23]; however, the optimal timing for cholecystectomy is still under debate.

No randomized trial, but four prospective trials (level III)[24–27] evaluated the optimal timing for cholecystectomy after biliary AP. Late cholecystectomy (8–12 weeks) was performed in one trial[25], and early laparoscopic cholecystectomy in three trials after ERC for mild AP[24,26,27]. In addition, one randomized trial compared ERC + ES + LC vs laparoscopic cholecystectomy[18], and one randomized trial compared ERC + ES vs ERC + ES + laparoscopic cholecystectomy[23] in patients with CBD stones. Since only one arm of these trials was evaluable for this analysis (ERC + ES + laparoscopic cholecystectomy), both trials were classified as prospective trials (level III).

Although laparoscopic cholecystectomy after AP is feasible, the operation is often more difficult and has an increased conversion rate to open surgery in all trials[24–26]. The conversion rates to open surgery are equal or even slightly lower for early laparoscopic cholecystectomy, and morbidity of early laparoscopic cholecystectomy after mild AP is generally low (Table 2). Similarly, conversion rates to open surgery were lower after early laparoscopic cholecystectomy in patients with symptomatic CBD stones (not exclusively biliary AP)[18,23].

Of note, open surgery for necrotizing AP is necessary in up to 20% of patients with AP dependent on the proportion of patients with severe AP[24,27], and cholecystectomy is routinely performed by most surgeons during this intervention without additional morbidity.

Table 2 Timing of cholecystectomy for biliary AP

Reference	n	Patient population	Pretreatment	Timing	Conversion rate	Morbidity
Uhl et al.[24]	35	Mild/moderate AP	No ERC	Early	5/35 (15%)	1/30 (3.3%)
	13	Necrotizing AP	ERC + ES		5/13 (48%)	2/8 (25%)
Schachter et al.[25]	19	Mild/moderate AP	ERC + ES	Late	2/19 (10.5%)[a]	–[c]
Tate et al.[26]	16	Mild/moderate AP	ERC + ES	Early	3/24 (12.5%)[b]	2/24 (8.3%)
	8	Severe AP				
	40	No pancreatitis	None	–	0/40	–
Schietroma et al.[27]	54	Mild/moderate AP	No ERC	Early	0/54	3/54 (6%)
	19	Severe AP	ERC + ES	Early	–[d]	1/19 (5.2%)
Boerma et al.[23]	56	Choledocholithiasis	ERC + ES	Late	9/44 (20%)	6/44 (14%)
Cuschieri et al.[18]	133	Choledocholithiasis	ERC + ES	Early	8/133 (6%)	17/133 (12.8%)

[a]Thirty-one per cent severe adhesions, bleeding or difficult dissection of the hilum
[b]LC was significantly more difficult than elective LC for chronic gallstone disease
[c]not provided in publication
[d]5 patients were treated by open cholecystectomy

Recommendations

1. Early LC after ES should be preferred in patients with mild to moderate AP (level C).

2. In patients with severe biliary AP who did not require surgery for necrotizing AP, cholecystectomy appears to be favourable after full recovery from AP (level C).

The role of surgery for severe acute pancreatitis

So far, no level I or II trial has evaluated the benefit of surgery for sterile or infected necrosis. One prospective (level III) trial[28] and one small prospective randomized trial (level II)[29] assessed the indication of antibiotic prophylaxis and surgery for infected necrosis, and one level II trial compared early versus late surgery for severe AP[30]. In addition, six prospective trials (level III) evaluated surgery for necrotizing AP[6,28,31–34]. Both publications of Beger et al. were included since the publication in 1991 provided information regarding the surgical complications of the original publication in 1988[31,35].

In two trials, patients with necrotizing AP underwent necrosectomy after failure of conservative treatment independent of infection of these necroses, and the outcome was separately analysed for patients with sterile and infected necrosis[31,33,35]. (Table 3). In the remaining four studies surgery was performed only for proven infection of necrosis, and outcomes of patients with sterile and infected necrosis were again separately analysed[6,28,32,34].

In order to evaluate whether all patients with necrotizing AP (sterile and infected necrosis) require surgery, we compared outcome data of patients with sterile necrosis who were operated[31,33,35] with those who were not operated[6,28,32,34].

Mier et al. randomized patients with an indication for surgery to either early (within 48–72 h, $n = 25$) or late necrosectomy (more than 12 days, $n = 15$)[30]. Of note, indication for surgery was defined as multi-organ failure (MOF) with clinical deterioration despite maximal intensive care. All patients received antibiotic prophylaxis, but infection of necrosis was never proven prior to surgery. Of the 15 patients in the group of late necrosectomy, three improved during a 12-day period of conservative treatment and did not require surgery. Unfortunately, these patients were excluded from the final analysis. The remaining 12 patients were operated. Although the difference in mortality between early (56%) and late (27%) surgery was not statistically significant, the authors terminated this study based on an odds ratio of 3.4 (95% CI 0.74–15.9).

In the first Nordback et al. trial[28], antibiotic treatment was started when surgery was indicated (proven infection of necrosis, MOF or recurrent inflammatory variables). Three of 25 patients (12%), who initially fulfilled criteria for surgery, recovered without surgery, and five patients (23%) died despite surgical treatment. In the follow-up trial, patients with sterile necrosis were randomized to the observation group or to receive prophylactic impenem[29]. Prophylactic imipenem resulted in a significantly lower need for surgery (infected necrosis). In the observation group, patients received imipenem treatment if infection of necrosis occurred. Surgery was performed only if antibiotic treatment failed; thus 64% of patients with infected necrosis in the control group did not require surgery due to imipenem treatment. Since follow-up data are not provided, it remains unclear whether these patients required surgery for infected necrosis at a later stage.

Recommendations

1. The detection of necrosis itself is not an absolute indication for surgery (level C). However, some patients will require surgery for reasons secondary to necrosis formation, although infection has not been proven.

2. Most patients with infected necrosis require surgery, but should primarily be treated with antibiotics, if possible (level B).

3. Surgery should preferentially be performed in the late phase of AP (level B).

Comparison of surgical techniques

Only one randomized trial has compared pancreatic resection vs continuous peritoneal lavage on 11 vs 10 patients[36]. Pancreas resection was associated with increased perioperative morbidity, and normal pancreatic parenchyma was unnecessarily removed. Since long-term outcome of patients is closely related to the amount of preserved pancreatic tissue, treatment policy has widely changed to limited necrosectomy[37]. Mainly two techniques aiming at maximal tissue preservation are currently used: first, the 'open packing' technique, in which repeated necrosectomies are performed at 48-h intervals until all necrosis has resolved and granulation tissue has developed. Thereafter, continuous lavage is often performed[6]. Second, a single necrosectomy with continuous postoperative lavage (8–10 L/day) through surgically placed drainages has been proposed by Beger et al.[35]. Since sterile necrosis *per se* does not appear to be an indication for surgery, we focus on patients with infected necrosis in this analysis.

Five prospective trials (level III) used 'open packing'[6,28,30,33,34], while two studies investigated the technique described by Beger et al. (level III)[32,35]. Complication rates after surgical treatment were high in all trials (Table 3). Of note, 25% of patients treated by the procedure reported by Beger et al. required one or more reoperations during the course of their disease for fistulas, intra-abdominal abscesses or bleeding.

'Open packing' is associated with a higher morbidity rate, mainly due to higher incidences of fistulas, bleeding and incisional hernias. In addition, mortality rates were slightly higher in the reports on 'open packing' (Table 3).

Table 3 Results from surgery for necrotizing pancreatitis

Reference	Indication for surgery	Group	n	Treatment	Fistula			Hernia	Bleeding	Abscess	Mortality
					Pancreas	GI	Total				
'Open packing' Bradley et al.[6]	Infected necrosis	i.n.	27	Surgery	–	–	–	–	–	–	4/27 (14.8%)
		s.n.	11	Conservative	–	–	–	–	–	–	0/11 (0%)
Tsiotos et al.[33]	Failure of conservative therapy	i.n.	57	Surgery	14/72 (19%)	19/72 (27%)	33/72 (46%)	12/72 (17%)	13/72 (18%)	9/72 (13%)	13/57 (22.8%)
		s.n.	15	Surgery							5/15 (33.3%)
Mier et al.[30]	Failure of conservative therapy	Early	25	Surgery	–	–	–	–	–	–	14/25 (56%)
		Late	11	Surgery	–	–	–	–	–	–	3/11 (27.3%)
Nordback et al.[28]	Infected necrosis, MOF, increase in inflammatory parameters		22	Surgery	2/22 (9%)	12/22 (55%)	14/22 (64%)	13/22 (59%)	3/22 (14%)	–	5/22 (22.7%)
			11[b]	Conservative	0/11 (0%)	0/11 (0%)	0/11 (0%)	0/11 (0%)	3/11 (27%)	–	0/11 (0%)
Kalfarentzos et al.[34]	Infected necrosis	i.n.	7	Surgery	n = 3[a]	n = 3[a]	n = 6[a]	2/7 (29%)	–	1/7 (14%)	1/7 (14.3%)
		s.n.	19	Conservative							1/19 (5.3%)
'Single Debridement' Buchler et al.[32]	Infected necrosis	i.n.	27[c]	Surgery	8/27 (29.6%)	0/27 (0%)	8/27 (29.6%)	–	2/27 (7.4%)	1/27 (3.7%)	7/27 (25.9%)
		s.n.	56[d]	Conservative							1/56 (1.8%)
Beger et al.[31,35]	Failure of conservative therapy	i.n.	37[c]	Surgery	–	–	11/95 (12%)	–	5/95 (5%)	12/95 (13%)	5/37 (14%)
		s.n.	52[c]	Surgery							3/52 (6%)

Table 3 (continued)

Reference	Indication for surgery	Group	n	Treatment	Fistula Pancreas	GI	Total	Hernia	Bleeding	Abscess	Mortality
Pooled data Indication for surgery	Sterile necrosis		67	Surgery[31,33]	–	–	–	–	–	–	8/67 (11.9%) (CI 5.3–22.2%)
			86	Conservative[6,32,34]	–	–	–	–	–	–	2/86 (2.3%) (CI 0.3–8.2%)
Pooled data Surgical technique	Infected necrosis[g]		138[f]	Open packing[6,29,30,33,34]	–	–	47/94 (50%) (CI 39.5–60.5%)	32/101 (32%) (CI 22.6–40.8%)	16/94 (17%) (CI 10.1–26.2%)	10/79 (12.7%) (CI 6.2–22.1%)	37/138 (26.8%) (CI 19.4–34.2%)
			64	Beger[31,32,35]	–	–	19/122 (15.6%) (CI 9.7–22.0%)	–	7/122 (5.7%) (CI 1.6–9.9%)	13/122 (10.7%) (CI 5.2–16.1%)	12/64 (18.8%) (CI 10.1–30.5%)

Pooled data of the trials listed in this table are presented at the bottom of the table (CI = 95% confidence interval)

[a] Data not separately provided for each patient; one patient may have had several fistulas

[b] Three patients with indication for surgery were treated conservatively due to response to antibiotic treatment

[c] 27/29 patients planned for surgical therapy were operated

[d] 1/57 patients planned for conservative treatment was operated

[e] 95 patients studied, but cultures are only available from 89 patients

[f] From Nordback trial only early necrosectomy included

[g] Only mortality rates were reported separately

i.n. = infected necrosis, s.n. = sterile necrosis, MOF = multi-organ failure

Recommendation

1. Single necrosectomy and postoperative lavage without planned re-laparo-
   tomies is less harmful and should be preferred for surgical treatment of
   necrotizing AP, when applicable (level C).

CONCLUSIONS

The treatment of AP remains challenging, and many aspects are still controversial. The level of evidence is often very low regarding well-based
recommendations on specific aspects of surgical treatment. In order to overcome the tradition to report only the own experience, we performed this
evidence-based analysis. A systematic review of the current literature provides
probably the best evidence for actual treatment modalities, and facilitates
defining the optimal treatment strategy for patients with AP.

The current indication of cholecystectomy for biliary pancreatitis has been
investigated in many studies. Cholecystectomy is indicated after any event of
biliary pancreatitis and symptomatic CBD stones. Early laparoscopic cholecystectomy should be performed in all patients with mild to moderate AP, while
delayed cholecystectomy seems to be favourable in patients with severe AP.

Only a few prospective trials on the surgical treatment of AP have been
published, but none of them was randomized. There is no doubt that better
diagnostics and improved conservative treatment modalities had a major
influence on the role of surgery for acute pancreatitis. Necrosis formation and
major deterioration of patient's general status, e.g. systemic inflammatory
response syndrome (SIRS), and development of organ failure, represented the
traditional indications for surgery in severe AP. However, it has become obvious
during the past two decades that early surgical interventions with extensive
resections are associated with very high morbidity and mortality rates.

The occurrence of pancreatic necrosis does not represent an absolute
indication for surgery. Whereas sterile necrosis can be treated conservatively
in most cases, infected necrosis with systemic inflammatory reactions that
cause sepsis are still a widely accepted indication for surgical necrosectomy.
However, a significant proportion of patients with infected necrosis can be
successfully treated with antibiotics. Further studies are needed to differentiate
between simple bacterial contamination of pancreatic necrosis and clinically
relevant systemic infection that is caused by infected pancreatic necrosis.

If the indication for surgery is given, the surgical intervention should be
delayed, after the acute phase of SIRS has been passed. Limited surgery with
organ-preserving necrosectomy should be preferred. So far, open surgery
represents the current standard. Experience with minimal invasive, endoscopic
and radiological interventions is still limited to small case-series.

Finally, it should be emphasized that the application of evidence-based
recommendations to an individual clinical case need to be performed in a
multidisciplinary manner by physicians experienced in AP. Thus, an important
factor, not always apparent in evidence-based studies, is that patients with
severe or complex diseases should be referred to a specialized centre.

References

1. Steinberg W, Tenner S. Acute pancreatitis. N Engl J Med. 1994;330:1198–210.
2. Lankisch PG. Epidemiology of acute pancreatitis. In: Malfertheimer P, editor. Acute Pancreatitis. Novel Concepts in Biology and Therapy, 1st edn. Berlin: Blackwell Science, 1999:145–53.
3. Bank S, Singh P, Pooran N, Stark B. Evaluation of factors that have reduced mortality from acute pancreatitis over the past 20 years. J Clin Gastroenterol. 2002;35:50–60.
4. Neoptolemos JP, Raraty M, Finch M, Sutton R. Acute pancreatitis: the substantial human and financial costs. Gut. 1998;42:886–91.
5. Soran A, Chelluri L, Lee KKW, Tisherman SA. Outcome and quality of life of patients with acute pancreatitis requiring intensive care. J Surg Res. 2000;91:89–94.
6. Bradley EL 3rd, Allen K. A prospective longitudinal study of observation versus surgical intervention in the management of necrotizing pancreatitis. Am J Surg. 1991;161:19–24.
7. Baron TH, Morgan DE. Acute necrotizing pancreatitis. N Engl J Med. 1999;340:1412–17.
8. London NJ, Neoptolemos JP, Lavelle J, Bailey I, James D. Contrast-enhanced abdominal computed tomography scanning and prediction of severity of acute pancreatitis: a prospective study. Br J Surg. 1989;76:268–72.
9. Clavien PA, Hauser H, Meyer P, Rohner A. Value of contrast-enhanced computerized tomography in the early diagnosis and prognosis of acute pancreatitis. A prospective study of 202 patients. Am J Surg. 1988;155:457–66.
10. Ranson JH, Rifkind KM, Turner JW. Prognostic signs and nonoperative peritoneal lavage in acute pancreatitis. Surg Gynecol Obstet. 1976;143:209–19.
11. Bradley EL 3rd. A clinically based classification system for acute pancreatitis. Summary of the International Symposium on Acute Pancreatitis, Atlanta, Ga, September 11 through 13, 1992. Arch Surg. 1993;128:586–90.
12. Zhu JF, Fan XH, Zhang XH. Laparoscopic treatment of severe acute pancreatitis. Surg Endosc. 2001;15:146–8.
13. Baron TH, Thaggard WG, Morgan DE, Stanley RJ. Endoscopic therapy for organized pancreatic necrosis. Gastroenterology. 1996;111:755–64.
14. Sackett DL. Rules of evidence and clinical recommendations on the use of antithrombotic agents. Chest. 1989;95:2–4S.
15. Chang L, Lo S, Stabile BE, Lewis RJ, Toosie K, de Virgilio C. Preoperative versus postoperative endoscopic retrograde cholangiopancreatography in mild to moderate gallstone pancreatitis: a prospective randomized trial. Ann Surg. 2000;231:82–7.
16. Suc B, Escat J, Cherqui D et al. Surgery vs endoscopy as primary treatment in symptomatic patients with suspected common bile duct stones: a multicenter randomized trial. French Associations for Surgical Research. Arch Surg. 1998;133:702–8.
17. Targarona EM, Ayuso RM, Bordas JM et al. Randomised trial of endoscopic sphincterotomy with gallbladder left in situ versus open surgery for common bileduct calculi in high-risk patients. Lancet. 1996;347:926–9.
18. Cuschieri A, Lezoche E, Morino M et al. EAES multicenter prospective randomized trial comparing two-stage vs single-stage management of patients with gallstone disease and ductal calculi. Surg Endosc. 1999;13:952–7.
19. Hammarstrom LE, Holmin T, Stridbeck H, Ihse I. Long-term follow-up of a prospective randomized study of endoscopic versus surgical treatment of bile duct calculi in patients with gallbladder in situ. Br J Surg.1995;82:1516–21.
20. Siegel JH VA, Cohen SA, Kasmin FE. Endoscopic sphincterotomy for biliary pancreatitis: an alternative to cholecystectomy in high-risk patients. Gastrointest Endosc. 1994;40:573–4.
21. Kaw M A-AY, Kaw P. Management of gallstone pancreatitis: cholecystectomy or ERCP and endoscopic sphincterotomy. Gastrointest Endosc. 2002;56:61–5.
22. Gislason HVM, Horn A, Hoem D et al. Endoscopic sphincterotomy in acute gallstone pancreatitis: a prospective study of the late outcome. Eur J Surg. 2001;176:204–8.
23. Boerma D, Rauws EA, Keulemans YC et al. Wait-and-see policy or laparoscopic cholecystectomy after endoscopic sphincterotomy for bile-duct stones: a randomised trial. Lancet. 2002;360:761–5.

24. Uhl W, Muller CA, Krahenbuhl L, Schmid SW, Scholzel S, Buchler MW. Acute gallstone pancreatitis: timing of laparoscopic cholecystectomy in mild and severe disease. Surg Endosc. 1999;13:1070–6.
25. Schachter P, Peleg T, Cohen O. Interval laparoscopic cholecystectomy in the management of acute biliary pancreatitis. Hepato-Pancreatico-Biliary Surg. 2000;11:319–22.
26. Tate JJ, Lau WY, Li AK. Laparoscopic cholecystectomy for biliary pancreatitis. Br J Surg. 1994;81:720–2.
27. Schietroma M, Carlei F, Lezoche E et al. Acute biliary pancreatitis: staging and management. Hepatogastroenterology. 2001;48:988–93.
28. Nordback I, Paajanen H, Sand J. Prospective evaluation of a treatment protocol in patients with severe acute necrotising pancreatitis. Eur J Surg. 1997;163:357–64.
29. Nordback I, Sand J, Saaristo R, Paajanen H. Early treatment with antibiotics reduces the need for surgery in acute necrotizing pancreatitis - a single-center randomized study. J Gastrointest Surg. 2001;5:113–18.
30. Mier J, Leon EL, Castillo A, Robledo F, Blanco R. Early versus late necrosectomy in severe necrotizing pancreatitis. Am J Surg. 1997;173:71–5.
31. Beger HG, Buchler M, Bittner R, Block S, Nevalainen T, Roscher R. Necrosectomy and postoperative local lavage in necrotizing pancreatitis. Br J Surg. 1988;75:207–12.
32. Buchler MW, Gloor B, Muller CA, Friess H, Seiler CA, Uhl W. Acute necrotizing pancreatitis: treatment strategy according to the status of infection. Ann Surg. 2000;232: 619–26.
33. Tsiotos GG, Luque-de Leon E, Soreide JA et al. Management of necrotizing pancreatitis by repeated operative necrosectomy using a zipper technique. Am J Surg. 1998;175:91–8.
34. Kalfarentzos FE, Kehagias J, Kakkos SK et al. Treatment of patients with severe acute necrotizing pancreatitis based on prospective evaluation. Hepatogastroenterology. 1999; 46:3249–56.
35. Beger HG. Operative management of necrotizing pancreatitis – necrosectomy and continuous closed postoperative lavage of the lesser sac. Hepatogastroenterology. 1991;38:129–33.
36. Schroder T, Sainio V, Kivisaari L, Puolakkainen P, Kivilaakso E, Lempinen M. Pancreatic resection versus peritoneal lavage in acute necrotizing pancreatitis. A prospective randomized trial. Ann Surg. 1991;214:663–6.
37. Tsiotos GG, Luque-de Leon E, Sarr MG. Long-term outcome of necrotizing pancreatitis treated by necrosectomy. Br J Surg. 1998;85:1650–3.

Acute pancreatitis II

Section IV
Longterm course and outcome

Chair: S. BANK and A.B. LOWENFELS

10
Prediction of outcome in acute pancreatitis: death and local complications

C. D. JOHNSON

INTRODUCTION

For the past 30 years a number of scoring systems and other features have been used to identify patients with acute pancreatitis who are at high risk of developing complications. The Atlanta symposium[1] defined severe acute pancreatitis as pancreatitis in which a complication was present. The various systemic and local complications of acute pancreatitis were also clearly defined in that consensus meeting. The available scoring systems have been used to predict the presence of severe pancreatitis, enabling a group of patients to be identified, with 'predicted severe acute pancreatitis', within 48 h of admission to hospital.

PREDICTIVE SCORES

Until now, attempts to predict outcome in acute pancreatitis[2,3] have been concerned with the definition of complications, and the early identification of patients at high risk of complications. The best known of the predictive systems are the Ranson criteria, the Glasgow criteria and the APACHE II score. John Ranson initially identified a list of risk factors from a patient population with acute alcohol-related pancreatitis[2]. Subsequently, a revised version was developed more suitable for patients with pancreatitis secondary to gallstones and other causes[3] (Table 1). The initial Glasgow criteria[4] were suitable for use in patients with pancreatitis from any aetiology, but were also subsequently modified to improve performance[5] (Table 2). Both of these systems require up to 48 h for full information to be collected.

A comparison of these scoring systems against the ability of a clinician to identify severely ill patients showed that, although initial clinical assessment was unreliable, by 48 h there was little to choose between clinical assessment and the two scoring systems[6]. However, the APACHE II score[7], originally

Table 1 Criteria for the Ranson scores. Exceeding the threshold of three or more criteria indicates predicted severe acute pancreatitis

	All causes[2]	Gallstone related[3]
At admission or diagnosis		
Age	>55 years	>70 years
White blood cell count	$>16 \times 10^9$/L	$>18 \times 10^9$/L
Blood glucose	>200 mg/100 ml	>220 mg/100 ml
Lactate dehydrogenase	>350 IU/L	>400 IU/L
Glutamic oxaloacetic transaminase	>250 SF units%	>250 SF units%
During initial 48 h		
Haematocrit fall	>10%	>10%
Blood urea-nitrogen rise	>5 mg/100 ml	>2 mg/100 ml
Serum calcium	<8 mg/100 ml	<8 mg/100 ml
Base deficit	> 4 mmol/L	> 5 mmol/L
Estimated fluid sequestration	> 6 L	>4 L
$P_{A}O_2$	< 60 mmHg	Not included

Table 2 Modified Glasgow score[5]. Presence of three or more positive criteria indicates predicted severe acute pancreatitis

Age	>55 years
White blood cell count	$>15 \times 10^9$/L
Blood glucose	>10 mmol/L
Plasma urea	>16 mmol/L
$P_{A}O_2$	<8 kPa
Plasma calcium	<2 mmol/L
Plasma albumin	<32 g/L
Lactate dehydrogenase	>600 IU/L

developed for use in general ITU patients, gives equivalent results to the pancreatitis specific scores, after an assessment period of 24 h[8] (Table 3).

These systems depend on measurement of disturbances of normal physiology, and it has only recently been appreciated that in many incidences a high score reflects the fact that the patient has already passed the threshold for organ failure as defined in the Atlanta criteria (Table 4). In a large multicentre trial which included patients with an APACHE II score > 6, which is a relatively low threshold, 44% of patients already had organ failure at the time of admission to the trial[9]. This observation invalidated the primary endpoint of the trial, which was to test for a reduction in the incidence of organ failure. A re-evaluation of complications in acute pancreatitis is therefore required, to enable clinical care and research activity to be directed most appropriately. There are a number of questions that require answers: What is the natural history of patients with organ failure on admission? Is initial organ failure a marker of severe pancreatitis? Is initial organ failure associated with later development of local complications? Can we identify patients with potentially fatal acute pancreatitis?

Table 3 The variables included in the APACHE II score (Acute Physiology, Age and Chronic Health Evaluation). Increasing deviation from normal values generates a numerical score. Addition of all components generates the APACHE II score. Higher scores indicate increasing severity of illness. Various thresholds have been used for predicted severe acute pancreatitis, ranging from >5 to >10. Total possible score = 70; patients with scores >10 are severely ill; scores >20 are associated with >80% mortality rate

Acute physiology
Score up to four points each for abnormal
    Temperature
    Arterial pressure
    Heart rate
    Respiratory rate
    P_{AO_2} or bicarbonate
    Arterial pH
    Plasma sodium
    Plasma potassium
    Creatinine
    Haematocrit
    White blood count
Score conscious level as 15 minus Glasgow Coma Score

Age
Score 2–6 for age bands 45 to >75 years

Chronic health
Pre-existing severe organ/system insufficiency or immunocompromised

After elective surgery	2
After emergency surgery or not operated	5

NATURAL HISTORY OF EARLY ORGAN FAILURE

A major drawback to the Atlanta classification of severe acute pancreatitis is the description of the presence of organ failure as an absolute indicator of severe pancreatitis. Accordingly, if at any time a patient satisfies one of the criteria in Table 4, the patient is deemed to have had a severe attack of pancreatitis, irrespective of the overall clinical outcome. All experienced clinicians will be familiar with patients who are admitted to hospital with evidence of hypoxaemia or oliguria, and who respond satisfactorily to aggressive resuscitation. These patients may recover rapidly, and have an otherwise uncomplicated course with resolution of symptoms within 4–5 days. However, according to the Atlanta classification they should be categorized as severe acute pancreatitis.

The spectrum of organ failure, particularly during the first week, has received relatively little attention. There is a widespread assumption that organ failure is potentially fatal, and while it is certainly the case that a patient who requires artificial ventilation, haemofiltration, and prolonged inotrope support is at a high risk of death, the same is not true of a patient with single organ failure that responds rapidly to appropriate treatment.

Table 4   Systemic complications (organ failure) as defined in the Atlanta consensus on severe acute pancreatitis

Cardiovascular	Systolic blood pressure <90 mmHh
Respiratory	Arterial P_{AO_2} <60 mmHg (<8 kPa)
Renal	Creatinine >2 mg/dL (>177 mmol/L) after rehydration
Coagulation	Platelets <10^5/mm^3, or fibrinogen <1 g/L, or fibrinogen degradation products >80 µg/ml
Metabolic	Calcium < 7.5 mg/dl (<1.87 mmol/L)
Gastrointestinal	Haemorrhage >500 ml/24 h
Systemic disturbance	Ranson or Glasgow scores >2; APACHE II score >7

Table 5   Systemic inflammatory response syndrome (SIRS) is present if any two of these features are found

Temperature	<35.5°C or >38°C
White blood count	>15 × 10^9/L
Respiratory rate	>20 breaths/min
Pulse rate	>100 beats/min

The confusion in this area may be related to the effects of the systemic inflammatory response syndrome (SIRS, Table 5), which is a frequent accompaniment to any serious inflammatory illness, including acute pancreatitis. Current thinking is that during the first week of acute pancreatitis patients may develop SIRS, in response to the pancreatitis. These patients with SIRS may respond to supportive treatment, but they are at risk of exacerbation of the illness by a further stimulus (such as repeated inflammation, endotoxin absorption, or infection) which can lead to progressive organ failure (and may contribute to extension of local complications).

Early deaths

It has been known for many years that approximately half the deaths in acute pancreatitis occur during the first week, and that these deaths are always the result of progressive multiple organ failure[10]. Later deaths are associated with local complications, particularly infected necrosis.

It can be argued, from this, that therapeutic effort and clinical trials should focus on those patients at gravest risk, that is those with progressive organ failure during the first week in hospital, and those who are likely to develop local complications, especially infected necrosis.

In 1990 the Glasgow group reported an association between changes in APACHE II score during the first week, and subsequent outcome[10]. They demonstrated that patients who recovered without complications had an improving APACHE II score, but patients who ultimately died had a progressively increasing score; patients who developed complications had APACHE II scores that persisted at an intermediate level (Figure 1). At the time it seemed self-evident that patients who died should show signs of deteriorating physiological status. Subsequently it has become apparent that these early changes in organ failure may be useful predictors of later outcome, particularly for the identification of patients with potentially fatal acute pancreatitis.

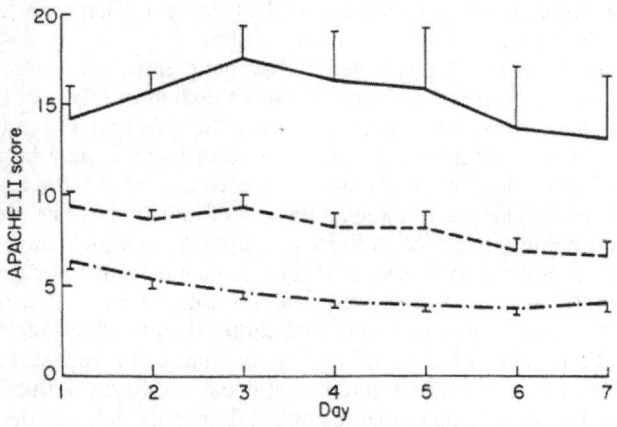

Figure 1 APACHE II scores during the first week of acute pancreatitis in patients who died (continuous), developed complications (dashed), or had mild pancreatitis (dotted) From Wilson et al.[10]

Early organ failure

Beger's group noted that, when organ failure was present in the first 72 h after onset of symptoms, the mortality rate was higher than in patients admitted to hospital without organ failure[11]. They commented that intractable organ failure is a frequent finding, again confirming the truism that if organ failure does not resolve, death will ensue.

The observation that organ failure present at the time of admission to hospital was a marker of severe disease[12,13] helped to focus attention on the presence of early organ failure as a marker of severity. These patients were much more likely to require intensive-care treatment than those patients admitted to the hospital without organ failure. However, the authors of these papers do not comment on the risk of ITU requirement in the much smaller group of patients who develop organ failure after admission.

In a study from Paris, which related the presence and severity of organ failure to the presence of infection in pancreatic necrosis[14], the authors noted that sterile necrosis was usually associated with reversible organ failure. These patients had a mortality rate of only 6%. However, this paper does not give any information on the duration of organ failure.

Organ failure – a dynamic process

A significant advance in our understanding of the dynamic nature of early organ failure in acute pancreatitis came with a publication from Glasgow which demonstrated clearly that organ failure present during the first week could be divided into two categories: organ failure which resolved, and organ failure which persisted beyond the first week[15]. This second group had a much higher (> 50%) mortality rate, whereas no deaths occurred in the 33 patients in whom organ failure resolved by the end of the first week. That report, however, provides no information about local complications.

It has been known for some years that pancreatic necrosis, especially infected pancreatic necrosis, is associated with a high mortality rate. Numerous publications have demonstrated the presence of infection in necrosis as a substantial factor in determining outcome. Accordingly it may be helpful to identify local complications early during the course of the disease, so that preventive strategies aimed at reducing the risk of infection can be used. This is the rationale behind trials of antibiotic prophylaxis, which have included patients with computed tomography (CT) evidence of pancreatic necrosis. In these studies, CT was used to identify patients with necrosis; that is, like the APACHE II score, CT was used to detect, rather than predict, the presence of complications. It is known that the severity of changes on early CT, obtained within the first 4 days of admission to hospital, can give some useful prognostic information. This can be quantified using a CT severity index as described by Balthazar et al.[16] (Table 6). Is it possible to relate changes in organ failure to the risk of infection of necrosis?

The available data are very limited. It is known that more extensive necrosis is more likely to become infected[17] Beger's group demonstrated that the presence of early organ failure was associated with more extensive necrosis[11]. Nearly 90% of their patients with early organ failure required necrosectomy, but that observation is biased by their use of persistent organ failure as an indication for necrosectomy. Le Mee and colleagues also confirmed the association between the presence of infection and persistence of organ failure, and the high mortality rate[14]. The association between persistent early organ failure and the subsequent risk of local complications has to our knowledge been investigated in only one report, published by our group in 2004[18].

PERSISTENT ORGAN FAILURE AND LOCAL COMPLICATIONS

In a database collected during a randomized controlled trial[9] we reviewed the detailed information available for 110 patients in whom a serious adverse event had been reported. Of these patients, 52 had persistent (> 48 h) organ failure during the first week of illness, and 27 patients had transient organ failure which resolved within 48 h. Subsequent evidence of local complications was found significantly more often in patients with persistent organ failure (80%) than in those with transient organ failure (29%) (Table 7). If it is accepted that the extent of pancreatic injury is largely determined early during the course of the disease, so that early evidence of hypoperfusion equates to the final extent

Table 6 CT severity index described by Balthazar[16]

Pancreatic infiltrates (CT grade)	
Normal pancreas	0
Oedematous pancreatitis	1
Plus mild extrapancreatic changes	2
Severe extrapancreatic changes including one infiltrate	3
Multiple/extensive extrapancreatic infiltrates	4
Necrosis	
None	0
< one-third	2
> one-third, < one-half	4
> half	6

CT severity index = CT grade + necrosis score (Scores correlate with outcome as shown)

CTSI	Complications (%)	Deaths (%)
0–3	8	3
4–6	35	6
7–10	92	17

Table 7 Relationship between organ failure and local complications, in 110 patients with documentation of a serious adverse event in a large clinical trial[18]. There was a significant association of persistent organ failure and local complications ($\chi^2 = 34.23$; d.f. = 2; $p < 0.001$)

	n	Local complications	No local complications	No data*
Persistent organ failure	52	27	8	17
Transient organ failure	27	7	17	3
No organ failure	31	2	27	2

*No data from 14 patients who died in the first week, and eight survivors with inadequate records to assess local complications. Local complications were necrosis or pseudocyst; early fluid collections were not considered as complications.

of necrosis[19], the observed association between persistent organ failure and subsequent evidence of local complications suggests that the persistence of organ failure for more than 48 h could be taken as a marker to select patients for contrast-enhanced CT examination. Local complications are unlikely to develop in patients with absent or transient organ failure (Table 7).

PERSISTENT ORGAN FAILURE AND DEATH

The improved knowledge of the natural history of organ failure discussed above, and the requirement for some hard criteria to define as early as possible a group of patients with potentially fatal acute pancreatitis, led us to examine our database for an association between persistent early organ failure and final outcome, i.e. fatal pancreatitis[18]. In 290 patients, with predicted severe acute pancreatitis, organ failure occurred during the first week in 174 patients.

Table 8 Relationship between presence and persistence of organ failure during the first week of acute pancreatitis, and death, in a large randomized clinical trial[18]

	Survived	Died	Total
No organ failure	113	3	116
Organ failure at entry			
Transient	59	1	60
Persistent	56	32	88
New organ failure within 7 days			
Transient	11	0	11
Persistent	11	4	15

Persistent early organ failure, lasting for more than 48h, had a mortality rate of 35%, compared with 3% in those with transient organ failure. The mortality among patients without organ failure was also 3% (Table 8).

This study has demonstrated that the association between organ failure and fatal outcome can be characterized early in the course of the disease. Using thresholds for organ failure consistent with the Atlanta criteria, and a practically useful time band of 48 h, we can identify a group of patients with persistent early organ failure. These patients have potentially fatal acute pancreatitis, with a mortality rate of 35%, and should be offered intensive support of failing systems, in a high-dependency or intensive-care setting.

DEFINITION OF SEVERITY

We also question whether the definitions of severity that have been current for the past 15 years are adequate. In our view the resolution of organ failure within 48 h reflects response to initial treatment, and resolution of the early SIRS. These patients usually recover without any evidence of local complications and with a very low mortality rate. Systemic complications (organ failure) in acute pancreatitis should only be taken as evidence of severe disease if the organ failure has persisted for more than 48 h.

SELECTING PATIENTS FOR CLINICAL TRIALS

For the past 15 years clinical trials of treatment in acute pancreatitis have used various markers of predicted severe acute pancreatitis. Especially for systemic therapies, patients have been selected on the basis of one of the pancreatitis scoring systems or APACHE II scores. Experience has shown that this selection inevitably includes large numbers of patients who already have organ failure[9]. Similarly, CT can identify patients with extensive pancreatic and peripancreatic changes. These patients by definition already have local complications. We have seen that organ failure may resolve with a relatively trouble-free recovery. Local complications include diverse conditions such as peripancreatic fluid infiltrates, pseudocyst, sterile necrosis and infected necrosis. With the exception of infected necrosis these conditions usually resolve with a low mortality rate, and in the case of fluid collections or limited sterile necrosis they may require no specific treatment.

There is a need to select for clinical trials those patients who are most severely ill, who have the highest risk of death. As noted above, initial clinical assessment and the presence of obesity will select patients at increased risk of death. Extremely high Ranson or APACHE II scores are also associated with high-risk groups. However, the addition to this initial clinical assessment of the dynamic component of organ failure seems desirable, as it would include patients with initial low scores who progress, and exclude those who are initially severely unwell but who respond rapidly to treatment.

PREDICTION OF DEATH

The focus on complications as a marker of severe disease has been confused by the failure to consider dynamic changes, and the relatively low threshold defined at Atlanta. Treatment of complications is often simply supportive, and the true aim of therapy is prevention of death. To study this problem, and to identify patients for aggressive treatment, it is necessary to identify patients at high risk of death.

During the 1990s, authors began increasingly to consider predictive factors for fatal outcome. Simple clinical assessment by an experienced observer early in the course of the disease misses two-thirds of patients who will subsequently die. However, the development of a clinical severity score staging system identified three categories with mortality rates of 7%, 23% and 67%[20]. Ranson demonstrated that higher scores in his scoring system were correlated with higher mortality rates[21]. Patients with three or four positive features had a mortality rate of 20%, rising to 40% with five or six features and 100% with seven or eight.

The greater flexibility and discrimination of the APACHE II score, and its ability to predict severe pancreatitis at 24 h at least as well as other systems requiring 48 h[8], are reasons for examining the ability of this system to predict fatal outcome. Larvin has reviewed his database[22] and found very few deaths with APACHE II scores up to 10. APACHE II scores >10 were associated with mortality rates in excess of 20%; scores greater than 16 have a mortality rate >35%. Thus initial assessment with APACHE II score will identify those individuals who are initially severely unwell with organ failure. In these individuals the organ failure is likely to persist, and a fatal outcome is likely.

Several other authors have observed an association between obesity (as determined by a body mass index (BMI) >30) with the incidence of complications[23–26]. Funnell and colleagues 23 pointed out the increased risk of death, and we have subsequently confirmed this in a series of 180 unselected patients with acute pancreatitis[24]. A simple clinical criterion of objectively measured obesity (BMI >30) was associated with a mortality rate of 25%. Local complications and organ failure were also more frequent in the obese patients.

Table 9 Currently available markers of potentially fatal acute pancreatitis suitable for selecting patients for clinical trials. Scoring systems are no longer needed to identify patients at risk of fatal outcome. Patients with age >70 years, obesity, or persistent organ failure are easily identified and include almost all high-risk patients

	Cutoff point	Mortality rate (%)
Clinical assessment	Subjective	?
Age	>70 years	17
Obesity	BMI >30	25
APACHE II score	>16	35
	>18	75
Ranson score	5–6	40
	7–8	100
Persistent organ failure	>48 h	35

Another easily available clinical feature associated with high mortality is increasing age. McKay and colleagues[27], in a population survey, demonstrated a 19% risk of death in patients >70 years old.

There are therefore a number of methods currently available for assessing high risk of death (Table 9). Patients who fall into any one of these groups must be considered to have potentially fatal acute pancreatitis. There are no prospective data available to determine whether these various features are independent, or whether they can be used in an additive fashion to increase the sensitivity of detection of patients with potentially fatal disease.

CONCLUSION

Recent improvements in the understanding of the natural history of acute pancreatitis require a re-evaluation of the definitions of severe pancreatitis. Organ failure present at the time of admission is common, and may reflect severe disease if it progresses, or persists for more than 48 h. However, resolution in response to initial treatment is associated with a lack of further complications. Transient early organ failure is rarely followed by death or local complications. By contrast, persistent early organ failure is a marker of a high-risk group for fatal acute pancreatitis, and for local complications.

References

1. Bradley EL III. A clinically based classification system for acute pancreatitis. Summary of the International Symposium on Acute Pancreatitis, Atlanta, Ga, September 11–13, 1992. Arch Surg. 1993;128:586–90.
2. Ranson JH, Rifkind KM, Roses DF, Fink SD, Eng K, Spencer FC. Prognostic signs and the role of operative management in acute pancreatitis. Surg Gynecol Obstet. 1974;139:69–81.
3. Ranson JH. Etiological and prognostic factors in human acute pancreatitis: a review. Am J Gastroenterol. 1982;77:633–8.

4. Imrie CW, Benjamin IS, Ferguson JC et al. A single-centre double-blind trial of Trasylol therapy in primary acute pancreatitis. Br J Surg. 1978;65:337–41.
5. Blamey SL, Imrie CW, O'Neill J, Gilmour WH, Carter DC. Prognostic factors in acute pancreatitis. Gut. 1984;25:1340–6.
6. Corfield AP, Cooper MJ, Williamson RC et al. Prediction of severity in acute pancreatitis: prospective comparison of three prognostic indices. Lancet. 1985;2:403–7.
7. Knaus WA, Draper EA, Wagner DP, Zimmerman JE. APACHE II: a severity of disease classification system. Crit Care Med. 1985;13:818–29.
8. Larvin M, McMahon MJ. APACHE-II score for assessment and monitoring of acute pancreatitis. Lancet. 1989;2:201–5.
9. Johnson CD, Kingsnorth AN, Imrie CW et al. Double blind, randomised, placebo controlled study of a platelet activating factor antagonist, lexipafant, in the treatment and prevention of organ failure in predicted severe acute pancreatitis. Gut. 2001;48:62–9.
10. Wilson C, Heath DI, Imrie CW. Prediction of outcome in acute pancreatitis: a comparative study of APACHE II, clinical assessment and multiple factor scoring systems. Br J Surg. 1990;77:1260–4.
11. Isenmann R, Rau B, Beger HG. Early severe acute pancreatitis: characteristics of a new subgroup. Pancreas. 2001;22:274–8.
12. Lankisch PG, Pflichthofer D, Lehnick D. No strict correlation between necrosis and organ failure in acute pancreatitis. Pancreas. 2000;20:319–22.
13. Lankisch PG, Pflichthofer D, Lehnick D. Acute pancreatitis: which patient is most at risk? Pancreas. 1999;19:321–4.
14. Le Mee J, Paye F, Sauvanet A et al. Incidence and reversibility of organ failure in the course of sterile or infected necrotizing pancreatitis. Arch Surg. 2001;136:1386–90.
15. Buter A, Imrie CW, Carter CR, Evans S, McKay CJ. Dynamic nature of early organ dysfunction determines outcome in acute pancreatitis. Br J Surg. 2002;89:298–302.
16. Balthazar EJ, Freeny PC, vanSonnenberg E. Imaging and intervention in acute pancreatitis. Radiology. 1994;193:297–306.
17. Vesentini S, Bassi C, Talamini G, Cavallini G, Campedelli A, Pederzoli P. Prospective comparison of C-reactive protein level, Ranson score and contrast-enhanced computed tomography in the prediction of septic complications of acute pancreatitis. Br J Surg. 1993; 80:755–7.
18. Johnson CD, Abu-Hilal M. Persistent organ failure during the first week as a marker of fatal outcome in acute pancreatitis. Gut. 2004;53:1340–4.
19. Block S, Maier W, Bittner R, Buchler M, Malfertheiner P Beger HG. Identification of pancreas necrosis in severe acute pancreatitis: imaging procedures versus clinical staging. Gut. 1986;27:1035–42.
20. Rabeneck L, Feinstein AR, Horwitz RI, Wells CK. A new clinical prognostic staging system for acute pancreatitis. Am J Med. 1993;95:61–70.
21. Ranson JH. Acute pancreatitis. Curr Probl Surg. 1979;16:1–84.
22. Larvin M. Assessment of clinical severity and prognosis. In: Beger HG et al., editors. The Pancreas. Oxford: Blackwell, 1998:489–502.
23. Funnell IC, Bornman PC, Weakley SP, Terblanche J, Marks IN. Obesity: an important prognostic factor in acute pancreatitis. Br J Surg. 1993;80:484–6.
24. Johnson CD, Toh SK, Campbell MJ. Combination of APACHE-II score and an obesity score (APACHE-O) for the prediction of severe acute pancreatitis. Pancreatology. 2004;4: 1–6.
25. Lankisch PG, Schirren CA. Increased body weight as a prognostic parameter for complications in the course of acute pancreatitis. Pancreas. 1990;5:626–9.
26. Porter KA, Banks PA. Obesity as a predictor of severity in acute pancreatitis. Int J Pancreatol. 1991;10:247–52.
27. McKay CJ, Evans S, Sinclair M, Carter CR, Imrie CW. High early mortality rate from acute pancreatitis in Scotland, 1984–1995. Br J Surg. 1999;86:1302–5.

11
Recovery after severe pancreatitis

V. KEIM

INTRODUCTION

The ability of the pancreas to regenerate after pancreatitis has been investigated for more than 100 years. As early as the end of the nineteenth century experiments were performed that suggest a regenerative capacity of the animal pancreas. The first available publication was from Martinotti[1], who in 1888 reported pancreatic ductal proliferation after pancreas resection. In an editorial from Osvaldo Tiscornia and David H. Dreiling, published in *Gastroenterology* in 1966[2], the authors summarized current knowledge on this topic and stated that no firm evidence was available concerning the situation in humans. They conclude that 'proof of pancreatic regeneration must await scientific evidence'. It is remarkable that nearly 40 years later the situation is still not completely clear. It is my aim to summarize the newer literature on this topic.

REGENERATION AFTER EXPERIMENTAL PANCREATITIS

The investigation of regeneration of the animal pancreas after induction of acute experimental pancreatitis has aroused considerable interest in recent years. Pancreatic repair after pancreatitis is complete after only 10–14 days[3]. Cholecystokinin (CCK) was identified as an essential hormone that regulates pancreatic growth after pancreatitis[4]. This hormone also stimulates mitogen-activated protein kinases, thyrosine kinases and phospholipase D[5–7]. The regeneration is accompanied by decrease of inflammatory cells and release of anti-inflammatory mediators[4]. There is a simultaneous, but transient, activation of fibroblasts and deposition of cellular matrix[8] that is removed in the later phase of recovery. Transforming growth factor-β seems to be one of the central regulatory steps of this process[9]. Proliferation of acinar cells is observed during the late phase of regeneration, most probably stimulated by the basic fibroblast growth factor, insulin-like growth factor and epidermal growth factor[10–12]. It is noticeable that activated fibroblasts stimulate acinar cell regeneration after caerulein pancreatitis through secretion of IGF-1[13,14]. Similar effects were described for matrix metalloproteinase-2[15].

PANCREATIC HYPERTROPHY AFTER RESECTION IN HUMANS

In contrast to the detailed knowledge concerning regeneration in experimental pancreatitis, only a few publications can be found that analyse the mechanisms of recovery in humans. In patients with pancreatic cancer the remnant pancreas was studied after pancreatic head resection[16]. In those subjects without recurrence of cancer the pancreas was measured by computed tomography. It was found that the gland did not change within 10 months, and after 21 months the residual pancreas was even smaller. This suggests that the human pancreas is unable to regenerate after resection. However, a significant bias could be that patients with resected pancreatic cancer very often suffer from recurrent disease though the malignant tumour is not (yet) visible in CT.

PANCREATIC FUNCTION AFTER PANCREATITIS IN HUMANS

By analysing publications from the last 30 years it is intriguing to find highly discrepant findings. Starting with 1972 the papers document a low or absent regenerative capacity[17-19], a recovery of the function in half of the patients[20-23] or a nearly normal function in all patients[24-27]. This makes it impossible to draw any firm conclusions from these data, or even to perform a meta-analysis. It only remains to analyse very carefully the details of these studies in order to identify parameters that probably explain why these findings are so discrepant.

VARIABLES THAT MIGHT DETERMINE THE DISCREPANT FINDINGS

Different variables may influence pancreatic function in patients with pancreatitis. In the available studies a variable percentage of patients suffering from chronic pancreatitis were included. It is well known that in these patients pancreatic function decreases with time[28]. In patients with alcoholic pancreatitis signs of chronic pancreatitis were already found at their first admission to hospital, so that a chronic pancreatitis is very likely in these subjects. It is therefore reasonable to assume that a certain impairment of pancreatic function existed before these patients were admitted to hospital. In consequence, reduced pancreatic function cannot be attributed to the most recent episode of pancreatitis.

An additional problem could be the inclusion of both severe and mild acute pancreatitis in the same study. Furthermore, in some patients surgery and/or necrosectomy was performed, and this procedure may reduce pancreatic tissue to a variable extent. Especially in patients operated very early after onset of disease, the necrotic parts of the gland cannot easily be distinguished from surviving tissue. Therefore, tissue was probably removed by the surgeon that carries the ability to regenerate, and this could lead to a significant pancreatic insufficiency. This is especially true for the older studies, as in these cases pancreatic surgery was performed in the majority of patients with pancreatitis, even in oedematous disease. Finally, the measurement of pancreatic function

Table 1 Variables that influence recovery from pancreatitis

Patients	Variable mix of biliary and alcoholic chronic pancreatitis, proportion of severe pancreatitis, small studies (<50 patients)
Treatment	No surgery, necrosectomy, resection
Diagnosis	ERP, secretin–caerulein-test, Lundh test, elastase, chymotrypsin, Pancreolauryl test
Follow-up	1 month–21 months

was performed by different techniques (Table 1) and the secretory capacity was analysed at different times after the episode of pancreatitis. Taken together, all these parameters will considerably influence findings in the respective patients. It is therefore not surprising to find rather inconsistent data.

META-ANALYSIS OR SINGLE IDEAL STUDY OF PANCREATIC REGENERATION?

Due to the unclear role and importance of the various parameters it seems to be not very helpful to perform a meta-analysis with these data. It is probably more useful to select those studies with clearly defined inclusion criteria. The first condition should be the exclusion of all patients with chronic pancreatitis and/ or chronic alcohol consumption. This could ensure that pancreatic function is not impaired before the attack of interest. In addition, only patients with the first episode of biliary pancreatitis should be eligible in whom bile duct stones were removed by ERCP. To prevent a recurrent acute pancreatitis the gallbladder should be removed within 3–4 weeks after pancreatitis, but no further surgery should be performed. Pancreatic function should be measured after 6–12 months by a highly reliable test, preferably the secretin–caerulein test. A review of the literature revealed that only the study published by Pareja et al.[29] met all these criteria. In a group of 48 patient suffering from acute biliary pancreatitis of differing severity pancreatic function was measured 1 year after the acute attack. It was found that pancreatic function (volume secretion, bicarbonate concentration, lipase secretion, lipase concentration, chymotrypsin secretion) was normal in almost all subjects (Figure 1). Only chymotrypsin secretion was abnormal in a few patients. This demonstrates that pancreatic function normalizes several months after an acute attack of pancreatitis.

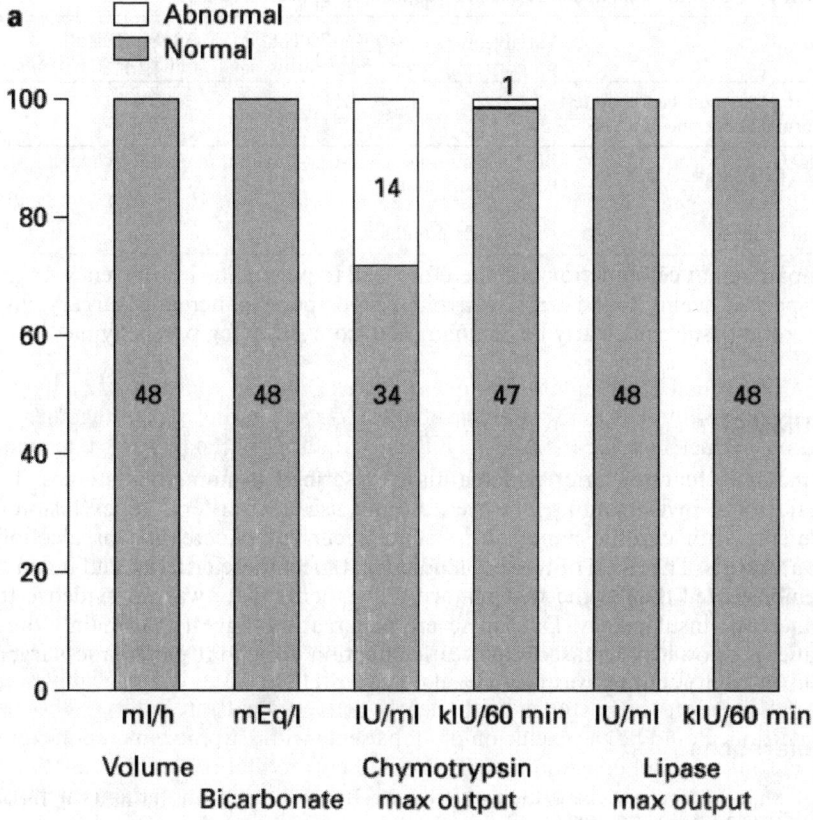

Figure 1 Pancreatic function in patients with biliary pancreatitis. A secretin–caerulein test was performed 1 year after the acute attack (from Pareja et al.[29])

RECOVERY IN SEVERE ACUTE PANCREATITIS: ROLE OF SURGERY

In another study[30] the same group of investigators focused on patients with severe pancreatitis (defined by Atlanta criteria) and analysed whether surgery may influence pancreatic recovery. There was no influence of severity on either exocrine or endocrine pancreatic function. It is remarkable, however, that primarily those patients who were subjected to surgery showed a reduced secretory capacity in the secretin–caerulein test (Table 2), as well as impaired endocrine function. This finding may suggest that surgery itself tends to reduce pancreatic function in the long term. This is in accord with a recent study by Zimmermann et al.[31], who observed large numbers of stellate cells in operative specimens from patients with acute pancreatitis. These cells secrete mediators that stimulate regeneration of acini, and the removal of this material could

Table 2 Pancreatic function in severe pancreatitis: role of necrosectomy

	Necrosectomy n = 12	No surgery n = 15
Normal secretin–caerulein test	42%	87%
Normal endocrine function	25%	75%

Data from Sabater et al.[30]

impair acinar cell function and therefore lead to pancreatic insufficiency. In this respect it seems to be wise to avoid or postpone pancreatic surgery until necrotic tissue can clearly be distinguished from surviving parenchyma.

SUMMARY

Pancreatic function after pancreatitis is described in numerous studies. The majority of investigations, however, did not use clear critera, i.e. exclusion of patients with chronic pancreatitis, acute recurrent pancreatitis or alcoholic pancreatitis. There are only a few studies that meet these criteria, and it can be demonstrated that in the vast majority of patients there was no evidence for pancreatic insufficiency. Data in severe pancreatitis suggest that mainly those patients showed decreased pancreatic function in whom pancreatic surgery and/or necrosectomy was performed.

References

1. Martinotti G. Sulla estirpazione del pancreas. Gior. d. r. Accad. di med. di Torino. 1888;3.s., xxxvi:348–60.
2. Tiscornia OM, Dreiling DA. Does the pancreatic gland regenerate? Gastroenterology. 1966;51:267–71.
3. Elsässer HP, Adler G, Kern HF. Replication and regeneration of the pancreas. In: Go VLW, Di Magno EP, Gardner JD, editors. The Pancreas: Biology, Pathobiology and Disease, 2nd edn. Raven: New York, 1993:75–86.
4. Pap A, Boros L, Hajnal F. Essential role of cholecystokinin in pancreatic regeneration after 60% distal resection in rats. Pancreas. 1991;6:412–18.
5. Rivard N, Lebel D, Laine J, Morisset J. Regulation of pancreatic tyrosine kinase and phosphatase activities by cholecystokinin and somatostatin. Am J Physiol. 1994;266: G1130–8.
6. Rivard N, Rydzewska G, Lods JS, Martinez J, Morisset J. Pancreas growth, tyrosine kinase, PtdIns 3-kinase, and PLD involve high-affinity CCK-receptor occupation. Am J Physiol. 1994;266:G62–70.
7. Rivard N, Rydzewska G, Morisset J. Cholecystokinin-induced pancreatic growth involves the high-affinity CCK receptor and concomitant activation of tyrosine kinase and phospholipase D. Ann NY Acad Sci. 1994;713:422–3.
8. Satake K, Yamamoto T, Umeyama K. A serial histologic study of the healing process after relapsing edematous acute pancreatitis in the rat. Surg Gynecol Obstet. 1987;165:148–52.
9. Menke A, Yamaguchi H, Gress TM, Adler G. Extracellular matrix is reduced by inhibition of transforming growth factor beta1 in pancreatitis in the rat. Gastroenterology. 1997;113:295–303.
10. Hoshi H, Logsdon CD. Direct trophic effects of fibroblast growth factors on rat pancreatic acinar cells *in vitro*. Biochem Biophys Res Commun. 1993;196:1202–7.

11. Vila MR, Nakamura T, Real FX. Hepatocyte growth factor is a potent mitogen for normal human pancreas cells *in vitro*. Lab Invest. 1995;73:409–18.
12. Logsdon CD. Stimulation of pancreatic acinar cell growth by CCK, epidermal growth factor, and insulin *in vitro*. Am J Physiol. 1986;251:G487–94.
13. Ludwig CU, Menke A, Adler G, Lutz MP. Fibroblasts stimulate acinar cell proliferation through IGF-I during regeneration from acute pancreatitis. Am J Physiol. 1999;276:G193–8.
14. Kihara Y, Tashiro M, Nakamura H, Yamaguchi T, Yoshikawa H, Otsuki M. Role of TGF-beta1, extracellular matrix, and matrix metalloproteinase in the healing process of the pancreas after induction of acute necrotizing pancreatitis using arginine in rats. Pancreas. 2001;23:288–95.
15. Ng EK, Barent BL, Smith GS, Joehl RJ, Murayama KM. Decreased type IV collagenase activity in experimental pancreatic fibrosis. J Surg Res. 2001;96:6–9.
16. Tsiotos GG, Barry MK, Johnson CD, Sarr MG. Pancreas regeneration after resection: does it occur in humans? Pancreas. 1999;19:310–13.
17. Bozkurt T, Maroske D, Adler G. Exocrine pancreatic function after recovery from necrotizing pancreatitis. Hepatogastroenterology. 1995;42:55–8.
18. Appelros S, Lindgren S, Borgstrom A. Short and long term outcome of severe acute pancreatitis. Eur J Surg. 2001;167:281–6.
19. Boreham B, Ammori BJ. A prospective evaluation of pancreatic exocrine function in patients with acute pancreatitis: correlation with extent of necrosis and pancreatic endocrine insufficiency. Pancreatology. 2003;3:303–8.
20. Tympner F, Domschke W, Rosch W, Koch H, Demling L. The function of the hydrokinetic and ekbolic pancreas after acute pancreatitis. Z Gastroenterol. 1976;14:684–7.
21. Olszewski S, Kinalska I, Dlugosz J, Stasiewicz J, Gabryelewicz A. The glucose tolerance, insulin response and pancreatic exocrine function in patients after acute pancreatitis. Endokrinologie. 1978;71:183–91.
22. Buchler M, Malfertheiner P, Block S, Maier W, Beger HG. Morphologic and functional changes in the pancreas following acute necrotizing pancreatitis. Z Gastroenterol. 1985;23:79–83.
23. Migliori M, Pezzilli R, Tomassetti P, Gullo L. Exocrine pancreatic function after alcoholic or biliary acute pancreatitis. Pancreas. 2004;28:359–63.
24. Angelini G, Pederzoli P, Caliari S et al. Long-term outcome of acute necrohemorrhagic pancreatitis. A 4-year follow-up. Digestion. 1984;30:131–7.
25. Glasbrenner, B, Büchler M, Uhl W, Malfertheiner P. Exocrine pancreatic function in the early recovery phase of acute oedematous pancreatitis. Eur J Gastroenetrol Hepatol. 1992;4:563–7.
25. Dominguez-Munoz JE, Pieramico O, Buchler M, Malfertheiner P. Exocrine pancreatic function in the early phase of human acute pancreatitis. Scand J Gastroenterol. 1995;30:186–91.
27. Seidensticker F, Otto J, Lankisch PG. Recovery of the pancreas after acute pancreatitis is not necessarily complete. Int J Pancreatol. 1995;17:225–9.
28. Ammann RW, Muellhaupt B. The natural history of pain in alcoholic chronic pancreatitis. Gastroenterology. 1999;116:1132–40.
29. Pareja E, Artigues E, Aparisi L, Fabra R, Martinez V, Trullenque R. Exocrine pancreatic changes following acute attack of biliary pancreatitis. Pancreatology. 2002;2:478–83.
30. Sabater L, Pareja E, Aparisi L et al. Pancreatic function after severe acute biliary pancreatitis: the role of necrosectomy. Pancreas. 2004;28:65–8.
31. Zimmermann A, Gloor B, Kappeler A, Uhl W, Friess H, Buchler MW. Pancreatic stellate cells contribute to regeneration early after acute necrotising pancreatitis in humans. Gut. 2002;51:574–8.

12
Recurrent acute pancreatitis

J. B. M. J. JANSEN and J. P. H. DRENTH

INTRODUCTION

The classification of pancreatitis is rather confusing, as clinical and histo-morphological criteria are frequently confounded. On the one hand pancreatitis is defined according to its clinical course, based on pain and complications; on the other hand, histo-morphological descriptions, such as inflammation, oedema, necrosis, fibrosis and calcifications, are frequently incorporated in the definition. In the majority of cases pancreatitis presents with intense pain for a relatively short duration of time, defined as *acute pancreatitis.*

Acute pancreatitis

Acute pancreatitis frequently runs a favourable clinical course, with quick recovery to a pain-free state, without further attacks. Histological data are not available for this condition, since patients quickly recover and pancreatic biopsies are not considered because of potentially serious complications. Morphological data obtained by contrast-enhanced computer tomography (CT) scanning show a reversible swelling of the pancreas. This course is defined as *acute oedematous pancreatitis.*

Acute necrotizing pancreatitis

About 25% of patients with acute pancreatitis have a complicated clinical course with multi-organ failure, infections and mortality. Post-mortem histo-logical data for these patients have demonstrated necrosis and fibrosis. Morphological data obtained by contrast-enhanced CT scanning demonstrate (peri)pancreatic infiltration with areas of impaired perfusion of contrast, corresponding with necrosis. It is thought that this subsequently leads to abscess formation. This condition is called *acute necrotizing pancreatitis.* Patients with this condition can have haemorrhages (ecchymosis) in one or both flanks (Grey Turner sign) or haemorrhage of the periumbilical region (Cullen sign), probably due to extravasation of pancreatic exudates. This form of acute acute necrotizing pancreatitis is called *acute haemorrhagic pancreatitis.*

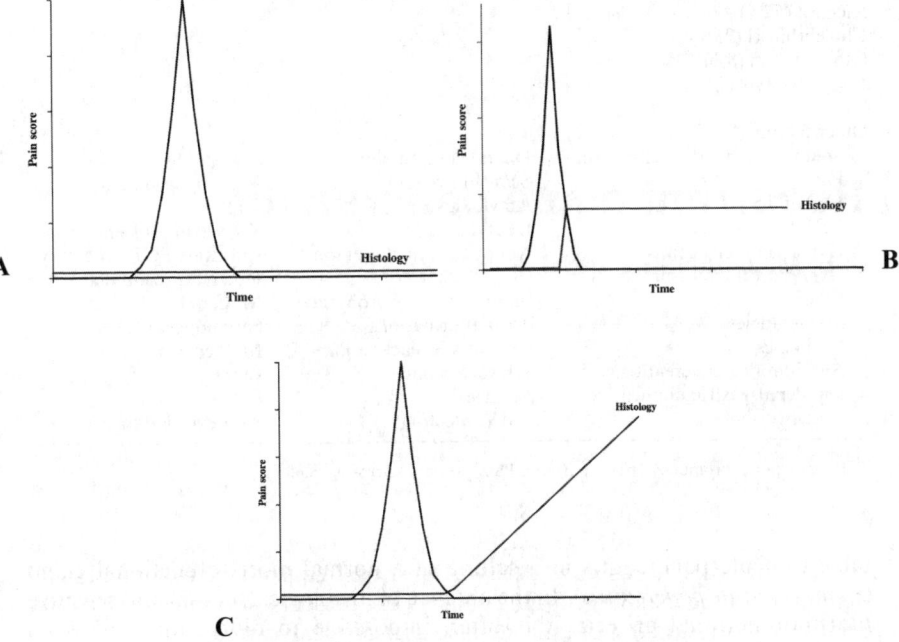

Figure 1 Possible methods of progression of histological abnormalities after a single attack of acute pancreatitis. **A**: Acute pancreatitis without histological abnormalities (acute oedematous pancreatitis with complete recovery). **B**: Acute pancreatitis with non-progressing histological abnormalities (acute necrotizing pancreatitis with complete recovery). **C**: Acute pancreatitis progressing to chronic pancreatitis

The underlying cause of the acute attack determines whether or not clinical signs and histo-morphological abnormalities actually progress (Figure 1).

DEFINITION

As indicated, progression of pancreatitis depends on the cause of the initial attack. Progression after a first attack is mostly characterized by further pain attacks. When attacks re-occur, problems with the definition become apparent. Most patients with recurrent pain attacks (type A pain), progress to continuous pain (type B pain)[1]. These patients have *chronic pancreatitis*, with matching histomorphological abnormalities and impaired exocrine and/or endocrine function. However, some of these patients with recurrent pain attacks do not progress to continuous pain. Repeated pain attacks may thus be a manifestation of chronic pancreatitis with characteristic histomorphological and functional abnormalities (*chronic recurrent pancreatitis*), but may also be attribu-

Table 1 Causes of recurrent acute pancreatitis[2]

Alcohol (57%)
Cholelithiasis (25%)
Other factors (8%)
Idiopathic (10%).

Other factors (8%)[3]:

Sphincter of Oddi dysfunction	Ductal compression	Hydatid liver disease
Pancreas divisum	Scorpion venom	Von Hippel-Lindau
Hereditary	Amyloidosis	TTP
CFTR mutations	Ductal ectasia	Wandering spleen
Hypertriglyceridaemia	Anomalous ductal union	Carnitine PCT deficiency
Hyperparathyroidism	Choledochocéle	Pancreatic candidiasis
ERCP	Inborn errors (porphyria)	M. Crohn
Malignancies	AV malformations	Sarcoidosis
Medicines	Hepatitis B reactivation	M. Wegener
Autoimmune pancreatitis	Schwachmann	Lupus
Duodenal/gastric duplication	Ascariasis	PSC
Kidney disease	CMV infection	Anorexia/bulimia

TTP, thrombotic thrombocytopenic purpura; PSC, primary sclerosing cholangitis

table to acute pancreatitis in a setting of a normal morphofunctional gland (*recurrent acute pancreatitis*). In the absence of histological, causal and sensitive morphofunctional criteria it is often impossible to differentiate between recurrent acute pancreatitis and chronic recurrent pancreatitis.

CAUSES

Causes of recurrent acute pancreatitis and chronic recurrent pancreatitis overlap considerably (Table 1). Insensitivity of morphofunctional criteria and lack of histological data, because of the considerable risk in obtaining pancreatic tissue, contribute to problems with the classification.

There is ongoing discussion whether chronic pancreatitis progresses from acute pancreatitis or whether chronic pancreatitis is already present at the time of the first attack of acute pancreatitis (Figure 2). Some authors were not able to find chronic lesions in patients who died after a first attack of alcoholic pancreatitis[4], whereas others were able to find lesions suggestive for chronicity of the disorder in a considerable number of patients who died after a first attack of alcoholic pancreatitis[5,6]. In an overview on this topic, Hanck and Singer concluded that it is probably safe to assume that the vast majority of alcoholic patients who present with a clinically 'acute' pancreatitis indeed have an underlying disease; namely a chronic alcohol-induced pancreatitis[7].

We therefore end up with three groups of patients with recurrent attacks of pancreatitis:

1. Patients with recurrent attacks of pancreatitis who do not develop chronic lesions.

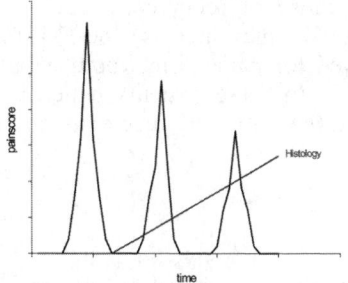
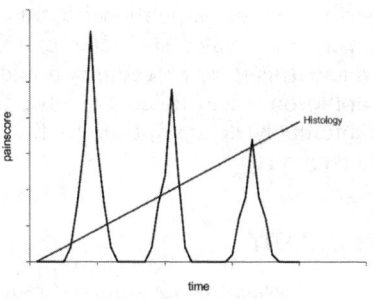

A   B

Figure 2 Does chronic pancreatitis always progress from acute pancreatitis, or is chronic pancreatitis already present during the first attack of acute pancreatitis? **A**: Chronic lesions developing after the first attack of acute pancreatitis. **B**: Chronic lesions already present before the first attack of acute pancreatitis

2. Patients with recurrent attacks of pancreatitis who have histological signs of chronic pancreatitis already present during the first attack.

3. Patients with recurrent attacks of pancreatitis who develop histological signs of chronic pancreatitis after the first or subsequent attacks of pancreatitis.

Causes of pancreatitis and genetic predisposition may play an important role in the development of chronic lesions in patients with recurrent attacks of acute pancreatitis.

For instance patients with choledocholithiasis may suffer from recurrent attacks of acute pancreatitis without histological signs of chronic pancreatitis[8], whereas acute alcoholic pancreatitis may progress to overt chronic pancreatitis even if patients stop consuming alcohol after the first attack[9]. We do not know whether patients with recurrent attacks of acute biliary pancreatitis, belonging to the first group, will ever develop chronic lesions, since these patients rapidly undergo surgery in order to remove the stones in an effort to prevent progression of the disease. Therefore, we can best conclude that, in patients with recurrent attacks of acute pancreatitis, chronic lesions are already present or may develop in the course of the disease, depending on the cause of the disease and genetic predisposition.

THERAPEUTIC OPTIONS

How should we approach patients with recurrent attacks of acute pancreatitis? Obvious causes for pancreatitis should be excluded by non-invasive methods (see Table 1). Hereafter, mainly sphincter of Oddi dysfunction, microcholedocholithiasis and idiopathic causes for recurrent acute pancreatitis remain. Since (micro)choledocholithiasis and sphincter of Oddi dysfunction may represent a considerable number of causes for recurrent attacks of acute pancreatitis[10], it can be argued, rather provocatively, that biliary sphincterotomy should be performed in patients with an unknown cause of recurrent attacks of pancreatitis. Since sphincter of Oddi manometry may increase the risk for pancreatitis, this procedure should be reserved for patients in whom biliary papillotomy has failed to solve the problem. In these patients pancreatic manometry is an option to find and treat the cause of recurrent acute pancreatitis.

SUMMARY

The classification of patients with pancreatitis is complicated by mixing up clinical and histomorphological features. Acute pancreatitis is defined as an attack of characteristic pain, with elevation of pancreatic enzymes in the serum. In the absence of other abnormalities this entity is defined as acute oedematous pancreatitis. The most common finding with radiological imaging is a swollen pancreas. When impaired perfusion of (peri)pancreatic infiltration with demarcation is found on contrast-enhanced CT imaging, with or without multi-organ failure, the entity is called acute necrotizing pancreatitis.

Recurrent attacks of acute pancreatitis may be observed with or without histomorphological and functional abnormalities. In the first case the entity is best defined as chronic recurrent pancreatitis; in the latter case the entity is defined as recurrent acute pancreatitis.

It may be argued that patients with recurrent pancreatitis of unknown origin, after testing by non-invasive methods, are best treated by biliary sphincterotomy. Manometry of the pancreatic sphincter can be performed in patients who fail to respond to biliary sphincterotomy. When there is increased pancreatic sphincter pressure pancreatic sphincterotomy can be performed.

References

1. Ammann RW. The natural history of alcoholic chronic pancreatitis. Intern Med. 2001; 40:368–75.
2. Gullo L, Migliori M, Pezzilli R et al. An update on recurrent acute pancreatitis: data from five European countries. Am J Gastroenterol. 2002;97:1959–62.
3. Lehman GE. Acute recurrent pancreatitis. Can J Gastroenterol. 2003;17:381–3.
4. Klöppel G et al. In: Gyr K, Singer M, Sarles H, editors. Pancreatitis: Concepts and Classifications. Amsterdam: Exerpta Medica, 1984:29–35.
5. Renner IG, Savage WT, Pantoja JL et al. Death due to acute pancreatitis. A retrospective analysis of 405 autopsy cases. Dig Dis Sci. 1985;30:1005–18.
6. Migliori M, Manca M, Santini D et al. Does acute alcoholic pancreatitis precede the chronic form or is the opposite true? A histological study. J Clin Gastroenterol. 2004;38: 274–5.
7. Hanck C, Singer M. Does acute alcoholic pancreatitis exist without preexisting chronic pancreatitis? Scand J Gastroenterol. 1997;32:625–6.
8. Hardt PD, Bretz L, Krauss A. Pathological pancreatic exocrine function and duct morphology in patients with cholelithiasis. Dig Dis Sci. 2001;46:536–9.
9. Fernandez-Cruz L, Navarro S, Castells A et al. Late outcome after acute pancreatitis: functional impairment and gastrointestinal tract complications. World J Surg. 1997;21: 169–72.
10. Coyle WJ, Pineau BC, Tarnasky PR et al. Evaluation of unexplained acute and recurrent acute pancreatitis using ERCP, sphincter of Oddi manometry and endoscopic ultrasound. Endoscopy. 2002;34:17–29.

Chronic pancreatitis I

Section V
Pathobiology of chronic pancreatitis

Chair: G. KLÖPPEL and D. WHITCOMB

13
Experimental models of pancreatic fibrogenesis

M. V. APTE and J. S. WILSON

INTRODUCTION

Pancreatic fibrosis, a characteristic histopathological feature of chronic pancreatitis, is no longer considered to be a mere end-product of chronic inflammation. Accumulating evidence supports the concept that pancreatic fibrosis is a dynamic process that may be reversible in its early stages. Thus, an understanding of the mechanisms responsible for the development of fibrosis has the potential to lead to the development of therapeutic strategies to prevent or retard the fibrotic process. Research in this field has been given significant impetus in recent years by the ability to isolate and culture pancreatic stellate cells (PSC), which are now established as key effector cells in pancreatic fibrogenesis[1-4].

PSC are resident cells of the pancreas and are situated at the base of acinar cells[1]. In health, PSC store vitamin A in lipid droplets within the cytoplasm and can be identified by immunostaining for stellate cell selective markers such as desmin (a cytoskeletal protein), glial fibrillary acidic protein (GFAP), and neuroectodermal proteins such as nestin, nerve growth factor (NGF) and neural cell adhesion molecule (NCAM). The biology of PSC, including their ability to proliferate, migrate and synthesize as well as degrade extracellular matrix (ECM) proteins, has now been well characterised[3,5-7]. Thus, in health, PSC are thought to play a role in maintenance of normal pancreatic ECM via a fine balance between synthesis and degradation. During pancreatic injury, PSC transform to an activated phenotype, most likely in response to factors such as proinflammatory cytokines, growth factors and oxidant stress. Activated PSC synthesize and secrete excess amounts of ECM proteins. The resulting imbalance between ECM synthesis and degradation can lead to the development of fibrosis within the gland.

The role of PSC in pancreatic fibrosis has been studied using two approaches – an *in-vitro* approach using cultured PSC and an *in-vivo* approach using pancreatic sections from patients with chronic pancreatitis and from animal models of pancreatic fibrosis. This chapter will review experimental models of pancreatic fibrogenesis that have sought to delineate the role of PSC in the fibrotic process, discuss the possible mechanisms responsible for activating PSC during pancreatic injury, and comment on current literature regarding potential antifibrotic strategies in the treatment of chronic pancreatitis.

EXPERIMENTAL MODELS

It must be acknowledged at the outset that animal models of pancreatic fibrosis probably do not accurately reflect the human condition in its entirety. However, given the limited availability of human pancreatic tissue, and the fact that human studies usually only allow a 'point-in-time' evaluation of pancreatic disease, experimental models remain a valuable tool. A major advantage of such models is the ability to perform time-course studies of the progression of pancreatitis and pancreatic fibrosis.

Over the past decade, a number of experimental models of pancreatic fibrosis have been described in the literature. A number of these (listed in Table 1) have examined one or more aspects of PSC function during the development of pancreatic injury. The majority are rat models, but mouse models have also been described. In general, the pattern of pancreatic fibrosis (as assessed by Sirius red staining for collagen) in these models is similar to that observed in human chronic pancreatitis (i.e. broad bands of predominantly periductal fibrosis as well as fine bands of collagen extending out between pancreatic acini[8] (Figure 1).

Of the models listed in Table 1, three are particularly relevant to alcohol-induced chronic pancreatitis. These include pancreatic injury produced in rats by: (a) intragastric administration of alcohol[9]; (b) oral ethanol feeding plus injections of cyclosporin A and caerulein[10]; and (c) oral ethanol administration with repeated episodes of caerulein pancreatitis[11]. Intragastric ethanol administration achieves high circulating ethanol levels (higher than *ad libitum* ethanol administration), but it must be noted that the 24-h administration of high doses of ethanol is 'unphysiological' (since it does not reflect the normal pattern of diet intake of humans or rodents) and the confounding effects of hypotension

Table 1 Experimental models of pancreatic fibrosis

Rat models
TNBS infusion into pancreatic duct
Intravenous DBTC injection
WBN/Kob spontaneous chronic pancreatitis
Severe hyperstimulation obstructive pancreatitis (SHOP)
Repeated injection of superoxide dismutase inhibitor
Cyclosporin + caerulein injection
Intragastric alcohol administration
Oral alcohol administration + cyclosporin + caerulein
Oral alcohol administration + repeated caerulein

Mouse models
Transgenic model – TGF-β_1 overexpression
Repeated caerulein injections

Note: The above list is not an exhaustive list of all animal models of chronic pancreatitis but is limited to those studies examining the role of PSC in pancreatic fibrogenesis.

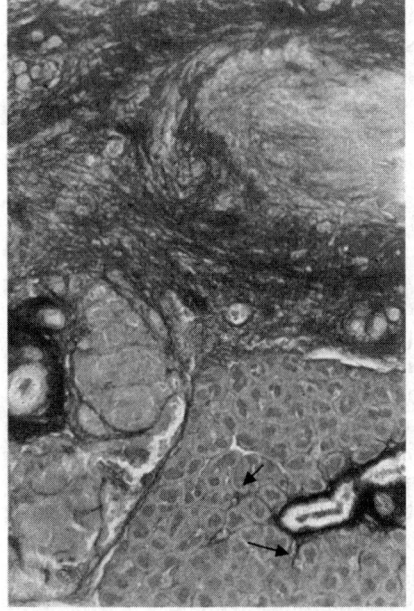 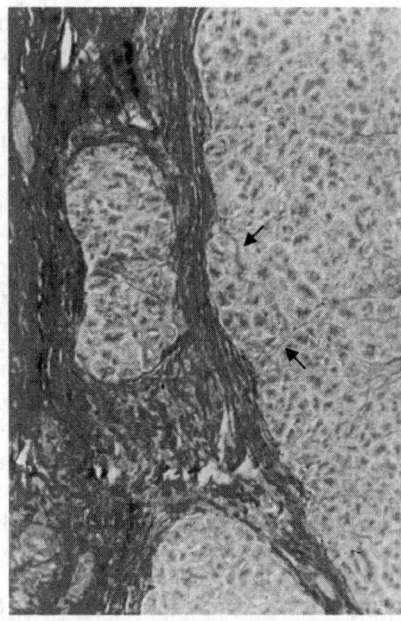

A   B

Figure 1   Sirius red staining for collagen in human chronic pancreatitis (**A**) and rat pancreatic fibrosis (**B**) demonstrating similarity in the pattern of fibrosis. Both rat and human sections exhibit broad bands of predominantly periductular fibrosis as well as fine bands of collagen in periacinar areas (arrows). Dark grey areas – broad bands of fibrosis (stained for collagen with sirius red); arrows – fine bands of collagen in periacinar areas

and shock in these animals cannot be discounted. The ethanol + cyclosporin A + caerulein model represents a model of pancreatic injury produced by multiple hits and has only been studied for a period of 2 weeks after injury. Although this model cannot be claimed to represent chronic pancreatitis, the authors report interesting findings with respect to PSC activation (as indicated by increased α smooth muscle actin expression) early in the course of injury. Most recently, Whitcomb and colleagues[11] have described acinar necrosis and fibrosis in rats fed an alcohol diet and subjected to repeated attacks of caerulein pancreatitis over a period of 4 weeks. Increased PSC proliferation and activation has been reported in this study.

Rat pancreatic fibrosis has also been produced by methods not involving alcohol administration. These include intraductal injection of trinitrobenzene sulphonic acid (TNBS)[8] or by intravenous injection of an organotin compound (dibutyltin chloride, DBTC)[12]. A strain of rats that develops spontaneous chronic pancreatitis and pancreatic fibrosis (WBN/Kob rats) has also been used to study PSC[13,14]. Mouse models used to date to assess the role of PSC in pancreatic fibrosis include a transgenic model of TGF-β_1 over-expression[15] and a model of pancreatic fibrosis produced by repeated injections of the secretagogue caerulein at supramaximal doses[16].

Pancreatic tissue from animal models of pancreatic fibrosis has been examined histologically using routine histological stains, immunohistochemistry and *in-situ* hybridization techniques. Dual staining (using Sirius red for collagen and immunostaining for α smooth muscle actin) of pancreatic sections has shown that there is co-localization of αSMA-positive staining with bands of fibrosis (collagen) suggesting the presence of activated PSC in fibrotic areas (this concurs with findings reported in human chronic pancreatitis)[8].

Serial frozen sections of the pancreas from the TNBS model of pancreatic fibrosis demonstrate increased staining for desmin and for platelet-derived growth factor receptor β (PDGFRβ) in areas of fibrosis (this finding concurs well with that described by Casini et al.[17] in human chronic pancreatitis)[8]. Increased desmin positivity suggests the presence of increased numbers of PSC in areas of fibrosis. The reason for this increase in PSC number may be local proliferation and/or migration of PSC to affected areas. Given that PDGF is a potent mitogen for PSC that also stimulates PSC migration, the observed increase in PDGFRβ staining in fibrotic areas suggests that the increase in PSC numbers in fibrotic areas may be mediated by PDGF via both increased local proliferation and increased migration of the cells. Using dual staining techniques (immunostaining for αSMA and *in-situ* hybridization for collagen mRNA), it has been demonstrated that activated PSC are a predominant source of collagen in TNBS-induced fibrosis.

Using the DBTC model of rat pancreatic fibrosis, Emmrich and colleagues[18] have conducted a time-course study demonstrating an early increase in the expression of desmin, GFAP and αSMA in the pancreas, that precedes the development of fibrosis in the gland.

Studies with transgenic mice overexpressing TGF-β have reported activation of PSC (increased αSMA expression) as early as 14 days after birth, which was found to persist up to 70 days of life[15]. The early activation of PSC was associated with increased expression of TGF-β and of the fibrillar collagens I and III. Persistence of activated PSC at day 70 was associated with increased expression of several profibrogenic growth factors (TGF-β, its downstream mediator connective tissue growth factor (CTGF) and fibroblast growth factor (FGF)) and increased deposition of collagen and fibronectin.

Taken together, the results of *in-vivo* studies to date indicate that PSC are activated early during the course of pancreatic injury and that these activated PSC are a major source of collagen in the fibrotic pancreas.

MECHANISMS OF PSC ACTIVATION

In order to identify the specific factors responsible for PSC activation during pancreatic injury, researchers have turned to *in-vitro* studies using cultured PSC. In general, the selection of putative activating factors for study has been based upon current knowledge of *in-vivo* events during pancreatic injury, such as the production of oxidant stress and the release of growth factors and cytokines including TGF-β, PDGF, tumour necrosis factor α (TNF-α) and the interleukins 1, 6 and 8 (IL-1, IL-6 and IL-8). In addition, factors that may have direct effects on PSC have also been examined. These include ethanol and its metabolites acetaldehyde and fatty acid ethyl esters (FAEE). PSC activation in response to the above factors *in vitro* has been assessed using one or more of a number of parameters of activation including cell proliferation, αSMA expression, ECM protein synthesis, matrix degradation via the production of matrix metalloproteinases, loss of vitamin A stores, cell migration, cytokine release and contractility.

Results of *in-vitro* studies may be summarised as follows:

1. PDGF is a potent proliferative and chemotactic factor for PSC[5,6,19]. These findings may explain the increased numbers of PSC observed in areas of pancreatic fibrosis – secondary to proliferation of local cells as well as recruitment of cells from surrounding areas to areas of injury in response to soluble chemotactic factors such as PDGF.

2. TGF-β is a potent profibrogenic factor for PSC inducing the synthesis of the ECM proteins collagen, laminin and fibronectin by the cells[5,6,19]. TGF-β also increases the secretion of the matrix metalloproteinase MMP2 by PSC[7]. MMP2 is known to degrade basement membrane collagen (collagen type IV) and it is thought that the destruction of normal collagen may facilitate the deposition of abnormal or fibrillar collagens[20]. TGF-β has also been found to induce the expression of PDGF receptor β on PSC, suggesting a synergistic action of the two growth factors on PSC[5].

3. The proinflammatory cytokines TNFα, IL-1, IL-6 and IL-8 activate PSC as assessed by one or more of the following activation indices – proliferation, αSMA expression and collagen synthesis[3,21].

4. In addition to activation by exogenous cytokines via paracrine pathways, it is now established that PSC may be activated by autocrine pathways since the cells can synthesize and secrete cytokines such as TGF-β and IL-1[22,23]. Moreover, the production of these cytokines can be stimulated by exogenous compounds such as ethanol, acetaldehyde and TGF-β itself[23]. These findings suggest that, once activated, PSC are capable of perpetuation of activation even in the absence of the initial trigger factors. This phenomenon may represent one of the mechanisms responsible for progression of chronic pancreatitis despite the cessation of the initial insult (e.g. alcohol excess).

5. Oxidant stress in PSC (produced via exposure to the pro-oxidant combination of ferrous sulphate and ascorbic acid) leads to PSC activation as indicated by increased αSMA expression and collagen synthesis[24].

6. Ethanol can directly activate PSC *in vitro*[24]. This effect is probably mediated by the oxidation of ethanol to acetaldehyde via alcohol dehydrogenase (ADH, a major ethanol-oxidizing enzyme found to be active in PSC) and the consequent generation of oxidant stress. It is notable that ethanol can cause activation of PSC from a quiescent state and does not require the cells to be preactivated to exert its stimulatory effects. This is an important finding suggesting that, *in vivo*, PSC activation may occur early during

chronic alcohol intake even in the absence of necroinflammation. Perpetuation of this activation may occur during ethanol-induced necroinflammatory episodes leading to the development of fibrosis.

Non-oxidative metabolites of ethanol, FAEE have not been reported to activate PSC but have been shown to induce specific signalling pathways within the cells[25].

7. A renin–angiotensin system in pancreatic tissue has been recently identified[26,27]. Furthermore, it has been shown that this system is up-regulated during acute pancreatitis[26,27]. Angiotensin II (produced by proteolytic cleavage of its precursor angiotensin I by angiotensin-converting enzyme) has been reported to induce proliferation of PSC[28,29]. Increased contractility of PSC in response to angiotensin II has also been reported[29]. However, further confirmation of the *in-vitro* effects of angiotensin II is needed, since the concentrations of the compound used in the studies by Reinehr et al.[29] and Hama et al.[28] varied widely, and the physiological relevance of such concentrations is unclear.

8. Increased pressure activates PSC as indicated by cell proliferation, αSMA expression, TGF-β production and collagen secretion by the cells[30]. These findings are relevant given that pancreatic interstitial pressure in chronic pancreatitis is significantly higher than that in normal pancreas[31]. PSC in culture were placed in a pressure loading apparatus and compressed helium gas was pumped into the chamber (without releasing any prepacked room air) to raise the internal pressure. The above observations are of considerable interest. However, it is difficult to discern (from the study) whether the observed effects are due to the helium gas itself rather than to increased pressure. Further studies in this area would be useful.

SIGNALLING PATHWAYS IN PSC

In recent years there has been increasing interest in the evaluation of signalling mechanisms that may mediate the observed effects of various factors on PSC. In general, cellular signalling involves ligand binding to specific receptors or direct effects of cellular stressors leading to a cascade of phosphorylation of signalling molecules. The phosphorylated effector protein of the pathway then translocates to the nucleus and influences the transcription of specific genes that regulate cellular function. It is hoped that the identification and characterization of responsible signalling molecules will allow the therapeutic targeting of specific pathways so as to prevent or reverse PSC activation and thereby prevent or retard the fibrotic process.

One of the major pathways that regulates cell functions such as protein synthesis, cell differentiation and cell division is the mitogen-activated protein kinase (MAPK) pathway[32]. Consequently, this pathway has been the focus of attention of a number of recent studies. It is now established that the effects of ethanol, acetaldehyde and oxidant stress (Figure 2) on PSC are mediated by activation of all three classes of the MAPK pathway – extracellular signal

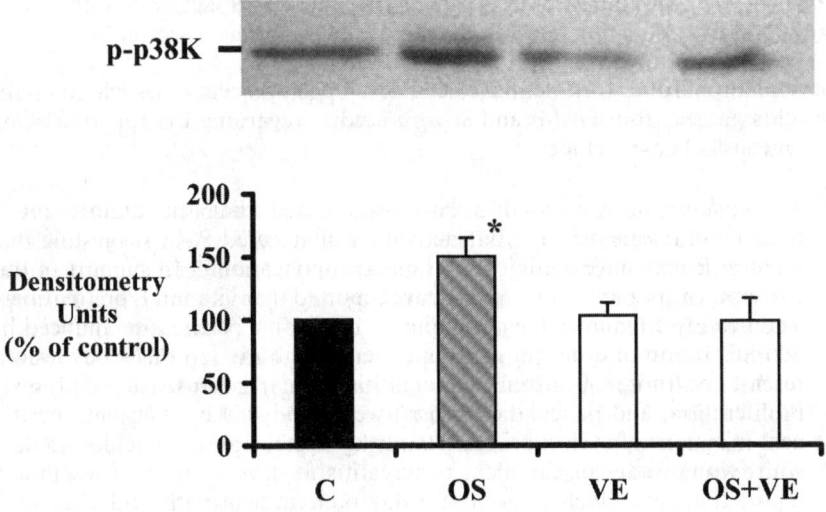

Figure 2 Activation of p38 MAP kinase in cutured pancreatic stellate cells exposed to oxidant stress (OS). The figure depicts a representative Western blot for the phosphorylated (activated) form of p38 kinase in PSC incubated with culture medium alone (C), the pro-oxidant mixture 10 μM $FeSO_4$/200 μM ascorbic acid (OS), 100 μM vitamin E (VE) and the pro-oxidant mixture + vitamin E (OS + VE). Densitometry of all Western blots ($n = 3$ separate cell preparations) demonstrated that oxidant stress induced p38 kinase activation and PSC. This induction was prevented in the presence of the antioxidant vitamin E (*$p < 0.01$; $n = 3$ separate cell preparations)

regulated kinase (ERK1/2), p38 kinase and c-jun amino terminal kinase (JNK)[19,33,34]. Most recently it has been demonstrated that ethanol and acetaldehyde also activate two signalling molecules upstream of the MAPK cascade, phosphatidylinositol 3-kinase (PI3K) and protein kinase C (PKC)[35].

It has been reported that PDGF-induced PSC proliferation is mediated by the ERK pathway[19], while PDGF-induced PSC migration is a function of the PI3K pathway[34]. However, it is important to note that crosstalk exists between PI3K and ERK, so that modulation of one pathway is usually associated with a change in the function of the other[34]. TGF-β has been shown to exert its profibrogenic effect on PSC via the intracellular signalling mediator SMAD2[36]. TGF-β is also known to increase its own mRNA expression in PSC in an autocrine manner, a process that has been shown to be regulated by the ERK pathway[36]. Recent studies have suggested a role for the peroxisome proliferator-activated receptor γ (PPARγ, a ligand-activated transcription factor which controls cellular growth and differentiation) in PSC activation[37,38]. Notably, the PPARγ ligand troglitazone has been reported to inhibit PDGF-induced and culture-induced activation of PSC[13].

POTENTIAL ANTIFIBROTIC STRATEGIES IN CHRONIC PANCREATITIS

Several antifibrotic strategies have been developed in recent years, based on the insights gained from *in-vivo* and *in-vitro* studies regarding the role of PSC in fibrogenesis. These include:

1. *Antioxidants*: *In-vitro* studies have established that the antioxidant α tocopherol (vitamin E) inhibits activation of cultured PSC, suggesting that vitamin E may have a clinical therapeutic application[24]. In support of this concept, Gomez and colleagues[39] have reported that vitamin E pretreatment significantly attenuates the development of chronic pancreatitis induced by administration of cyclosporin A and caerulein to rats. In this study lesions resembling those of chronic pancreatitis (acinar necrosis, myofibroblast proliferation, and pancreatic fibrosis) were produced by daily intraperitoneal injections of cyclosporin A (20 mg/kg diluted 1:4 in saline) for 15 days with two episodes of caerulein pancreatitis at days 1 and 8. The authors report that rats which received a 4-day pretreatment with oral vitamin E (600 mg/kg per day by gavage) and ongoing daily treatment with vitamin E throughout the course of the study, exhibited significantly decreased oxidant stress, collagen content and myofibroblast numbers within the pancreas. Although these findings are encouraging, it must be noted that the cyclosporin A + caerulein protocol employed produces a mild form of pancreatic injury (as acknowledged by the authors themselves) and that vitamin E treatment has only been assessed in a protocol involving pretreatment. Further studies assessing the efficacy of vitamin E in severe pancreatic injury and, in particular, in established disease would be useful and more relevant to the clinical situation.

2. *Anti-TGF-β strategies*: It is now well established that TGF-β is a potent profibrogenic cytokine for PSC. Up-regulation of TGF-β expression at both mRNA and protein levels has been demonstrated in chronic pancreatitis[39–41]. Therefore, strategies to reduce TGF-β production, or to inhibit its activity, would reasonably be expected to have beneficial antifibrotic effects. In this regard, Menke et al.[42] have reported that administration of TGF-β neutralizing antibodies significantly inhibits the increase in pancreatic ECM protein content induced during acute caerulein pancreatitis in rats. In this study anti-TGF-β antibodies were administered intravenously 30 min before the start of the caerulein infusion and then 24 and 48 h after the start of the infusion. However, it should be noted that the model employed was not of chronic pancreatitis, and the efficacy of treatment after onset of disease was not assessed. Of somewhat more clinical relevance is a more recent report of the beneficial effects of a herbal medicine Saiko-keishi-to (TJ-10) using the WBN/Kob rat model of spontaneous chronic pancreatitis[41]. In this model chronic pancreatitis develops over a period of 20–24 weeks after birth. TGF-β mRNA levels peak at 12 weeks while maximal fibrosis is observed at 16 weeks. Treatment with TJ-10 (80 mg/kg by gavage daily) from 4 to 24 weeks significantly decreased the rate of development of pancreatic fibrosis. This

was associated with a decrease in the expression of TGF-β, fibronectin, collagen type III and αSMA within the pancreas, compared to untreated controls. TJ-10 also significantly reduced inflammation in the pancreas. Taken together, these findings suggest that the antifibrotic effects of TJ-10 may be mediated via decreased PSC activation secondary to decreased TGF-β expression. Additional postulated mechanisms include decreased proinflammatory cytokine levels (secondary to inhibition of inflammation) and reduced oxidant stress (since components of TJ-10 are known to act as free radical scavengers).

3. *Modulation of signalling pathways*: As noted earlier, a number of signalling pathways have now been identified as regulators of PSC activation. Although specific inhibitors of these pathways such as wortmannin (PI3 kinase inhibitor), calphostin C (PKC inhibitor), U01226 (ERK inhibitor) and SB203580 (p38 kinase inhibitor) have been found to inhibit PSC activation *in vitro*, these compounds have not yet been assessed in *in-vivo* models of pancreatic fibrosis. However, the modulation of PPARγ has recently been investigated in an *in-vivo* model[13] (adequate PPARγ expression has been reported to be essential for maintenance of PSC quiescence[37]). Troglitazone (a PPARγ ligand) was found to exert significant antifibrotic effects in the WBN/Kob model of spontaneous chronic pancreatitis. In this study WBN/Kob rats were fed rat chow containing troglitazone (0.2%) from 4 weeks of age for a period of 3–6 months. The rate of pancreatic fibrosis was significantly reduced in treated animals and this was associated with decreased proliferation and αSMA expression in PSC.

4. *Angiotensin inhibition*: In view of the observations noted earlier regarding the pro-proliferative effect of angiotensin II on PSC, a recent *in-vivo* study has examined the effects of the angiotensin-converting enzyme inhibitor (captopril) and an angiotensin II receptor antagonist (losartan) on alcohol-induced pancreatic fibrosis[14]. This study involved intragastric ethanol administration to rats for 4 weeks and treatment with either captopril (60 mg/kg per day) or losartan (3 mg/kg per day) in the liquid diet. The treatments were commenced 3 days before the commencement of feeding of the ethanol diet. The authors report that both captopril and losartan significantly blunted the ethanol-induced increase in αSMA expression, TGF-β expression and, importantly, interlobular and intralobular fibrosis within the pancreas.

5. *Vitamin A supplementation*: Loss of cytoplasmic vitamin A stores is a consistent feature of PSC activation. However, until recently the role of vitamin A in the maintenance of PSC quiescence had not been examined. McCarroll et al.[43] have now demonstrated that supplementation of vitamin A (retinol 10 μM) in the culture medium can significantly inhibit the proliferation of PSC and also prevent PSC activation induced by culture on plastic or by exposure to ethanol, as indicated by reduced αSMA expression (Figure 3) and inhibition of ECM protein (collagen, fibronectin and laminin) production by PSC. It is tempting to speculate that vitamin A

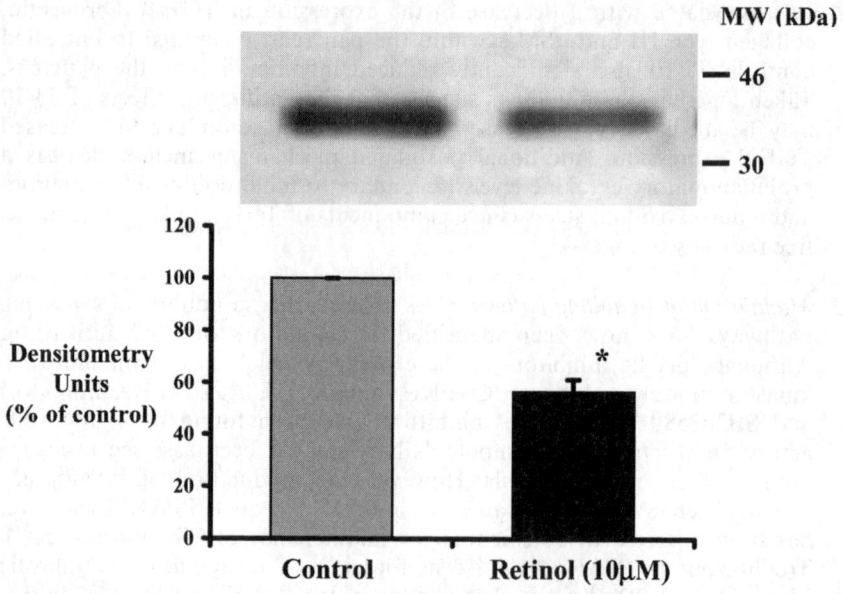

Figure 3 Effect of retinol supplementation on PSC activation as assessed by a smooth muscle actin expression. The figure shows a representative Western blot for αSMA expression in PSC incubated for 48 h with either culture medium alone (Control) or retinol 10 μM. Densitometry of all Western blots ($n = 3$ separate cell preparations) showed a significant decrease in αSMA expression in PSC incubated with retinol compared to controls (*$p < 0.01$; $n = 3$ separate cell preparations)

may be an effective antifibrotic agent in chronic pancreatitis via its specific effect on PSC. However, it is to be noted that the therapeutic window for this compound is likely to be narrow, because excess vitamin A has been reported to cause fibrosis, at least in the liver[44,45]. Studies of the effects of vitamin A supplementation on experimental models of pancreatic fibrosis are needed.

In summary, an understanding of the mechanisms responsible for pancreatic fibrosis is essential for the development of treatment strategies to prevent or retard the process. The limited availability of human pancreatic tissue makes human studies difficult. Experimental models of pancreatic fibrosis are a reasonable and valuable alternative. These models enable detailed studies of the induction and progression of pancreatic injury and also lend themselves to testing the efficacy of antifibrotic agents in pancreatic fibrosis. It must be noted that most treatment regimens shown to be beneficial in experimental models of pancreatic fibrosis have been instituted before or at the time of induction of injury. Since pretreatment is usually not an option in the clinical situation, it is important that researchers endeavour to also assess treatment protocols under conditions of established disease.

References

1. Apte MV, Haber PS, Applegate TL et al. Periacinar stellate shaped cells in rat pancreas – identification, isolation, and culture. Gut. 1998;43:128–33.
2. Bachem MG, Schneider E, Gross H et al. Identification, culture, and characterization of pancreatic stellate cells in rats and humans. Gastroenterology. 1998;115:421–32.
3. Schneider E, Schmid-Kotsas A, Zhao J et al. Identification of mediators stimulating proliferation and matrix synthesis of rat pancreatic stellate cells. Am J Physiol Cell Physiol. 2001;281:C532–43.
4. Apte MV, Wilson JS. Stellate cell activation in alcoholic pancreatitis. Pancreas. 2003;27:316–20.
5. Apte MV, Haber PS, Darby SJ et al. Pancreatic stellate cells are activated by proinflammatory cytokines: implications for pancreatic fibrogenesis. Gut. 1999;44:534–41.
6. Phillips PA, Wu MJ, Kumar RK et al. Cell migration: a novel aspect of pancreatic stellate cell biology. Gut. 2003;52:677–82.
7. Phillips PA, McCarroll JA, Park S et al. Pancreatic stellate cells secrete matrix metalloproteinases – implications for extracellular matrix turnover. Gut. 2003;52:275–82.
8. Haber P, Keogh G, Apte M et al. Activation of pancreatic stellate cells in human and experimental pancreatic fibrosis. Am J Pathol. 1999;155:1087–95.
9. Tsukamoto H, Towner SJ, Yu GS, French SW. Potentiation of ethanol-induced pancreatic injury by dietary fat. Induction of chronic pancreatitis by alcohol in rats. Am J Pathol. 1988;131:246–57.
10. Gukovsky I, Lugea A, Cheng J, French B, Riley EN, French SW. Model of chronic alcoholic pancreatitis. Gastroenterology. 2002;122:A93.
11. Deng X, Wang L, Elm MS et al. Chronic alcohol consumption accelerates fibrosis in response to cerulein-induced pancreatitis in rats. Am J Pathol. 2005;166:93–106.
12. Merkord J, Weber H, Sparmann G, Jonas L, Hennighausen G. The course of pancreatic fibrosis induced by dibutyltin dichloride (DBTC). Ann NY Acad Sci. 1999;880:231–7.
13. Shimizu K, Shiratori K, Kobayashi M, Kawamata H. Troglitazone inhibits the progression of chronic pancreatitis and the profibrogenic activity of pancreatic stellate cells via a PPAR gamma-independent mechanism. Pancreas. 2004;29:67–74.
14. Uesugi T, Froh M, Gabele E et al. Contribution of angiotensin II to alcohol-induced pancreatic fibrosis in rats. J Pharmacol Exp Ther. 2004;17:17.
15. Vogelmann R, Ruf D, Wagner M, Adler G, Menke A. Effects of fibrogenic mediators on the development of pancreatic fibrosis in a TGF-beta1 transgenic mouse model. Am J Physiol – Gastrointest Liver Physiol. 2001;280:G164–72.
16. Neuschwander-Tetri BA, Burton FR, Presti ME et al. Repetitive self-limited acute pancreatitis induces pancreatic fibrogenesis in the mouse. Dig Dis Sci. 2000;45:665–74.
17. Casini A, Galli A, Pignalosa P et al. Collagen type I synthesized by pancreatic periacinar stellate cells (PSC) co-localizes with lipid peroxidation-derived aldehydes in chronic alcoholic pancreatitis. J Pathol. 2000;192:81–9.
18. Emmrich J, Weber I, Sparmann GH, Liebe S. Activation of pancreatic stellate cells in experimental chronic pancreatitis in rats. Gastroenterology. 2000;118:A166.
19. Jaster R, Sparmann G, Emmrich J, Liebe S. Extracellular signal regulated kinases are key mediators of mitogenic signals in rat pancreatic stellate cells. Gut. 2002;51:579–84.
20. Friedman SD. The cellular basis of hepatic fibrosis. N Engl J Med. 1993;328:1828–35.
21. Mews P, Phillips P, Fahmy R et al. Pancreatic stellate cells respond to inflammatory cytokines: potential role in chronic pancreatitis. Gut. 2002;50:535–41.
22. Shek FW, Benyon RC, Walker FM et al. Expression of transforming growth factor-β1 by pancreatic stellate cells and its implications for matrix secretion and turnover in chronic pancreatitis. Am J Pathol. 2002;160:1787–98.
23. Apte M, Keating J, Phillips P et al. Endogenous expression of proinflammatory cytokines and nerve growth factor by pancreatic stellate cells – implications for fibrosis and neural changes in chronic pancreatitis. J Gastroenterol Hepatol. 2001;16:A114.
24. Apte MV, Phillips PA, Fahmy RG et al. Does alcohol directly stimulate pancreatic fibrogenesis? Studies with rat pancreatic stellate cells. Gastroenterology. 2000;118:780–94.
25. Masamune A, Kikuta K, Satoh M, Suzuki N, Shimosegawa T. Fatty acid ethyl esters activate activator protein-1 and mitogen-activated protein kinases in rat pancreatic stellate cells. Pancreatology. 2004;4:311.

26. Leung PS, Chan WP, Nobiling R. Regulated expression of pancreatic renin–angiotensin system in experimental pancreatitis. Mol Cell Endocrinol. 2000;166:121–8.
27. Ip SP, Kwan PC, Williams CH, Pang S, Hooper NM, Leung PS. Changes of angiotensin-converting enzyme activity in the pancreas of chronic hypoxia and acute pancreatitis. Int J Biochem Cell Biol. 2003;35:944–54.
28. Hama K, Ohnishi H, Yasuda H et al. Angiotensin II stimulates DNA synthesis of rat pancreatic stellate cells by activating ERK through EGF receptor transactivation. Biochem Biophys Res Commun. 2004;315:905–11.
29. Reinehr R, Zoller S, Klonowski-Stumpe H, Kordes C, Haussinger D. Effects of angiotensin II on rat pancreatic stellate cells. Pancreas. 2004;28:129–37.
30. Watanabe S, Nagashio Y, Asaumi H et al. Pressure activates rat pancreatic stellate cells. Am J Physiol Gastrointest Liver Physiol. 2004;287:G1175–81.
31. Jalleh RP, Aslam M, Williamson RC. Pancreatic tissue and ductal pressures in chronic pancreatitis. Br J Surg. 1991;78:1235–7.
32. Lopez-Ilasaca M. Signaling from g-protein-coupled receptors to mitogen-activated protein (MAP)-kinase cascades. Biochem Pharmacol. 1998;56:269–77.
33. McCarroll JA, Phillips PA, Park S et al. Pancreatic stellate cell activation by ethanol and acetaldehyde: is it mediated by the mitogen-activated protein kinase signaling pathway? Pancreas. 2003;27:150–60.
34. McCarroll JA, Phillips PA, Kumar RK et al. Pancreatic stellate cell migration: role of the phosphatidylinositol 3-kinase(PI3-kinase) pathway. Biochem Pharmacol. 2004;67:1215–25.
35. McCarroll J, Phillips P, Santucci N, Pirola R, Wilson J, Apte M. Alcoholic pancreatic fibrosis: role of the phosphatidylinositol-3 kinase (PI3-k) and protein kinase c (PKC) pathways in pancreatic stellate cells. J Gastroenterol Hepatol. 2004;18:A245.
36. Ohnishi H, Miyata T, Yasuda H et al. Distinct roles of Smad2-, Smad3-, and ERK-dependent pathways in transforming growth factor-beta1 regulation of pancreatic stellate cellular functions. J Biol Chem. 2004;279:8873–8.
37. Masamune A, Kikuta K, Satoh M, Sakai Y, Satoh A, Shimosegawa T. Ligands of peroxisome proliferator-activated receptor-gamma block activation of pancreatic stellate cells. J Biol Chem. 2002;277:141–7.
38. Masamune A, Kikuta K, Satoh M, Suzuki N, Shimosegawa T. Protease-activated receptor-2-mediated proliferation and collagen production of rat pancreatic stellate cells. J Pharmacol Exp Ther. 2004;14:14.
39. Gomez JA, Molero X, Vaquero E, Alonso A, Salas A, Malagelada JR. Vitamin E attenuates biochemical and morphological features associated with development of chronic pancreatitis. Am J Physiol Gastrointest Liver Physiol. 2004;287:G162–9.
40. van Laethem JL, Deviere J, Resibois A et al. Localization of transforming growth factor beta 1 and its latent binding protein in human chronic pancreatitis. Gastroenterology. 1995;108:1873–81.
41. Su SB, Motoo Y, Xie MJ, Taga H, Sawabu N. Antifibrotic effect of the herbal medicine Saiko-keishi-to (tj-10) on chronic pancreatitis in the WBN/Kob rat. Pancreas. 2001;22:8–17.
42. Menke A, Yamaguchi H, Gress TM, Adler G. Extracellular matrix is reduced by inhibition of transforming growth factor beta1 in pancreatitis in the rat. Gastroenterology. 1997;113:295–303.
43. McCarroll JA, Phillips PA, Santucci N, Pirola R, Wilson J, Apte M. Vitamin A induces quiescence in culture-activated pancreatic stellate cells – potential as an anti-fibrotic agent? Pancreas. 2003;27:396.
44. Leo MA, Lieber CS. Alcohol, vitamin a, and beta-carotene: adverse interactions, including hepatotoxicity and carcinogenicity. Am J Clin Nutr. 1999;69:1071–85.
45. Kapp P, Bely M, Nemesanszky E. Ultrastructural findings in the liver due to long-term retinol (isotretinoin) treatment. Significance of the perisinusoidal (Ito) cells. Orv Hetil. 2004;145:173–9.

14
Gene mutations as a cause of chronic pancreatitis

D. C. WHITCOMB

INTRODUCTION

The limited medical and surgical advances in the treatment of chronic pancreatitis reflect our knowledge and approach to this disease. On the other hand, treatment failure may be inevitable because of what chronic pancreatitis actually is. Advanced chronic pancreatitis should be defined as a hopeless condition in which the pancreas is destroyed by inflammation and fibrosis, and there is no chance of regression or regeneration. Currently, our diagnostic efforts are aimed at detecting and staging the pathological changes within the pancreas and our therapeutic interventions are directed at replacing lost function (e.g. pancreatic enzymes), and attempting to control pain with medicine, drainage procedures, nerve interruption or partial gland resection.

If advanced chronic pancreatitis is a hopeless condition, our laboratory and clinical efforts should be targeted at understanding the molecular and pathological mechanisms of the disease. The first problem in developing therapeutic or preventative strategies is in understanding the aetiology of chronic pancreatitis. The second problem is to understand the modifying factors that determine disease progression, since hopeless, advanced chronic pancreatitis usually begins as mild chronic pancreatitis.

What do we actually know about chronic pancreatitis? First, we know that something happens within a person that causes a normal pancreas to progressively deteriorate into an end-stage, sclerotic pancreatic remnant over some period of time (Figure 1). Historically, this progression has been documented through autopsy studies and surgical biopsies leading to definitions of chronic pancreatitis based on histology[1,2]. Therefore, our clinical efforts reflect this historical perspective and are directed at predicting histology in living subjects using CT, ERCP, MRCP or pancreatic function tests.

Our research group is also concerned that investigative studies comparing tissue from normal pancreases with tissue from subjects with chronic pancreatitis using arrays, proteomics or other techniques will never lead to an understanding of aetiology, mechanism of progression or substantially improve prognosis (Figure 1)[3]. Comparative molecular and gene expression studies on pancreatic tissue will define histology, not aetiology.

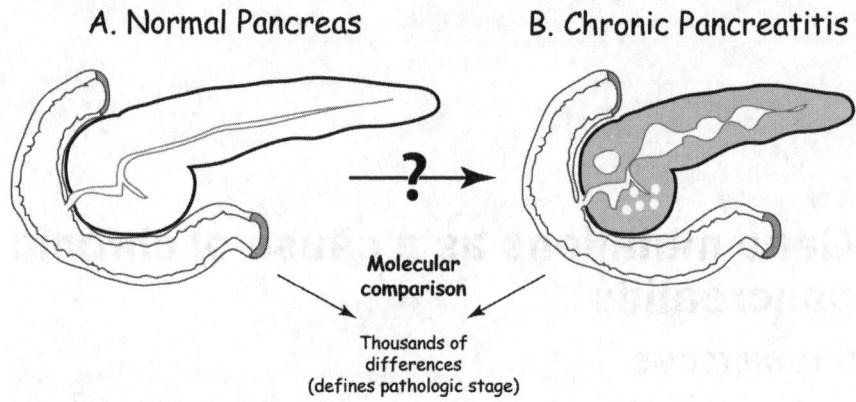

Figure 1 Comparison studies and aetiology. Comparison of tissue form normal pancreas (**A**) with end-stage chronic pancreatitis (**B**) is valuable for defining the histological and pathological features. Addition of molecular techniques provides information on thousands of differences between **A** and **B**. However, these approaches are more valuable in defining molecular pathology and staging than for determining etiology or prognosis. (From Whitcomb[3] with permission)

Human genetic studies revolutionized our understanding of the aetiology and prognosis of chronic pancreatitis. The initial breakthrough came in 1996 with the genetic linkage studies in hereditary pancreatitis kindreds[4,5] and the molecular identification of mutations in the cationic trypsinogen gene (*PRSS1*) of these families[6]. Combining our knowledge of pancreatic physiology and mechanisms controlling intrapancreatic trypsin activity has provided the clues to understanding chronic pancreatitis as a complex disease[3]. The new insights into the molecular mechanisms of acute and chronic pancreatitis have forced us to rethink the organization of information and development of new models for testing new hypotheses. In discussing the topic of 'Gene mutations as a cause of chronic pancreatitis' for the Falk Symposium, I will focus on three areas: (1) the SAPE model of chronic pancreatitis in which chronic pancreatitis is viewed as a process that begins when the immune system is triggered, (2) five lines of evidence showing that recurrent acute pancreatitis leads to chronic pancreatitis, and (3) factors that modify the immune response determine the rate of fibrosis and other complications in chronic pancreatitis.

THE SAPE MODEL: CHRONIC PANCREATITIS IS A PROCESS THAT BEGINS WHEN THE IMMUNE SYSTEM IS TRIGGERED BY ACUTE PANCREATITIS

We initially investigated families with hereditary pancreatitis to complement our animal and clinical studies into the pathogenesis of alcoholic chronic pancreatitis. We learned that all types of chronic pancreatitis had similar histological features (cf. ref. 7), and that animals fed alcohol for months did

Table 1 Evidence that chronic pancreatitis follows acute pancreatitis

Type of evidence	References
1. Clinical evidence	13–15
2. Pathological evidence	16–18
3. Aetiological evidence*	2, 20, 50
4. Genetic studies*	6, 26, 32
5. Animal studies	36, 39

* Evidence discussed in this chapter.

not develop chronic pancreatitis – despite ongoing acinar cell stress and injury[8,9]. Furthermore, most subjects who drink excessive alcohol do not develop end-stage chronic pancreatitis. We concluded that multiple environ-mental and genetic risk factors must be converging in those individuals with chronic pancreatitis, and that understanding of the interaction of risk factors would require organization of all known risk factors converging in *each person* according to mechanistic categories. This led to development of the TIGAR-O risk/aetiology classification system[2] (modified in Table 2, column 3). Next, it became apparent that most of the risk factors for chronic pancreatitis were far more common than was chronic pancreatitis; that different risk factors were important at different times in the process leading to chronic pancreatitis; that the process must begin at some point in time; and that the triggering event triggered the immune system, which was responsible for the inflammation and fibrosis characteristic of chronic pancreatitis histology. This led to development of the SAPE model hypothesis.

Disease modelling – the SAPE model hypothesis

If one attempts to model the progressive features of chronic pancreatitis it is imperative to have an activated immune system inside the pancreas. We therefore developed the SAPE model hypothesis to classify and organize all of the many factors that influence the development and progression of chronic pancreatitis focusing on the immune system[10]. The model was thus structured to recognize the multiple roles and mediators of the immune system in the development of fibrosis, which include both proinflammatory and anti-inflam-matory components (e.g. TGF-β) and multiple cell types (e.g. T cells, macro-phages, stellate cells). Finally, it recognized that the initiation of the process leading to chronic pancreatitis required recruitment and activation of inflam-matory cells, an event that is known to occur with an episode of acute pancreatitis. This Sentinel Acute Pancreatitis Event (SAPE) is used to designate a specific injury to the pancreas that is sufficient to be the initial activator of the immune system (from a modelling perspective), regardless of whether or not the first episode of acute pancreatitis in a specific patient is recognized clinically. In this model the SAPE immediately changes susceptibility risk factors (which may have been present for years) into aetiological factors (Figure 2). The SAPE hypothesis model, in itself, does not prove that acute pancreatitis is required for

Table 2 Aetiologies of acute, recurrent acute and chronic pancreatitis

Acute[50]	Recurrent acute[20]	Chronic[2]
Paediatric	**Toxic–metabolic**	**Toxic–metabolic**
Idiopathic	*Alcohol*	Alcoholic
Systemic disease	*Hypertriglyceridaemia*	Tobacco smoking
Trauma	*Hypercalcaemia*	Hypertriglyceridaemia
Structural	Medications	Hypercalcaemia
Medications	Toxins	Chronic renal failure
Infections		
Metabolic	**Mechanical**	**Idiopathic**
Familial	Choledocholithiasis	Tropical
	Periampullary obstruction	
Adult	*Congenital malformation*	**Genetic**
Gallstones		*PRSS1*
Alcohol	**Miscellaneous**	*SPINK1*
Idiopathic	Vascular	*CFTR*
Medications	Infectious	
Hyperlipidaemia	*Hereditary*	**Autoimmune**
Hypercalcaemia	*Tropical*	
Trauma	*Cystic fibrosis*	**Recurrent** and severe acute
Tumour		pancreatitis associated
Familial	**Suspected**	chronic pancreatitis
	SOD	
	Divisum	**Obstructive**
	Autoimmune	

Italicized aetiologies from the acute and recurrent acute columns represent aetiologies that cannot be easily removed. Paediatric aetiologies are from 1276 cases listed in descending order of frequency[50]. Recurrent acute is modified from Somogyi[20]. SOD, sphincter of Oddi dysfunction. Chronic pancreatitis is the TIGAR-O classification system used by the Midwest Multicenter Pancreatic Study Group[2].

Figure 2 (opposite)   The SAPE hypothesis model. **A**: Normal pancreas. If the subject is a heavy alcohol user the acinar cells are under metabolic and oxidative stress (*), but the histology remains relatively normal. Alcohol increases the risk of crossing the acute pancreatitis threshold (bold line crossing the dashed line). **B**: Acute pancreatitis with pancreatic injury and infiltration of proinflammatory cells. The first, or 'sentinel' Acute Pancreatitis Event (SAPE) is a critical step because it initiates the inflammatory process that results in both injury and later fibrosis. **C**: Late acute pancreatitis is dominated by anti-inflammatory cells that limit further injury by proinflammatory cells and products, and promote healing. This includes activation of stellate cells which produce collagen, etc. In the absence of recurrent acute pancreatitis, acinar cell toxins (e.g. high-dose alcohol) or factors that activate the immune system, the pancreas may eventually return to normal-appearing histology – except for some residual inflammatory cells that are primed to respond to any future injury. **D**: Recurrent acute pancreatitis, acinar cell injury or other factors that activate an acute inflammatory response (Th1) are immediately countered by an anti-inflammatory counter response (T reg) which, among other things, drives fibrosis. This vicious cycle results in both continued injury (top) and further fibrosis (bottom) leading to (**E**) extensive acinar cell loss and sclerosis (right) that is characteristic of chronic pancreatitis. Both genetic factors and environmental factors play a role in this process by increasing susceptibility to acute pancreatitis, altering the severity and duration of acute pancreatitis, and altering the healing processes that drive fibrosis. Alcohol is especially important because it acts at multiple steps in this process. (From Whitcomb[12] with permission)

SAPE Hypothesis Model

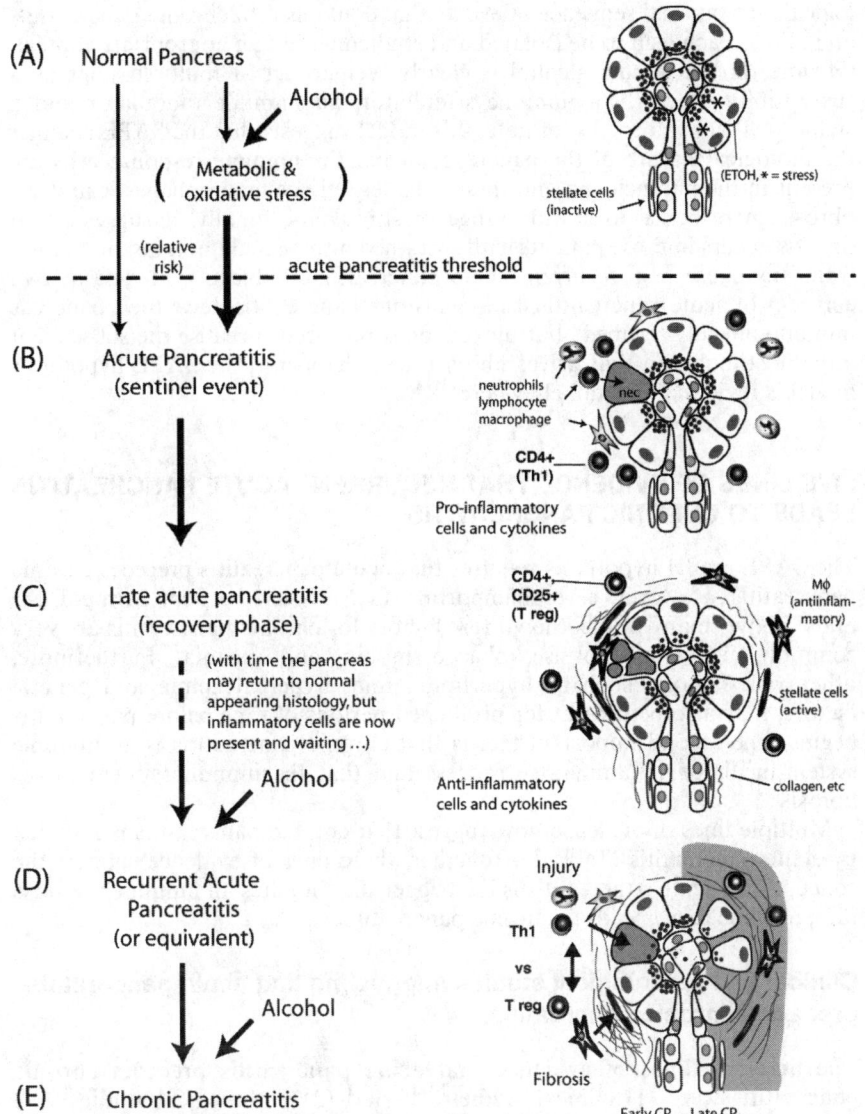

(A) Normal Pancreas

Alcohol

(Metabolic & oxidative stress)

stellate cells (inactive)

(ETOH, * = stress)

(relative risk)

acute pancreatitis threshold

(B) Acute Pancreatitis (sentinel event)

neutrophils lymphocyte macrophage

nec

CD4+ (Th1)

Pro-inflammatory cells and cytokines

(C) Late acute pancreatitis (recovery phase)

(with time the pancreas may return to normal appearing histology, but inflammatory cells are now present and waiting ...)

Alcohol

CD4+, CD25+ (T reg)

Mφ (antiinflammatory)

stellate cells (active)

collagen, etc

Anti-inflammatory cells and cytokines

(D) Recurrent Acute Pancreatitis (or equivalent)

Alcohol

Injury

Th1

vs

T reg

Fibrosis

(E) Chronic Pancreatitis (early to late)

Early CP   Late CP

the development of chronic pancreatitis (see next section), but it does provide a logical and rational sequence of events that could lead to chronic pancreatitis, and allows each step to be isolated and studied within an appropriate context. Of note, in this model alcohol is clearly seen to act at multiple steps as a susceptibility factor, an immune stimulator, an immune modulator and a stellate cell activator. Also of note, this model suggests that the SAPE changes the biological nature of the pancreas so that the immune response cells are present in the parenchyma and these cells (e.g. tissue macrophages) can drive fibrosis in response to a wide range of stimulants. Finally, it suggests that fibrosis occurs in those patients with sustained or repeated immune stimulation from any cause (e.g. recurrent acute pancreatitis). Subjects with one or two episodes of acute pancreatitis, as in gallstone pancreatitis, have their pancreas immunologically 'primed', but fibrosis does not occur because the subsequent immunostimulation that drives fibrosis never happens. The SAPE hypothesis model is reviewed in detail elsewhere[11,12].

FIVE LINES OF EVIDENCE THAT RECURRENT ACUTE PANCREATITIS LEADS TO CHRONIC PANCREATITIS

The SAPE model hypothesis requires that acute pancreatitis precedes chronic pancreatitis. However, several important facts should be kept in mind. As noted above, many of the known risk factors for chronic pancreatitis are very common, such as alcohol use, tobacco smoking and uraemia[2]. Furthermore, other risk factors, such as hyperlipidaemia, hypercalcaemia and genetic factors, may also be present for prolonged periods of time before pancreatitis begins. The second important fact is that chronic pancreatitis is an immune system-mediated inflammatory process and that the immune system drives fibrosis.

Multiple lines of evidence now suggest that chronic pancreatitis is initiated by acute pancreatitis (Table 1). Together, these lines of evidence support the concept that acute pancreatitis is the trigger that initiates an immune response that, in some cases, leads to chronic pancreatitis.

Clinical and pathological studies suggesting that acute pancreatitis precedes chronic pancreatitis

The first two lines of evidence that acute pancreatitis precedes chronic pancreatitis were (1) clinical studies[13–15] and (2) pathological studies[16–18]. These observations remain very useful but cannot *prove* that acute pancreatitis comes first. The reason, of course, is that patients with both acute and chronic pancreatitis are not biopsied *before* the onset of symptoms or biopsied early and late in the course of the disease. The old concept that acute pancreatitis in alcoholics, for example, only follows early chronic pancreatitis[1] is based on little data and cannot be proved or disproved for the reasons stated above. The pathological evidence is discussed in detail elsewhere in this volume.

Aetiological evidence for a link between acute and chronic pancreatitis

The third line of evidence that acute pancreatitis precedes chronic pancreatitis is more compelling than the first two lines of evidence. If acute pancreatitis is the initiating factor leading to chronic pancreatitis, then we would predict that the aetiologies of the two conditions are similar. Table 2 highlights lists of aetiologies for acute, recurrent acute and chronic pancreatitis (modified from recent reviews). We must also remember that one of the clinical priorities of treating patients with acute pancreatitis is to address the underlying aetiology to prevent another attack[19,20]. This may include a review and discontinuation of medications suspected of causing pancreatitis or removing the gall bladder if gallstones are suspected. Other aetiologies, such as alcoholism, structural abnormalities (e.g. pancreas divisum), some metabolic problems, family history and idiopathic causes, are more difficult to eliminate! Aetiologies of acute pancreatitis that cannot easily be addressed are italicized in Table 2 in the acute pancreatitis column (column 1). Failure or inability to remove these aetiologies predisposes the patient to recurrent acute pancreatitis. Likewise, the aetiologies of recurrent acute pancreatitis that cannot be eliminated are similar to the aetiologies associated with chronic pancreatitis. Thus, the common aetiologies of untreated acute pancreatitis, recurrent acute pancreatitis and chronic pancreatitis argue that acute pancreatitis *can* lead to chronic pancreatitis.

Genetic evidence that acute pancreatitis leads to chronic pancreatitis

The fourth line of evidence is genetic. The three genes with mutations that clearly predispose to chronic pancreatitis (*PRSS1, SPINK1* and *CFTR*) will all be briefly considered. A more detailed discussion is provided in recent reviews by the author[3,12]. The first mutated gene, *PRSS1*, was discovered in families with hereditary pancreatitis; an unusual form of acute and chronic pancreatitis that runs in families following an autosomal dominant pattern. The first mutation (R122H) eliminated an autolysis site so that prematurely activated trypsinogen could not be inactivated inside the acinar cell, and would therefore lead to zymogen activation, pancreatic injury and pancreatitis[6]. This provided compelling evidence that acute pancreatitis is associated with unregulated trypsinogen activation, and that the high risk of chronic pancreatitis in these subjects follows recurrent acute pancreatitis. Interestingly, the trypsinogen mutations associated with an increased risk of recurrent acute and chronic pancreatitis are gain-of-function mutations usually close to the domains governing enzyme activation or trypsin inhibition. These sites are normally regulated by calcium, with low calcium levels preventing trypsin-mediated trypsinogen activation and facilitating trypsin autolysis. High calcium levels promote trypsinogen activation and prevent inactivation[3,21]. These findings also support the growing evidence that elevated calcium levels inside the pancreas lead to trypsinogen activation and acute pancreatitis[22-25].

The second major gene with mutations associated with chronic pancreatitis is serine protease inhibitor, Kazal type 1 (*SPINK1*), also known as pancreatic secretory trypsin inhibitor (PSTI). SPINK1 is a specific trypsin inhibitor that is produced in the acinar cells and that provides the first line of defence against premature trypsin activation[6,26]. Mutations in *SPINK1* are associated with chronic pancreatitis in children[26], some families[27] and tropical pancreatitis[28]. However, as a trypsin inhibitor, it appears that loss of SPINK1 function should lead to more trypsin activity, zymogen activation, pancreatic injury and acute pancreatitis.

The third major gene with mutations associated with chronic pancreatitis is the cystic fibrosis transmembrane conductance regulator gene (*CFTR*). CFTR is a regulated anion channel expressed in may epithelial cells and is found on the luminal surface of the proximal pancreatic duct cells[29]. Two severe *CFTR* gene mutations (CFTR^{sev}/CFTR^{sev}) eliminate CFTR function and therefore disrupt ion secretion in the epithelial cells using CFTR as an anion channel. The clinical syndrome, cystic fibrosis, is characterized by progressive dysfunction of the pancreas, lungs, intestines and other epithelial cell lined organs[30]. If one of the alleles has a milder mutation (e.g. CFTR^{sev}/CFTR^{mild}) there will be some retained CFTR function and a limited disease profile that can include acute pancreatitis[30]. This is important because the pancreatic histology in cystic fibrosis is chronic pancreatitis (implying injury) rather than agenesis or atrophy (implying obstruction). In 1998 two research groups reported that *CFTR* mutations were also common in patients with chronic pancreatitis[31,32], suggesting that impaired duct function could predispose to recurrent acute and chronic pancreatitis. Patients with pancreas divisum, which adds resistance to duct flushing, also have recurrent acute pancreatitis in the context of *CFTR* mutations[33]. Thus, the loss of CFTR function results in the loss of effective trypsin flushing. In addition, newer models of duct cell physiology suggest that bicarbonate secretion is CFTR-mediated[34]. Therefore loss of CFTR function may provide a double risk to the pancreas by impairing the rapid removal of activated enzymes from the duct and through loss of alkalinization of the duct fluid which protects the pancreas by maintaining prematurely activated trypsin in a trypsinogen conformation[3,21].

Based on a clear understanding of the biology of trypsin, SPINK1 and CFTR it is clear that mutations in these genes actually predispose to acute pancreatitis rather than chronic pancreatitis. The reason that a subset of these subjects progress to chronic pancreatitis is considered below.

Animal studies suggest that recurrent acute pancreatitis leads to chronic pancreatitis

Development of good animal models of chronic pancreatitis has been a major problem in the past[35]. As noted above, laboratory animals with long-term alcohol feeding alone fail to develop typical chronic pancreatitis. The many animal models that have been developed to help understand various aspects of chronic pancreatitis are reviewed elsewhere in this book, but several common features are worth noting. First, there must be an injury to the pancreas to initiate the immune response[36], and secondly the fibrosis appears to be driven by TGF-β[36] by acting on pancreatic stellate cells[37,38]. The role of alcohol in potentiating the fibrosis following recurrent caerulein-induced pancreatitis is striking, as demonstrated by a new Wistar rat model using the Lieber–DeCarli alcohol feeding protocol[39]. This new model may be especially important in examining the features of chronic alcoholic pancreatitis in rats since these animals develop inflammatory cell infiltration, cytokine expression profiles, fat necrosis, and fibrosis. Further discussion is beyond the scope of this chapter, but these studies demonstrate that in a rat model recurrent acute pancreatitis (three episodes) leads to all of the essential features of chronic pancreatitis.

Combined risk for recurrent acute pancreatitis

A detailed review of the factors that predispose to recurrent acute pancreatitis suggests that some individuals have combinations of factors that each weaken the mechanism protecting the pancreas from premature trypsinogen activation or sustained trypsin activation. Inadequate protection from trypsin leads to recurrent episodes of trypsin-mediated pancreatic injury when environmental or metabolic stresses overwhelm the residual protective barriers and cross the threshold necessary to initiate acute pancreatitis. Figure 3 illustrates two subjects with different global genetic and environmental risks. The low-risk person faces the same variable pancreatic stresses of life as a person with multiple underlying risk factors. However, premature trypsin activation is adequately handled in the low-risk person, while pancreatic injury and acute pancreatitis occurs repeatedly in the high-risk person.

Taken together, acute pancreatitis is *an event* that is initiated by an injury to the pancreas that results in inflammation of the pancreas. Chronic pancreatitis is a *process* linked to recurrent acute pancreatitis or other immune system stimulants. As seen in Table 2, the major aetiologies of acute pancreatitis that

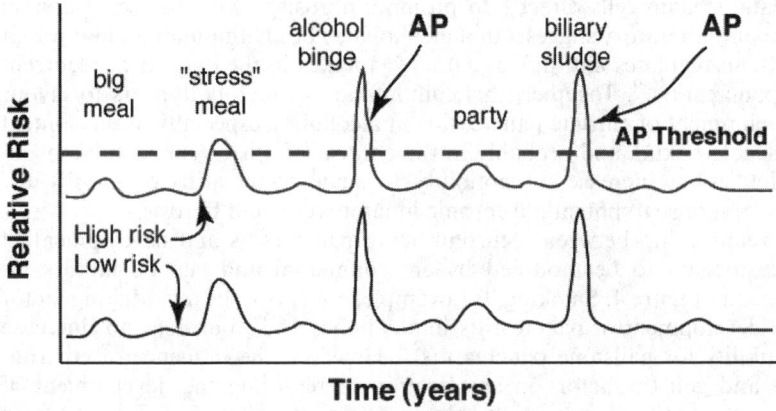

Figure 3 Risk of acute pancreatitis and frequency of acute pancreatitis. Patients with genetic mutations in genes protecting the pancreas from trypsinogen activation or other forms of injury are at high risk of acute pancreatitis (AP) with metabolic or environmental stresses that may activate an amount of trypsin within the pancreas that individuals with normal protective mechanisms can accommodate without crossing the threshold that leads to injury and acute pancreatitis. (From Whitcomb[12] with permission)

cannot be treated or prevented can lead to recurrent acute pancreatitis, and a subset of patients with recurrent acute pancreatitis develop chronic pancreatitis. Furthermore, the major genetic susceptibility factors for chronic pancreatitis actually cause acute pancreatitis. However, recurrent pancreatitis alone is not always sufficient to cause fibrosis, which is the hallmark of chronic pancreatitis. We hypothesize that environmental and genetic modifying factors strongly influence the rate and extent of pancreatic fibrosis or healing.

FACTORS THAT MODIFY THE IMMUNE RESPONSE DETERMINE THE RATE OF FIBROSIS AND OTHER COMPLICATIONS IN CHRONIC PANCREATITIS

Experience with hereditary pancreatitis kindreds and clinical experience with patients with recurrent acute pancreatitis and chronic pancreatitis suggest that a subset of patients with recurrent acute pancreatitis do not develop chronic pancreatitis. Fibrogenesis is an immune-mediated process that normally occurs during later stages of an inflammatory process, and is driven by anti-inflammatory cytokines such as TGF-β[36,39,40].

We noted that only a small subset of alcoholic patients develop chronic pancreatitis. However, alcohol, at some level, is clearly associated with the majority of cases of chronic pancreatitis in adults. Alcohol, as noted above and in animal models, increases susceptibility to acute pancreatitis[41,42]. However, alcohol also produces acinar cell injury through generation of toxic free fatty acid ethyl esters (FAEE)[8,43,44], mitochondrial injury[9] oxidative stress[9] which leads to the release of cytokine and chemokines[45,46] that can stimulate any active immune cells within the vicinity. Furthermore, alcohol may stimulate pancreatic stellate cells directly to promote fibrosis[47]. Finally, recent animal work in our laboratory suggests that alcohol may be an immunomodulator that potently up-regulates anti-inflammatory cytokines in the context of recurrent acute pancreatitis[39]. Together, this combination of factors appears to favour the development of chronic pancreatitis in alcoholics, especially in the context of tobacco smoking and probably in the context of other genetic polymorphisms that either increase susceptibility to acute pancreatitis or modify the immune response to potentiate chronic inflammation and fibrosis.

The relationship between recurrent acute pancreatitis and development of fibrosis appears to be modified by environmental and genetic factors, as illustrated in Figure 4. Smoking, for example, appears to be a modifying factor for the development of pancreatitis in alcoholics[2,48,49], but does not increase susceptibility for gallstone pancreatitis[49]. However, the influence of environmental and genetic factors in accelerating or retarding the development of chronic pancreatitis in subjects with recurrent acute pancreatitis has not been adequately explored.

Taken together, the best model of chronic pancreatitis appears to reflect the convergence of three domains of risk (Figure 5) as a complex disorder[3]. In the first domain are the metabolic and environmental factors that increase the risk of trypsinogen activation. In the second domain are factors that are mutated or altered to limit the capability of the pancreas to respond to injury. The

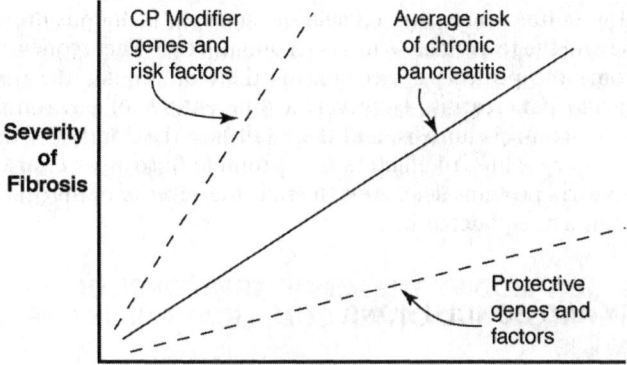

GENES IN CHRONIC PANCREATITIS

Figure 4 Relationship between recurrent acute pancreatitis, fibrosis and modifying factors. Animal models suggest that there should be a direct relationship between episodes of recurrent acute pancreatitis (RAP) and the severity of fibrosis (average risk). However, the clinical observation that some patients with alcoholic or hereditary recurrent acute pancreatitis develop severe fibrosis with a relatively limited number of pancreatitis attacks, while others appear to be resistant to fibrosis, suggests that there are important CP-modifer genes and environmental risk factors (shifting the curve to the left) or protective factors (shifting the curve to the right). (From Whitcomb[12] with permission)

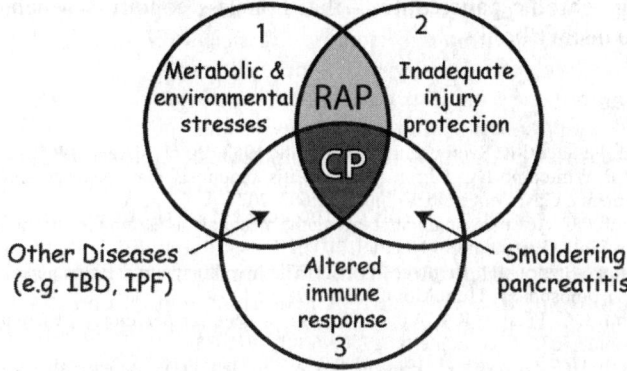

Figure 5 Three domains of chronic pancreatitis risk. Chronic pancreatitis is modeled as a complex trait in which one or more factors must be present in each of at least three domains before chronic pancreatitis develops. The three major genes with mutations that increase susceptibility to chronic pancreatitis (*PRSS1*, *SPINK1* and *CFTR*) are all in the domain of 'inadequate injury protection' and lead to recurrent acute pancreatitis (RAP) in the presence of a sufficiently strong metabolic or environmental stressor. Only the subset of patients with an altered immune response favouring fibrosis develop chronic pancreatitis (CP), but this response requires RAP to direct it to the pancreas rather than other organs. (Modified from Whitcomb[3] with permission)

threshold for acute pancreatitis reflects the strength of the insulting factor in domain one and the resistance to injury in domain two. The frequency of insults that overcome the protective mechanisms therefore equals the frequency of recurrent acute pancreatitis. However, a different set of environmental and genetic factors controls fibrosis, and these fall into the domain of the immune response to injury. Thus, the factors that promote fibrosis or retard reabsorption of the matrix proteins determine the rate and severity of fibrosis in patients with recurrent acute pancreatitis.

SUMMARY AND CONCLUSIONS

Within this chapter I attempted to lay the groundwork for how our group is approaching the question of which gene mutations cause chronic pancreatitis. Our working model suggests that there are three classes of genes that will be very important, and they will fall into three domains that are also influenced by environmental factors – namely stressors, protectors, and response modifiers. To date, most of the recent genetic progress has been made in understanding susceptibility to acute pancreatitis – which we now understand is a major, but not exclusive, prerequisite for chronic pancreatitis. We believe that a global understanding of all risk factors in each individual patient must be the goal of physicians in the future. This information should then be used to strategically alter the changeable risk and response factors for the individual patient. By acting early and wisely we can halt the pathological process of recurrent pancreatic injury and fibrosis. Thus, we may be able to prevent the development of end-stage chronic pancreatitis – that hopeless condition which should be confined to history books.

References

1. Sarles H. Pancreatitis: Symposium of Marseille, 1963. Basel: Karger, 1965.
2. Etemad B, Whitcomb DC. Chronic pancreatitis: diagnosis, classification, and new genetic developments. Gastroenterology. 2001;120:682–707.
3. Whitcomb DC. Advances in understanding the mechanisms leading to chronic pancreatitis. Nat Clin Pract Gastroenterol Hepatol. 2004;1:1.
4. Le Bodic L, Bignon JD, Raguenes O et al. The hereditary pancreatitis gene maps to long arm of chromosome 7. Hum Mol Genet. 1996;5:549–54.
5. Whitcomb DC, Preston RA, Aston CE et al. A gene for hereditary pancreatitis maps to chromosome 7q35. Gastroenterology. 1996;110:1975–80.
6. Whitcomb DC, Gorry MC, Preston RA et al. Hereditary pancreatitis is caused by a mutation in the cationic trypsinogen gene. Nature Genet. 1996;14:141–5.
7. Shrikhande SV, Martignoni ME, Shrikhande M et al. Comparison of histological features and inflammatory cell reaction in alcoholic, idiopathic and tropical chronic pancreatitis. Br J Surg. 2003;90:1565–72.
8. Pfützer RH, Tadic SD, Li HS et al. Pancreatic cholesterol esterase, ES-10 and FAEESIII gene expression are increased in pancreas and liver, but not in brain or heart with long-term ethanol feeding in rats. Pancreas. 2002;25:101–6.
9. Li HS, Zhang JY, Thompson BS et al. Rat mitochondrial ATP synthase ATP5G3: cloning and upregulation in pancreas after chronic ethanol feeding. Physiol Genom. 2001;6:91–8.
10. Whitcomb DC. Hereditary pancreatitis: new insights into acute and chronic pancreatitis. Gut. 1999;45:317–22.

11. Schneider A, Whitcomb DC. Hereditary pancreatitis: a model for inflammatory diseases of the pancreas. Best Pract Res Clin Gastroenterol. 2002;16:347–63.
12. Whitcomb DC. Value of genetic testing in management of pancreatitis. Gut. 2004;53:11.
13. Comfort M, Gambill D, Baggenstoss A. Chronic relapsing pancreatitis. Gastroenterology. 1946;6:239–85.
14. Ammann RW, Muellhaupt B. Progression of alcoholic acute to chronic pancreatitis. Gut. 1994;35:552–6.
15. Ammann RW, Muellhaupt B, Group ZPS. The natural history of pain in alcoholic chronic pancreatitis. Gastroenterology. 1999;116:1132–40.
16. Kloppel G, Maillet B. Pathology of acute and chronic pancreatitis. Pancreas. 1993;8:659–70.
17. Renner IG, Savage WT, Pantoja JL, Renner VJ. Death due to acute pancreatitis: a retrospective analysis of 405 autopsy cases. Dig Dis Sci. 1985;30:1005–18.
18. Seligson U, Cho JW, Ihre T, Lundh G. Clinical course and autopsy findings in acute and chronic pancreatitis. Acta Chir Scand. 1982;148:269–74.
19. Uhl W, Warshaw A, Imrie C et al. IAP Guidelines for the surgical management of acute pancreatitis. Pancreatology. 2002;2:565–73.
20. Somogyi L, Martin SP, Venkatesan T, Ulrich CD II. Recurrent acute pancreatitis: an algorithmic approach to identification and elimination of inciting factors. Gastroenterology. 2001;120:708–17.
21. Bennett WS, Huber R. Structural and functional aspects of domain motions in proteins. CRC Crit Rev Biochem. 1984;15:291–384.
22. Sutton R, Criddle D, Raraty MG, Tepikin A, Neoptolemos JP, Petersen OH. Signal transduction, calcium and acute pancreatitis. Pancreatology. 2003;3:497–505.
23. Frick TW, Fernandez, del CC, Bimmler D, Warshaw AL. Elevated calcium and activation of trypsinogen in rat pancreatic acini. Gut. 1997;41:339–43.
24. Lerch MM, Gorelick FS. Early trypsinogen activation in acute pancreatitis. Med Clin N Am. 2000;84:549–63.
25. Kruger B, Albrecht E, Lerch MM. The role of intracellular calcium signaling in premature protease activation and the onset of pancreatitis. Am J Pathol. 2000;157:43–50.
26. Witt H, Luck W, Hennies HC et al. Mutations in the gene encoding the serine protease inhibitor, kazal type 1 are associated with chronic pancreatitis. Nature Genet. 2000;25:213–6.
27. Pfützer RH, Barmada MM, Brunskil APJ et al. SPINK1/PSTI polymorphisms act as disease modifiers in familial and idiopathic chronic pancreatitis. Gastroenterology. 2000;119:615–23.
28. Rossi L, Pfützer RL, Parvin S et al. SPINK1/PSTI mutations are associated with tropical pancreatitis in Bangladesh: a preliminary report. Pancreatology. 2001;1:242–5.
29. Marino CR, Matovcik LM, Gorelick FS, Cohn JA. Localization of the cystic fibrosis transmembrane conductance regulator in pancreas. J Clin Invest. 1991;88:712–16.
30. Stern RC. The diagnosis of cystic fibrosis. N Engl J Med. 1997;336:487–91.
31. Sharer N, Schwarz M, Malone G et al. Mutations of the cystic fibrosis gene in patients with chronic pancreatitis. N Engl J Med. 1998;339:645–52.
32. Cohn JA, Friedman KJ, Noone PG, Knowles MR, Silverman LM, Jowell PS. Relation between mutations of the cystic fibrosis gene and idiopathic pancreatitis. N Engl J Med. 1998;339:653–8.
33. Gelrud A, Sheth S, Banerjee S et al. Analysis of cystic fibrosis gene product (CFTR) function in patients with pancreas divisum and recurrent acute pancreatitis. Am J Gastroenterol. 2004;99:1557–62.
34. Whitcomb DC, Ermentrout DB. A mathematical model of the pancreatic duct cell generating high bicarbonate concentrations in pancreatic juice. Pancreas. 2004;29:E30–40.
35. Steinberg W, Tenner S. Acute pancreatitis. N Engl J Med. 1994;330:1198–210.
36. Van Laethem J, Robberecht P, Resibois A, Deviere J. Transforming growth factor beta promotes development of fibrosis after repeated courses of acute pancreatitis in mice. Gastroenterology. 1996;110:576–82.
37. Bachem MG, Schneider E, Gross H et al. Identification, culture, and characterization of pancreatic stellate cells in rats and humans. Gastroenterology. 1998;115:421–32.
38. Apte MV, Haber PS, Applegate TL et al. Periacinar stellate shaped cells in rat pancreas: identification, isolation, and culture. Gut. 1998;43:128–33.

39. Deng X, Wang L, Elm MS et al. Chronic alcohol consumption accelerates fibrosis in response to cerulein-induced pancreatitis in the rat. Am J Pathol. 2005 (In press).
40. Muller-Pillasch F, Menke A, Yamaguchi H et al. TGFbeta and the extracellular matrix in pancreatitis. Hepatogastroenterology. 1999;46:2751–6.
41. Katz M, Carangelo R, Miller LJ, Gorelick F. Effect of ethanol on cholecystokinin-stimulated zymogen conversion in pancreatic acinar cells. Am J Physiol. 1996;270:G171–5.
42. Pandol SJ, Periskic S, Gukovsky I et al. Ethanol diet increases the sensitivity of rats to pancreatitis induced by cholecystokinin octapeptide. Gastroenterology. 1999;117:706–16.
43. Werner J, Saghir M, Warshaw AL et al. Alcoholic pancreatitis in rats: injury from nonoxidative metabolites of ethanol. Am J Physiol Gastrointest Liver Physiol. 2002;283:G65–73.
44. Werner J, Laposata M, del Fernandez CC et al. Pancreatic injury in rats induced by fatty acid ethyl ester, a nonoxidative metabolite of alcohol. Gastroenterology. 1997;113:286–94.
45. Han B, Logston CD. NFκB activation is required for CCK stimulation of chemokine expresion in rat acinar cells. Pancreas. 1998;17:438.
46. Gukovskaya AS, Gukovsky I, Zaninovic V et al. Pancreatic acinar cells produce, release, and respond to tumor necrosis factor-alpha. Role in regulating cell death and pancreatitis. J Clin Invest. 1997;100:1853–62.
47. Apte MV, Phillips PA, Fahmy RG et al. Does alcohol directly stimulate pancreatic fibrogenesis? Studies with rat pancreatic stellate cells. Gastroenterology. 2000;118:780–94.
48. Talamini G, Bassi C, Falconi M et al. Alcohol and smoking as risk factors in chronic pancreatitis and pancreatic cancer. Dig Dis Sci. 1999;44:1301–11.
49. Morton C, Klatsky AL, Udaltsova N. Smoking, coffee and pancreatitis. Am J Gastroenterol. 2004;99:31–8.
50. Whitcomb DC, Lowe ME. Pancreatitis: acute and chronic. In: Walker WA, Goulet O, Kleinman RE, Sherman PM, Shneider BL, Sanderson IR, editors. Pediatric Gastrointestinal Disease: Pathophysiology, Diagnosis, Management. Hamilton (ON): BC: Decker; 2004:1584–97.

Chronic pancreatitis I

Section VI
Clinical diagnosis and classification

Chair: P. BANKS and L. GULLO

15
To define chronic pancreatitis

M. SARNER

For 40 years chronic pancreatitis has been held to be a condition in which persisting and permanent inflammatory damage to the pancreas has occurred[1,2]. In the context of evolving classification systems for chronic pancreatitis there have been various minor revisions of this definition but the basic tenet – that there is *irreversible* pancreatic damage – has remained unchanged.

Two questions arise: is this definition clinically useful and secondly, is it possible to tell if the changes identified are really irreversible?

For example, a patient with chronic abdominal pain, diabetes, steatorrhoea, abnormal imaging, abnormal histology and abnormal function testing has chronic pancreatitis. However, the diagnosis turns out to be autoimmune pancreatitis or an obstructed pancreas and appropriate treatments (steroids or clearing the obstruction) produce resolution of the clinical picture with the pancreas being restored. Was this chronic pancreatitis?

Persistence or permanence, these are the questions. Is it possible to say at a single point in time that a lesion or lesions will never repair and is causing symptoms? A damaged pancreas is not necessarily a symptomatic one – extensive calcification can be seen in asymptomatic patients.

Persistence of lesions can be easily determined by repeated study, but to achieve a clinically useful definition there needs to be an easy way to determine irreversibility.

The definition of disease is important, not only to ensure that the label placed on the patient is correct, enabling answers to the basic questions concerning diagnosis, prognosis and treatment, but also an agreed definition is crucial for homogeneity of study groups. This means that the defining characteristics have to be agreed, and this may be difficult in chronic pancreatitis.

The difficulties rest with the modalities used to study the organ at present. In chronic pancreatitis diagnosis usually stands or falls on the information obtained from imaging, function testing and histology. These are not mutually exclusive, and information from all three may be required before a definite diagnosis can be made.

Regrettably, imaging techniques cannot necessarily determine the permanence of a lesion or its clinical impact. A disrupted pancreas, as shown by imaging, may recover in some cases and even modern techniques such as multi-sliced CT scanning, endoscopic ultrasound or pancreatic magnetic resonance imaging are as yet not sufficiently sophisticated to provide diagnosis at a cellular level.

Function testing remains disappointing. Advanced cases are easy to diagnose but lesions indicating damage but not failure of the pancreas are difficult to define by function tests alone. Perhaps new technology will help here, combining imaging and function testing as in secretin-stimulated MRCP[3].

Histology, showing characteristic changes of acinar cell atrophy, tubular complexes, inflammatory cell infiltrate, changes in pancreatic nerves and subsequent fibrosis, is the gold standard, but obtaining histology is an invasive technique and the change may be patchy and so sampling error is possible.

The clinical definition is that chronic pancreatitis is said to be present when there is a combination of abdominal pain, steatorrhoea and/or diabetes, together with appropriate abnormal investigations. However, the certainty of permanence may be difficult to determine without long-term follow-up.

The situation is made more difficult in respect of the various causes which produce pancreatic inflammatory disease. For example, are obstructing lesions certain to cause chronic disease? Does calcification indicate irreversibility? If inflammation is located by means of sampling does this mean that it will never resolve or that it will certainly progress? Only long-term follow-up will answer these questions.

Imaging alone is not enough. For example in chronic obstructive pancreatitis there may well be uniform main pancreatic duct dilation, but if the obstruction is removed then recovery can occur. In autoimmune pancreatitis, pancreatic insufficiency can certainly occur, but spontaneous or steroid-induced recovery is well known and so, by definition of irreversibility, this cannot be chronic pancreatitis. In addition, that variety of pancreatic tumour which on investigation turns out to be an inflammatory mass which resolves can be added to these two other examples of 'chronic' pancreatitis – chronic obstructive and auto-immune, since these can all show a complete recovery, thus denying this diagnosis if permanence of the lesion is the hallmark.

The three established diagnostic pillars – imaging, function testing and histology – can leave the clinician in the uncomfortable situation of having normal pancreatic function but a grossly abnormal ductogram or, alternatively, a normal pancreatic ductogram in a patient with abdominal pain, abnormal function tests and a biopsy showing inflammation. Does this patient have permanent disease? Now that the human genome has been sequenced it is possible to study those genes which have been identified as being expressed in chronic pancreatitis. These may serve as disease markers but the widespread application of these techniques has not yet occurred. This is certainly a growth area and now subject to intensive research which may provide answers in the future[4].

Essential to the diagnosis of irreversible disease is permanent damage to the duct epithelium. If the basement membrane of the duct epithelium is intact then structure and function will recover[5]. However, if there is a breach to the basement membrane, that is to say immune staining for type IV collagen or laminin shows a breach in continuity, then there will be low bicarbonate output and probable, but not certain, failure of recovery. There is a rat model for this. Otsuki[6] has instilled two different agents into the main pancreatic duct of the rat using a reversible model (3% sodium taurocholate) and an irreversible model using oleic acid. Following instillation of these fluids, a labelling index in the epithelial cells of the MPD can be used to assess cell proliferation. In reversible pancreatitis tubular complexes surrounded by fibrosis are seen after 3 days, but after 7 days newly formed acinar cells are observed and, after 2 weeks, the lobular architecture has returned. In contrast, using the oleic acid model, irreversible pancreatitis can be seen after 3 days; there is an initial inflammatory cell infiltrate with oedema and necrosis, and by day 7 this has turned into haemorrhage with an inflammatory cell infiltrate and tubular complexes. After 2 weeks almost all of the exocrine pancreatic tissue has been replaced by fat. In the reversible model, type IV collagen can be seen as a discontinuous line after 3 days, but after a month the line has become continuous and there is recovery. However, in the irreversible model, the discontinual nature of the collagen line persists and this represents failure of recovery.

Examination of the epithelial cells of the main pancreatic duct shows that they can express a transcription factor known as pancreatic duodenal homeobox-1 (PDX-1) and the cells expressing this factor are thought to be marker cells that can regain multipotency to differentiate into any pancreatic cell type, i.e. a pancreatic stem cell[7]. Regeneration of the pancreas after pancreatitis involves proliferentiation and differentiation of these cells; therefore recovery or not may depend on the degree of damage to the duct epithelium containing these PDX-1 cells and their persistence or loss.

In addition, there is the turnover of extracellular matrix, reflecting the difference between synthesis and degradation of extracellular matrix proteins[8]. In reversible pancreatitis pancreatic matrix metalloproteinase 2 and matrix metalloproteinase 9 (MMP2/MMP9) increase slightly and transiently with type IV collagen in the reversible model recovering completely after 28 days. However, in the irreversible model, MMP2 and MMP9 increase significantly and type IV collagen does not recover. In summary, the earliest changes begin at the cellular level, particularly in the ductal basement membranes and the extracellular matrix.

Gross damage to the acinar cell has to occur before there is any abnormality of function testing; damage at the individual cellular level will not produce imaging abnormalities unless the change is very substantial. Thus, short of an invasive biopsy to enable sophisticated studies such as those detailed above, it can be very difficult to determine irreversibility. Of course, imaging techniques do not stand still, and endoscopic ultrasound, multi-sliced CT and MRCP secretin studies are advancing. They are increasingly sensitive at picking up lesser degrees of damage compared with the past performance of function testing or ERCP, but will still have difficulties in defining permanence.

It may be that in due course a combination of histology, particularly looking at ductular basement membrane structures, plus very sensitive imaging techniques and genetic studies will be able to determine the presence or absence of pancreatic inflammatory disease that is irreversible. Irreversibility may be determined by serial function testing using derivatives of MR scanning but, at present, function testing is insufficiently sensitive to define lesser degrees of damage.

The current hypothesis is that there is an initial insult, of whatever cause, which produces intra-pancreatic enzyme release. There is a resulting disruption of the ducts and possible destruction of the totepotential pancreatic stem cells. The balance between synthesis and degradation in the extracellular matrix is set towards degradation and eventually this produces autolysis and subsequent fibrosis. At this stage chronic pancreatitis can safely be diagnosed. Clinical significance depends upon the classical symptoms of malabsorption, diabetes and abdominal pain.

In conclusion, chronic pancreatitis can be defined as a condition of many causes in which there is a combination of impairment of function, abnormal imaging and histological change which can never return to normal. These changes are of clinical significance if there are associated symptoms; that is to say abdominal pain, malabsorption and diabetes mellitus.

References

1. Sarles H. Pancreatitis. Symposium of Marseille, 1963. Basel: Karger, 1965.
2. Sarner M, Cotton PB. Definitions of acute and chronic pancreatitis. Clin Gastroenterol. 1984;13:865–70.
3. Prasad SR, Sahani D, Saini S. Clinical applications of magnetic resonance cholangiopan-creatography. J Clin Gastroenterol. 2001;33:362–6.
4. Friess H, Kleeff J, Buchler MW. Molecular pathophysiology of chronic pancreatitis – an update. J Gastrointest Surg. 2003;7:943–5.
5. Bockman DE, Muller M, Buchler M, Friess H, Beger HG. Pathological changes in pancreatic ducts from patients with chronic pancreatitis. Int J Pancreatol. 1997;21:119–26.
6. Otsuki M. Chronic pancreatitis. Pancreatology. 2004;4:28–41.
7. Taguchi M, Yamaguchin T, Otsuki M. Induction of PDX-1 positive cells in the main duct during regeneration after acute necrotizing pancreatitis in rats. J Pathol. 2002;197:638–46.
8. Kennedy RH, Bockman DE, Uscanga L, Choux R, Grimaud JA, Sarles H. Pancreatic extracellular matrix alterations in chronic pancreatitis. Pancreas. 1987;2:61–72.

16
Diagnosis of early stages of chronic pancreatitis using computed tomography

P. C. FREENY

INTRODUCTION

The 1983 Cambridge Symposium proposed that chronic pancreatitis be defined as 'a continuing inflammatory disease of the pancreas characterized by irreversible morphological change, and typically causing pain and/or permanent loss of function'[1]. The generally accepted features that substantiate the diagnosis rely upon (a) typical patient history, b) abnormal pancreatic function tests, and (c) morphological abnormalities depicted by imaging studies such as ERCP or MRCP, CT, and EUS.

Chronic pancreatitis can be subclassified as early-stage or late-stage disease[2]. Late-stage disease implies that the patient has shown both clinical and morphological progression of disease and that the functional and morphological abnormalities are permanent and irreversible. At this stage the clinical and imaging diagnosis is relatively straightforward since most patients have persistent pain, significantly altered function, and morphological changes depicted by CT, ERCP or MPCP, or EUS of abnormal parenchyma, abnormal main pancreatitc duct and/or ductal calcifications. However, despite multiple international symposia addressing the problem, currently there is no universally accepted definition, or method of diagnosis, of early-stage chronic pancreatitis. The presence of permanent or irreversible change (Cambridge Symposium definition) requires that patients must manifest the abnormal morphological and function changes over some time interval. Ammann believes that the diagnosis of early-stage chronic pancreatitis, in patients without histological confirmation of the diagnosis, should be reserved for patients who subsequently progress to late-stage disease (personal communication, 2004). Using either definition, one might conclude that the diagnosis of early-stage disease can be made only after some interval of time, rather that at a specific point in time; notably, at the time of the patient's initial clinical presentation.

DIAGNOSIS OF EARLY-STAGE CHRONIC PANCREATITIS

The manifestations of early-stage chronic pancreatitis are caused by recurring episodes of an acute inflammatory process involving the pancreas. If it is assumed that patients with early-stage chronic pancreatitis do not manifest any of the typical abnormal morphological changes of late-stage disease (abnormal parenchyma or main pancreatic duct and/or ductal calcifications), then this would preclude the use of imaging modalities (CT, ERCP, EUS) for diagnosis of early-stage disease. Only the findings of an acute inflammatory process of the pancreas would be present at this early or initial stage of the disease and a specific diagnosis of chronic pancreatitis could not be made. EUS, however, may be an exception to this statement, since some recent work suggests that EUS may show abnormalities before ERCP, CT, or function tests become abnormal[3].

The CT diagnosis of chronic pancreatitis relies on depiction of a combination of abnormalities that reliably have been shown to indicate the presence of the disease. These include pancreatic duct dilation, intraductal calcifications, heterogeneous parenchyma, focal or diffuse gland enlargement, or diffuse gland atrophy[4].

The Cambridge Symposium classified the imaging findings of chronic pancreatitis, as they relate to ERCP, CT, and EUS, according to the *severity of the findings* (normal, mild, moderate and severe) but not according to the *stage* of the disease (early-stage or late-stage)[5]. The CT findings of chronic pancreatitis as defined by the Cambridge Symposium are listed in Table 1. Of these findings, intraductal calcification is the only specific finding of chronic pancreatitis, since the other features can be seen in other inflammatory and neoplastic pancreatic diseases. Furthermore, if one accepts that pancreatic ductal calcifications are a manifestation of late-stage disease, then there are really no CT features that are specific for the diagnosis of early-stage disease.

We have evaluated a series of 100 patients who had the diagnosis of chronic pancreatitis confirmed on the basis of typical clinical symptoms (attacks of pain) and abnormal pancreatic exocrine (secretin–caerulein test) or endocrine (glucose tolerance test) function tests. The clinical severity of the disease was classified as mild, moderate, or severe using a 1–10-point scoring system (Table 2).

Mild disease was present if the score was between 1 and 3. In this category there were 14 patients. If one selects the patients with the most clinically mild disease (pain score 0–1, exocrine function test score 1–2, and no diabetes or other complications) there were only three patients. Interestingly, there was very poor correlation between the clinical score and the severity of the morphological abnormalities. All three patients had a CT score of severe, two had severe ERCP changes, while one had a normal ERCP.

There were nine patients with a clinical score of 3 who had pain scores of 0–2, exocrine function test scores of 1–2, no diabetes, and a complication score of 0–1. There also was poor correlation with imaging modalities. CT severity was normal in three, moderate in three, and severe in three, while ERCP severity was normal in one, moderate in four, and severe in four.

Table 1 Cambridge classification of pancreatic morphology in chronic pancreatitis

Changes	ERCP	CT
Normal	MPD normal No abnormal LSB	MPD 2 mm Normal gland size, shape Homogeneous parenchyma
Equivocal	MPD normal <3 abnormal LSB	One of the following: MPD 2–4 mm, gland enlarged <2× normal, heterogeneous parenchyma
Mild	MPD normal >3 abnormal LSB	Two or more signs for diagnosis MPD 2–4 mm diameter Slight gland enlargement Heterogeneous parenchyma
Moderate	MPD abnormal LSB abnormal	Small cysts <10 mm MPD irregularity Focal acute pancreatitis Gland contour irregularity
Severe		

Any of the above changes plus one or more of the following:
Cyst >10 mm
Intraductal filling defects
Calculi
MPD obstruction, stricture
Severe MPD irregularity
Contiguous organ invasion

MPD, main pancreatic duct; LSB, lateral side branch ducts.

Focal change: less than one-third of gland involved.

Table 2 Clinical and functional scoring system (Score: 1–10)

Exocrine function (S-C test): 1–3 score
1. Mild (preservation of >80% normal function)
2. Moderate (preservation of >50% but <80% of normal function)
3. Severe (loss of >50% normal function)

Endocrine function (GTT): 0–2 score
0. No diabetes
1. Latent diabetes (abnormal GTT; no exogenous insulin requirement)
2. Manifest (abnormal GTT; exogenous insulin required)

Abdominal pain: 0–3 score
0. No pain
1. Mild (intermittent pain)
2. Moderate (intermittent pain requiring analgesics)
3. Severe (continuous pain requiring analgesics)

Biliary (hepatic) function abnormalities (SGOT, AP, BR): 0–2 score
0. Normal
1. Abnormal liver enzymes
2. Abnormal liver enzymes and BR >2 mg/100 ml

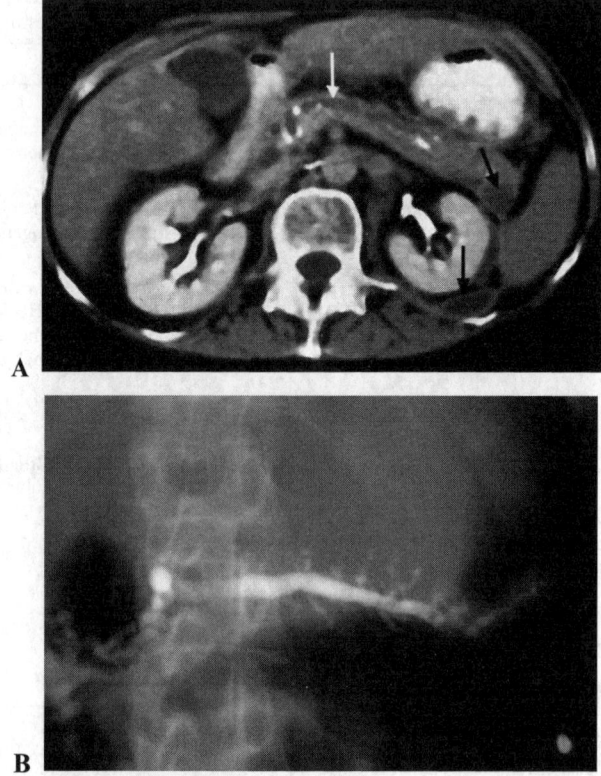

Figure 1 Severe chronic pancreatitis. **A:** CT shows a dilated pancreatic duct (white arrow) containing calcifications. A small pseudocyst is seen in the tail and extending posterior to the left kidney (black arrows). **B:** ERCP shows dilated pancreatic duct and lateral side branches. The pseudocyst in the tail does not fill during ERCP

While the clinical score of 3, mild disease, does not necessarily indicate early-stage disease, this is the closest that we can get to looking at the correlation between the clinical severity of the disease and the severity of the morphological changes as depicted by CT or ERCP. In the total group of 14 patients with mild disease (clinical score of 3), CT was classified as normal in three, moderate in four and severe in seven, while ERCP was normal in two, moderate in four and severe in eight. Thus, morphological findings tend to upstage patients with clinically mild disease.

The lack of correlation between morphology and clinical severity in patients with clinically mild disease is not entirely understood. However, several authors have proposed possible explanations. DiMagno and co-workers first observed that uninvolved parenchyma may in fact compensate partially for the involved portions of the gland[6]. Braganza et al., in a 1982 paper entitled 'Relationship between pancreatic exocrine function and ductal morphology', also suggested that 'the overall patchy nature of the disease, or the variable

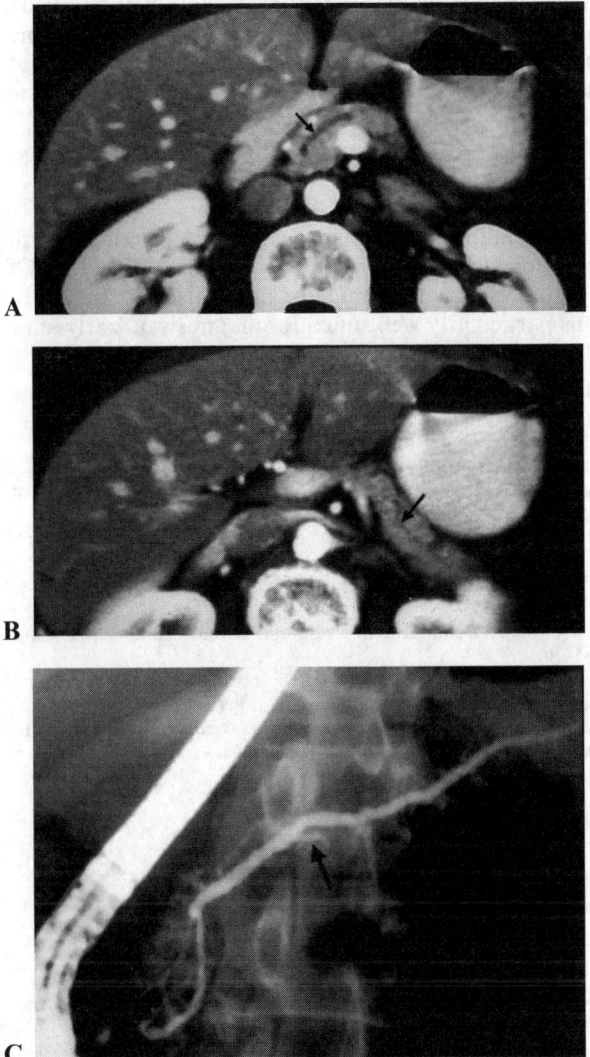

Figure 2 Moderate chronic pancreatitis. **A, B**: CT shows a normal pancreas and pancreatic duct (arrows). **C**: ERCP shows mild irregularity of the walls of the main duct and focal dilation of lateral side branches (arrow)

affectation of acinar and ductular structures' may explain the disparity between observed morphology and measured pancreatic exocrine function[7]. It may also be that the morphological changes of chronic pancreatitis as depicted by ERCP or CT simply precede the functional changes by some time interval.

SUMMARY

While imaging modalities are highly sensitive in depicting the morphological abnormalities associated with chronic pancreatitis, CT and ERCP show poor correlation in patients with clinically mild disease. In addition, neither modality seems particularly well suited for diagnosis of 'early-stage' disease.

References

1. Sarner M, Cotton P. Classification of pancreatitis. Gut. 1984;25:756–9.
2. Ammann RW, Akovbiantz A, Largiader F, Schueler G. Course and outcome of chronic pancreatitis. Longitudinal study of a mixed medical–surgical series of 254 patients. Gastroenterology, 1984;86:820–8.
3. Raimondo M, Wallace M. Diagnosis of early chronic pancreatitis by endoscopic ultrasound. Are we there yet? J Pancreas. 2004;5:1–7.
4. Luetmer P, Stephens D, Ward E. Chronic pancreatitis: reassessment with current CT. Radiology. 1989;171:353–7.
5. Sarner M, Cotton P. Definitions of acute and chronic pancreatitis. Clin Gastroenterol. 1984;13:865–70.
6. DiMagno E, Malagelada J-R, Go V. The relationship between pancreatic ductal obstruction and pancreatic secretion in man. Mayo Clin Proc. 1979;54:157–62.
7. Braganza J, Hunt L, Warwick F. Relationship between pancreatic exocrine function and ductal morphology. Gastroenterology. 1982;82:1341–7.

Chronic pancreatitis II

Section VII
Controversial issues of therapy

Chair: P. LAYER and J. MOSSNER

17
Mechanisms of pain in chronic pancreatitis

F. S. LEHMANN and C. BEGLINGER

INTRODUCTION

Chronic pancreatitis (CP) is characterized by an ongoing, inflammatory process of the exocrine pancreas which often leads to exocrine insufficiency[1]. In the United States, CP has a prevalence of 26.4 cases per 100 000 population[2]. Morphologically, the most prominent features are atrophy of the exocrine pancreatic tissue, parenchymal fibrosis and ductal strictures. Chronic alcohol abuse is the most common cause of CP, but the disease is also associated with a number of other disorders including duct obstruction from tumours and strictures, hypercalcaemia, hyperlipidaemia and genetic mutations[3]. In many patients the cause of CP is unknown. Complications of CP include pancreatic pseudocysts (10–25%), as well as biliary (30%) and duodenal (10–25%) obstruction[1].

Recurrent upper abdominal pain is the most relevant clinical symptom of CP. The deep and penetrating pain occurs frequently during the night and may increase after eating, thus further contributing to weight loss by fasting[4]. The pain often has considerable consequences for patients in terms of work loss, addiction to analgesics and narcotics as well as hospitalizations. In 27–67% of patients with alcoholic CP, surgical intervention is necessary because of medically intractable pain[5].

Pain is highly variable and different pain patterns have been described. In patients with CP, pain is often difficult to assess, because its evaluation may be clouded by underlying personality disorders and by alcohol or drug addiction. Patients often present with intermittent pain that ranges from mild to moderate to severe[4], but pain may also be absent, frequent or persistent and may increase or decrease over time. In general, only a few patients with CP are completely painfree[6]. In alcoholic CP less than 10% of cases have no pain, whereas patients with the late-onset type of idiopathic CP and in tropical CP often have a mild and painless clinical course[4]. Controversy exists as to whether the pain decreases or disappears after several years when the disease 'burns itself out' in late stages. Several studies suggest that the progressive loss of exocrine function several years after diagnosis, the occurence of severe duct abnormalities and/or calcifications and abstinence from alcohol may be accompanied by a reduction or a complete relief of pain. An editoral by diMagno outlined that the pain eventually decreases in 75% of patients with or without surgery[7]. In the study by Ammann et al., progression to pain relief was observed in all patients with advanced CP forming the basis for the 'burn-out theory'[5]. This theory remains, however, highly controversial, and some studies even indicate that the likelihood of spontaneous pain relief is low. In the study of Lankisch et al., pain relief did not occur in the majority of patients, even after long-term observation of more than 10 years[6]. In that study the percentage of patients with pain decreased with the appearance of pancreatic insufficiency, calcifications, pancreatic duct abnormalities and cessation of alcohol use, but the majority of patients were still faced with persisting attacks of pain[6]. In the study by Malfertheiner et al., 89% of patients with CP still had pain despite the occurrence of pancreatic calcifications[8]. In previous studies, cessation of alcohol use was accompanied in only about 50% of patients by a significant decrease of severity of pain[9,10].

MECHANISMS OF PAIN

The pathophysiology of pain in CP is only incompletely understood. Several hypotheses have been proposed regarding the generation and continuation of chronic pain in CP, and it seems likely that the pain is caused by more than one mechanism. The existence of different concepts is reflected in the various therapeutic approaches for pain relief in these patients. The potential mechanisms causing pain in CP are summarized in Table 1 (modified from Di Sebastaino et al.[1]) and will be discussed in the following sections.

Extrapancreatic causes of pain

Extrapancreatic disorders such as bile duct and duodenal stenosis have been suggested as factors causing pain in CP[1]. Symptomatic bile duct or duodenal obstruction are observed in 5–10% of patients with CP, mainly in those with large-duct disease, and may be caused by extensive pancreatic fibrosis and inflammation or by the development of a pseudocyst in the head of the gland[2]. In 1991 Becker and Mischke described a pathological condition named 'groove

Table 1 Mechanisms of pain in chronic pancreatitis

1. Extrapancreatic causes
2. Pancreatic pseudocysts
3. High pancreatic pressure
4. Pancreatic ischaemia
5. Pancreatic fibrosis
6. CCK-mediated feedback
7. Acute inflammation
8. Alterations of pancreatic nerves
9. Neuroimmune interactions

Modified from Di Sebastiano et al.[1]

pancreatitis', which was found to be present in 19.5% of 600 patients with CP[11]. Groove pancreatitis is characterized by the formation of a scar plate between the head of the pancreas and the duodenum. The interstitial scarring may lead to disturbance of the motility of the duodenum, unilateral or concentric stenosis of the C-loop of the duodenum, and tubular stenosis of the common bile duct. Aetiology and clinical symptoms of groove pancreatitis are similar to those found in other types of CP.

Pancreatic pseudocysts

Pseudocysts of the pancreas can cause intense pain in CP, and their treatment by resection, external or internal drainage usually reduces the clinical symptoms. In the study by Reimer Jensen et al., 87% of patients with CP and pseudocysts had moderate or even severe pain[12]. Pseudocysts are found in 10–25% of patients with CP, and in two-thirds of them, the cyst develops in the body or tail of the pancreas. Morphologically, pancreatic pseudocysts are defined as collections of pancreatic secretions surrounded by non-epithelial fibrous walls of granulation tissue. Pseudocysts in CP have a much lower rate of spontaneuous resolution than in acute pancreatitis and therefore often require invasive treatment.

High pancreatic pressure

Several studies suggest that increased intrapancreatic and intraductal or parenchymal pressure are common causes for pain in CP, although the mechanisms by which increased pressure may cause pain are not known[13–18]. The pressure within the pancreas depends both on the exocrine pancreatic secretion and on the impedance to its outflow. Obstruction to the pancreatic main and side ducts by single or multiple strictures, calculi, or increased viscosity of pancreatic juice may lead to increased ductal and interstitial pressure. In clinical studies both ductal and interstitial pressures have been shown to be increased in CP[13–19]. In normal pancreatic tissue the intraductal pressure as determined by ERCP ranges between 10 and 16 mmHg, whereas it is increased to between 18 and 48 mmHg in patients with CP[4]. The parenchymal pressure assessed during surgery ranges between 3 and 11 mmHg in control subjects and between 17 and 21 mmHg in patients with CP.

In several studies published by Ebbehoj et al., a direct relationship between pain intensity and intraductal pancreatic pressure before and after decompressive surgery was demonstrated[13–18]. Pancreatic pressure was assessed by percutaneous or intraoperative fine-needle puncture. Patients whose pressure remained low after surgery were painfree, whereas those with recurrent pain had increased intrapancreatic pressure. The significance of increased pressure as cause for pain in CP is further supported by endoscopic and surgical data suggesting that duct compression improves pain in 50–85% of patients.

It is now generally accepted that an increased ductal pressure and dilation of the pancreatic duct are typical findings in painful CP. However, a clear-cut relationship between intensity of pain and pressure as described by Ebbehoj et al., or between pain and degree of ductal distension could not be confirmed in subsequent studies[8,12,19]. Manes et al. studied 12 patients with CP undergoing surgery and five controls with cancer of the pancreatic tail[19]. Although the authors confirmed that the pancreatic pressure was significantly higher in CP than in controls, pain score and pancreatic pressure were not correlated. In the studies by Reimer Jensen et al.[12] and Malfertheiner et al.[8], no significant correlation between the degree of pain and morphological changes (duct obstruction and dilation) could be demonstrated. In addition, many patients still had significant pain after pancreatic duct drainage, suggesting that additional mechanisms are involved in the pathogenesis of pain in CP. Problems of data interpretation of the pressure hypothesis are summarized in Table 2.

Table 2 Interpretation of results from pressure hypothesis

Influence of increased pressure	Problems with data interpretation
Obstruction/plugs, stones, structural changes increase pressure	Not all patients benefit from decompression procedures
Increased pressure in ducts and tissue: pain?	30% of patients treated with decompression exhibit recurrences
Decompression of dilated ducts can relieve pain	Structural changes do not correlate with pain
Does painful CP burn out?	Pancreatic pressure does not correlate with pain

Pancreatic ischaemia: compartment syndrome

Ischaemia could be an additional mechanism causing pain in CP. Experimental evidence indicates that increased pancreatic pressure correlates with decreased blood flow in cats with CP[20,21]. In this feline model, surgical incision of the gland and ductal drainage significantly improved blood flow. Thus, pain may develop when increased pancreatic pressure produces a compartment syndrome that induces ischaemia. The existence of a compartment syndrome, which is proposed by the inverse relationship of blood flow and tissue pressure, could explain why the abdominal pain gets worse after eating and why patients often show a significant pain relief after drainage operations.

Pancreatic fibrosis

Intralobular and perilobular fibrosis belong to the typical histological features of CP. The pathogenesis of pancreatic fibrogenesis is unclear, and it is also not known whether fibrosis by itself may produce pain. It has been postulated that fibrosis leads to increased intraductal pressure and thereby to pain during the course of CP. Perivascular pancreatic stellate cells may be the link between

Table 3 Interpretation of results from pancreatic fibrosis

Influence of increased fibrosis?	Problems with data interpretation
Intralobular/perilobular fibrosis leads to irreversible scarring	Degree of pancreatic fibrosis has no influence on pain generation
Fibrosis leads to increased pressure tissue: pain?	Degree of fibrosis does not correlate with pain
Pathogenesis of fibrogenesis is unclear	

fibrosis and pain. These cells seem to be stimulated during fibrosis in CP, and may cause microvascular ischaemia and pain[22]. In contrast to this hypothesis, intensity of pain and degree of fibrosis were not correlated in the study by Di Sebastiano et al.[23]. According to that study the degree of pancreatic fibrosis would have no significant impact on pain in CP. The interpretation of results of the fibrosis hypothesis is summarized in Table 3.

Inhibition of CCK-mediated negative feedback

Under physiological conditions, exocrine pancreatic secretion is regulated by a negative feedback mechanism. A CCK-releasing peptide induces the release of CCK, which in turn stimulates pancreatic exocrine secretion including trypsin. The CCK-releasing peptide in the duodenum is normally denatured by pancreatic trypsin, thus inhibiting the exocrine pancreatic function by a negative feedback. It has been speculated that inhibition of the normal negative feedback mechanism could cause pain in CP. In patients with CP and exocrine insufficiency, basal CCK concentrations are significantly higher than in normal healthy subjects[24]. In CP, damage of the parenchymal tissue leads to reduced secretion of trypsin, which in turn lacks for sufficiently denaturing the CCK-releasing peptide. This would result in an ongoing stimulation of the exocrine pancreas and thus induce the development of pain. This concept is supported by the observation that, in some CP patients, pain relief was achieved after high oral doses of pancreatic enzymes. Thus, oral administration of pancreatic enzymes would induce appropriate denaturing of the CCK-releasing peptide, thereby reducing the release of CCK, the stimulation of the exocrine pancreas, and finally the increased intraductal pressure and pain[1,3].

The significance of the CCK-mediated feedback in the pathogenesis of pain in CP has been questioned for several reasons. (1) In many patients with painful CP, pancratic enzymes have no effect on pain relief. (2) Induction of pancreatic secretion by CCK is not associated with pain in CP. (3) Octreotide, which significantly inhibits pancreatic secretion, does not influence the intensity of pain in most CP patients[1].

Alterations of pancreatic nerves

Bockman et al. demonstrated a significant increase in the number and mean diameter of pancreatic nerve fibres in tissues from patients with CP[25]. The mean area of tissue served per nerve was considerably less than in controls. The authors assumed that both sensory and motor nerve fibres were equally affected. The histological findings could be due to a real increase in neural components or the consequence of a continuous degeneration of pancreatic parenchyma. The increased number and diameter of intralobular and inter-lobar nerve bundles in CP has been confirmed in subsequent studies[26]. In the ultrastructural analysis of CP tissue samples, individual nerve fibres were damaged, and there was evidence of oedema in the nerve bundles[25]. The histological and ultrastructural alterations seemed to be located mainly within the pancreatic head. This is consistent with the observation that more than 90% of patients were painfree after duodenum-preserving pancreatic head resection[25]. Nerve growth factor (NGF) and its high-affinity receptor tyrosine kinase A (TrkA) have been implicated in the pathogenesis of intrapancreatic nerve growth and pain generation in CP. NGF and TrkA are overexpressed in CP, and are mainly found in ductal cells, acinar cells, in the perineurium and in intrapancreatic ganglion cells[27]. The expression levels of NGF and TrkA were positively correlated with pain in these patients.

In CP, growth-associated protein 43 (GAP-43), a marker for neuronal activation, is significantly increased in the majority of pancreatic nerve fibres (axons of postganglionic parasympathetic neurons and fibres of extrinsic neurons) and intrinsic neurons compared to the low-level expression of GAP-43 in the normal human pancreas[23]. These findings suggest plastic changes of the intrinsic nervous system during CP. Data from Di Sebastiano and Fink indicate that the level of GAP-43 expression not only depends on the duration of the disease, but is also directly correlated with individual pain scores[23,28].

In the study by Bockman et al., foci of inflammatory cells were found around pancreatic nerves and ganglia[25]. Electron microscopic analysis revealed not only disrupted and damaged perineural sheaths, but also invasion by lymphocytes. The close spatial relation of nerves and immune cells in the chronically inflamed pancreas suggests that neuroimmune mechanisms are involved in the pathogenesis of inflammation and pain in CP. The normal perineurium forms a continuous barrier between the nerve and its suroundings, and thus provides a protected microenvironment within the nerve bundle which persists for up to 21 h after death[29]. When the perineural sheath is severely damaged it can no longer maintain its barrier function. It may therefore allow free access of bioactive substances such as activated enzymes or inflammatory mediators to the unprotected nerves, thereby causing stimulation of pain. Consistent with the current concept, di Sebastiano et al. found a direct correlation between the degree of perineural inflammation and the pain intensity[23].

Neuroimmune interaction

In a recently published study, Di Sebastiano et al. observed a significant increase in IL-8 mRNA expression in CP tissue samples[30]. IL-8 was found

Table 4 Interpretation of results related to neuroimmune interactions

Findings	Problems with data interpretation
Alterations in pancreatic nerve	No functional data available
Evidence for damaged pancreatic nerves	Insufficient database
Changes in peptidergic innervation	Neuroimmune crosstalk poorly defined
Expression of cytokines/growth factors	No experimental model available to test the hypothesis
Alterations correlated with clinical scores	

mainly in macrophages around pancreatic nerves, as well as in acinar and ductal cells. IL-8 mRNA expression and the inflammatory score were positively correlated. The close spatial relation of IL-8-positive immune cells and pancreatic nerves further supports the concept of a possible link between neuropeptides and inflammatory mediators. In different models of pain and inflammation, cytokines including IL-1 and IL-8 have been shown to interact with neuropeptides such as substance P (SP). However, the exact mechanisms of the neuroimmune crosstalk, the interaction of inflammatory cells and nerves in CP need to be further investigated.

In normal human pancreas, nerves contain several neuropeptides including neuropeptide Y (NPY), peptide histidine isoleucine (PHI), SP, calcitonin gene-related protein (CGRP) and vasoactive intestinal peptide (VIP). Several of these peptides belong to the family of pain neurotransmitters. This was the rationale to examine the distribution and intensity of these neurosubstances in painful CP compared to normal pancreatic tissue. Several studies have shown that there was a significantly increased expression of SP and CGRP in the chronically inflamed pancreas[26]. In contrast, the changes in VIP, NPY and PHI were only modest. The selective up-regulation of SP and CGRP was mainly observed in those intralobular and interlobular nerve bundles which were previously found to be increased in number and diameter.

SP and CGRP, which interact in a complex manner, are not only potent immunomodulators but also, as previously discussed, regarded as pain neuro-transmitters. In addition, SP stimulates fibroblasts and could be involved in the fibrotic process in CP. The observation of an overexpression of SP and CGRP provides further evidence for a direct involvement of pancreatic nerves in the pathogenesis of pain in CP. Brain-derived neurotrophic factor (BDNF) is a member of the neurotrophic factor family and may play an important role in peripheral and central pain modulation. The exact mechanisms by which BDNF influences pain are not known.

Using immunohistochemistry and Western blot analysis, Zhu et al. could demonstrate that BDNF was significantly increased in CP tissue samples and that the expression levels of BDNF were positively correlated with pain intensity and pain frequency[31]. In the normal pancreas, BDNF can be detected in the cytoplasm of most ductal cells and (weakly) in most acinar cells, islet cells, nerve fibres and ganglia cells. In CP tissue, immunostaining of BDNF is present (intensely) in most cells of ductular complexes and in the perineurium of enlarged cells, as well as (moderately) in degenerating acinar and islet cells, most enlarged nerve fibres and intrinsic pancreatic ganglia cells (moderate)[31]. It has been speculated, that BDNF may also be present in the dorsal root ganglia and in the spinal horn, and that it may there be involved in central sensory modulation. This would explain why peripheral nerve blockage cannot always sufficiently suppress pain in CP patients[32,33]. The role of BDNF in CP is still unclear, but it has been implicated in the pathogenesis of nerve repair, regeneration and sprouting, as well as in peripheral and central pain regulation. Limitations of data interpretation of the neuroimmune interaction concept are summarized in Table 4.

SUMMARY

Recurrent upper abdominal pain is the most relevant clinical symptom of CP. The pain in CP is difficult to assess, and different patterns have been described. The pathogenesis of pain in these patients is complex and not fully understood. Several hypotheses have been proposed regarding the generation and continuation of chronic pain in CP, but none of these concepts has so far been proven. It also seems likely that the pain is caused by more than one mechanism. The importance of each mechanism needs to be defined. A better understanding of the pathophysiology of pain will hopefully offer new options for effective treatment. An experimental model of CP, which mimics the human disease, needs to be developed. The answer to several important questions such as (1) what is the role of increased pressure, (2) what is the role of the immune system, and (3) why does pain disappear in some patients, is still lacking.

References

1. Di Sebastiano P, di Mola FF, Bockman DE, Friess H, Buchler MW. Chronic pancreatitis: the perspective of pain generation by neuroimmune interaction. Gut. 2003;52:907–11.
2. Steer ML, Waxman I, Freedman S. Chronic pancreatitis. N Engl J Med. 1995;332:1482–90.
3. Warshaw AL, Banks PA, Fernandez-Del Castillo C. AGA technical review: treatment of pain in chronic pancreatitis. Gastroenterology. 1998;115:765–76.
4. Glasbrenner B, Adler G. Evaluating pain and the quality of life in chronic pancreatitis. Int J Pancreatol. 1997;22:163–70.
5. Ammann RW, Muellhaupt B, and the Zurich Pancreatitis Study Group. The natural history of pain in alcoholic chronic pancreatitis. Gastroenterology. 1999;116:1132–40.
6. Lankisch PG, Lohr-Happe A, Otto J, Creutzfeldt W. Natural course in chronic pancreatitis. Pain, exocrine and endocrine pancreatic insufficiency and prognosis of the disease. Digestion. 1993;54:148–55.
7. DiMagno EP. Toward understanding (and management) of painful chronic pancreatitis. Gastroenterology. 1999;116:1252–7.
8. Malfertheiner P, Buchler M, Stanescu A, Ditschuneit H. Pancreatic morphology and function in relationship to pain in chronic pancreatitis. Int J Pancreatol. 1987;2:59–66.
9. Little JM. Alcohol abuse and chronic pancreatitis. Surgery. 1987;101:357–60.
10. Hayakawa T, Kondo T, Shibata T, Sugimoto Y, Kitagawa M. Chronic alcoholism and evolution of pain and prognosis in chronic pancreatitis. Dig Dis Sci. 1989;34:33–8.
11. Becker V, Mischke U. Groove pancreatitis. Int J Pancreatol. 1991;10:173–82.

12. Reimer Jensen A, Matzen P, Malchow-Moller A, Christoffersen I and the Copenhagen Pancreatitis Study Group. Pattern of pain, duct morphology, and pancreatic function in chronic pancreatitis. A comparative study. Scand J Gastroenterol. 1984;19:334–8.
13. Ebbehoj N. Pancreatic tissue fluid pressure and pain in chronic pancreatitis. Dan Med Bull. 1992;39:128–33.
14. Ebbehoj N, Borly L, Madsen P, Svendsen LB. Pancreatic tissue pressure and pain in chronic pancreatitis. Pancreas. 1986;1:556–8.
15. Ebbehoj N, Borly L, Bulow J, Rasmussen SG, Madsen P. Evaluation of pancreatic tissue fluid pressure and pain in chronic pancreatitis. A longitudinal study. Scand J Gastroenterol. 1990;25:462–6.
16. Ebbehoj N, Borly L, Madsen P, Matzen P. Pancreatic tissue fluid pressure during drainage operations for chronic pancreatitis. Scand J Gastroenterol. 1990;25:1041–5.
17. Ebbehoj N, Borly L, Bulow J et al. Pancreatic tissue fluid pressure in chronic pancreatitis. Relation to pain, morphology and function. Scand J Gastroenterol. 1990;25:1046–51.
18. Ebbehoj N, Borly L, Bulow J, Henriksen JH, Heyeraas KJ, Rasmussen SG. Evaluation of pancreatic tissue fluid pressure measurements intraoperatively and by sonographically guided fine-needle puncture. Scand J Gastroenterol 1990;25:1097–102.
19. Manes G, Buchler M, Pieramico O, Di Sebastiano P, Malfertheiner P. Is increased pancreatic pressure related to pain in chronic pancreatitis? Int J Pancreatol. 1994;15:113–17.
20. Reber HA, Karanjia ND, Alvarez C et al. Pancreatic blood flow in cats with chronic pancreatitis. Gastroenterology. 1992;103:652–9.
21. Karanjjia ND, Widdison AL, Leung F, Alvarez C, Lutrin FJ, Reber HA. Compartment syndrome in experimental chronic obstructive pancreatitis: effect of decompressing the main pancreatic duct. Br J Surg. 1994;81:259–64.
22. Wells RG, Crawford JM. Pancreatic stellate cells: the new stars of chronic pancreatitis? Gastroenterology. 1998;115:491–3.
23. Di Sebastiano P, Fink T, Weihe E et al. Immune cell infiltration and growth-associated protein 43 expression correlates with pain in chronic pancreatitis. Gastroenterology. 1997;112:1648–55.
24. Slaff JI, Wolfe MM, Toskes PP. Elevated fasting cholecystokinin levels in pancreatic exocrine impairment: evidence to support feedback regulation. J Lab Clin Med. 1985;105:282–5.
25. Bockman DE, Buchler M, Malfertheiner P, Beger HG. Analysis of nerves in chronic pancreatitis. Gastroenterology. 1988;94:1459–69.
26. Buchler M, Weihe E, Friess H et al. Changes in peptidergic innervation in chronic pancreatitis. Pancreas. 1992;7:183–92.
27. Friess H, Zhu ZW, di Mola FF et al. Nerve growth factor and its high-affinity receptor in chronic pancreatitis. Ann Surg. 1999;230:615–24.
28. Fink T, di Sebastiano P, Buchler M, Beger HG, Weihe E. Growth-associated protein-43 and protein gene-product 9.5 innervation in human pancreas: changes in chronic pancreatitis. Neuroscience. 1994;63:249–66.
29. Soderfeldt B. Olsson Y, Kristensson K. The perneurium as a diffusion barrier to protein tracers in human peripheral nerve. Acta Neuropathol. 1973;25:120–6.
30. Di Sebastiano P, di Mola FF, di Febbo C et al. Expression of interleukin 8 (IL-8) and substance P in human chronic pancreatitis. Gut. 2000;47:423–8.
31. Zhu ZW, Friess H, Wang L, Zimmermann A, Buchler MW. Brain-derived neurotrophic factor (BDNF) is upregulated and associated with pain in chronic pancreatitis. Dig Dis Sci. 2001;46:1633–9.
32. Ihse I, Zoucas E, Gyllstedt E, Lillo-Gil R, Andren-Sandberg A. Bilateral thoracoscopic splanchnicectomy: effects on pancreatic pain and function. Ann Surg. 1999;230:785–90.
33. Maher JW, Johlin FC, Pearson D. Thoracoscopic splanchnicectomy for chronic pancreatitis pain. Surgery. 1996;120:603–9.

18
Chronic pancreatitis: controversies in pain therapy, medical therapeutic options

J. MÖSSNER

INTRODUCTION

Symptomatic therapy of chronic pancreatitis is based on several theories (Table 1). Abstinence from alcohol improves social reintegration and compliance, and may mitigate the further course of the disease and decrease the complication rate. Abstinence from smoking may retard the progress of arteriosclerosis and prevent complications of smoking such as lung cancer. Therapy of pain is based on its supposed pathogenesis. Pathogenesis of pain is multifactorial. Therapy of pain should be causal whenever possible. Medical pain therapy can be effected by different routes of application of drugs (oral, sublingual, intravenous, transdermal, epidural, intrathecal, and blockage of plexus coeliacus). Interventional endoscopy may improve pain by drainage of bile duct stenosis or pancreatic duct stenosis, drainage of pseudocysts or endoscopic removal of pancreatic duct stones after disintegration by extracorporeal shock waves.

Cure of the disease is still not possible; ten years after primary diagnosis up to 50% of all patients have already died. Causes of death are rarely multiorgan failure or sepsis due to acute relapses of the disease, complications of surgery or late complications of diabetes, but rather diseases due to the 'lifestyle' of most of these patients. Due to smoking, and possibly decreased immune capacity as a consequence of alcoholism, patients are at increased risk of developing lung cancers and cancers of the upper gastrointestinal tract. These patients are at increased risk of coronary heart disease, alcohol-related accidents, and complications of inadequate insulin therapy. Furthermore, there is some risk of developing pancreatic cancer due to decades of chronic organ inflammation. This risk is especially relevant in patients with early-onset idiopathic or hereditary chronic pancreatitis.

Pain and exocrine pancreatic insufficiency are the leading symptoms of chronic pancreatitis. It is generally accepted that enzyme therapy should be started in patients with chronic pancreatitis when faecal fat excretion exceeds 15 g/day or when weight loss is present[1]. However, treatment of pain seems to

Table 1 Symptomatic treatment of chronic pancreatitis

Measure	Aim
Alcohol stop	Social reintegration. Improvement of compliance. Retardation for disease progression? Reduction of complication rate?
Nicotine stop	Retardation of arteriosclerosis. Improvement of pain?
Medical treatment of pain: oral, sublingual; intravenous; transdermal; peridural; intrathecal; plexus coeliacus blockade	Freedom from pain
Interventional endoscopy Bile duct drainage	Improvement of pain. Improvement of cholestasis. Prevention of secondary biliary cirrhosis. Prevention of cholangitis. Treatment of pruritus
Pancreatic duct drainage	Freedom from pain. Retardation of chronic destructive inflammation?
Pseudocyst drainage Endoscopic transgastral, duodenal, papillary	Freedom from pain. Prevention of rupture
Pancreatic stone removal ESWL + endoscopic stone extraction	Freedom from pain. Retardation of chronic inflammation?
Treatment of exocrine insufficiency Porcine pancreatic extracts (acid protected microtablets, pellets). Conventional porcine pancreatic extracts in cases of lack of gastric acid (fungal lipase?). (Genetically constructed microbial acid resistant lipase?). Fat-soluble vitamins. Diet	Improvement of maldigestion
Treatment of endocrine insufficiency Insulin	
Surgery	Improvement of pain. Treatment of complications. Suspicion of cancer. Retardation of disease progression?

be much more cumbersome[2]. This may partly be due to the multifactor causes of pain in chronic pancreatitis (Table 2). Furthermore, the pathomechanism of pain is still poorly understood.

The concept of treatment of pain by exogenous application of pancreatic enzymes is based on two assumptions: (1) putting the pancreas at rest by inhibition of pancreatic enzyme secretion reduces pain; and (2) exogenous

Table 2 Pathogenesis of pain in chronic pancreatitis

Inflammatory mass of pancreatic head → duodenal ± bile duct compression
Inflammatory infiltration of retroperitoneum
Pseudocyst → compression of adjacent organs
Pancreatic duct obstruction by scars or stones/protein precipitates → elevation of ductal pressure
Inflammatory infiltration of sensory nerves
Pancreatic ischaemia due to arteriosclerosis
Extrapancreatic causes: gastric, duodenal ulcer
Meteorism due to maldigestion
Psychological causes of pain due to alcoholism

---

application of pancreatic enzymes inhibits pancreatic enzyme secretion by a negative feedback mechanism. However, inhibition of pancreatic secretion by octreotide was not effective in decreasing pain[3]. In a Japanese multicentre study the cholecystokinin (CCK) antagonist loxiglumide was compared with placebo[4]. In a 4-week trial loxiglumide was effective in lowering pain. One may speculate whether this pain-decreasing effect was due to inhibition of secretion by CCK.

NEGATIVE FEEDBACK INHIBITION OF PANCREATIC ENZYME SECRETION: STUDIES IN ANIMALS

Both CCK and secretin play important roles in the regulation of exocrine pancreatic secretion. Inhibition of pancreatic enzyme secretion by the presence of pancreatic proteases in the duodenum via a negative feedback has been demonstrated in various animals such as rats[5-11], chicken[12] and pig[13]. In rats this negative feedback control is clearly mediated via CCK[8,9,14,15]. CCK is probably released by protease-sensitive proteins originating either from duodenal mucosa[16-18] or pancreatic juice[19]. In the duodenal mucosa diazepam-binding inhibitor[16] and in the pancreatic secretions monitorpeptide has been described as CCK-releasing peptides[19]. Secretin is probably also released by protease-sensitive proteins[8,20].

Regulation of pancreatic secretion is rather complex and different among species, and involves both hormones and nerves. Gut peptide hormones may act directly at acinar and duct cells or indirectly via stimulation or inhibition of release of neurotransmitters. Somatostatin, pancreatic polypeptide, and calcitonin-gene-related peptide play key roles in inhibition of pancreatic secretion[21].

NEGATIVE FEEDBACK INHIBITION OF PANCREATIC ENZYME SECRETION: STUDIES IN HUMANS

The findings in humans, however, are still controversial. Some groups reported feedback inhibition of human pancreatic enzyme secretion[20,22-25], and bicarbonate secretion[20] by proteases such as trypsin and chymotrypsin and a mediation via CCK[26-28] and secretin[20]. However, the mechanisms of this putative negative feedback, and whether it does play a role in humans, is still not known. Furthermore, some degree of inhibition might be regulated independently from proteases by the intraduodenal concentration of bile acids[26]. There are reports supporting the concept of a negative feedback as they could demonstrate a stimulation of pancreatic enzyme secretion by intraduodenal application of protease inhibitors[29-31]. However, this feedback could also be an atropine-sensitive pathway rather than CCK[29,30]. Other studies neglected the existence of a negative feedback inhibition in humans. In these studies pancreatic enzymes did not exert a negative feedback on pancreatic secretions when nutrients were absent[32]. However, in these studies pancreatic enzymes were infused in the jejunum not in the duodenum. Some authors claim that the putative negative feedback mechanism in humans is operative only in the duodenum. In other studies inhibition of intraduodenal trypsin did not stimulate pancreatic secretion[33].

We demonstrated in healthy volunteers that intrajejunal application of low concentrations of porcine pancreatic extracts, as well as intraduodenal application of very high concentrations, stimulated rather than inhibited endogenous pancreatic enzyme secretion, whereas intraduodenal perfusion with an identical concentration of pure trypsin inhibited pancreatic secretion[34,35]. In these experiments the acid protection of porcine pancreatic extracts was removed to ensure that the duodenum was perfused with active proteases. We postulated that the high protein content of porcine pancreatic extracts overwhelmed a potential inhibitory effect of proteases. These studies have been confirmed by others who observed an increase of plasma CCK after adding porcine pancreatic extracts to a meal[36]. It is well known that fat digestion, which releases free fatty acids, is required for CCK release. Thus, another study could demonstrate that intraduodenal perfusion of tetrahydrolipstatin, an irreversible lipase inhibitor, reduces not only fat-stimulated lipase activity in the duodenum, but also amylase and trypsin secretion and plasma CCK[37].

Slaff et al.[25] used another brand of porcine pancreatic extracts as compared to our studies and reported an inhibitory effect on pancreatic secretion. However, they studied pancreatic function after discontinuation of oral enzyme therapy. Burton et al.[38] measured pancreatic enzyme secretion in the human transplanted pancreas. Addition of six capsules of pancrelipase (150 000 units of proteases) to a 300-ml Lundh meal reduced meal-stimulated amylase secretion in the allograft. It would be interesting to compare the activity of proteases in relation to the protein content in their study with our studies which demonstrated the opposite, i.e. stimulation of pancreatic enzyme secretion by porcine pancreatic extracts. Dominguez-Munoz et al.[39] compared two different brands of porcine pancreatic extracts, enteric-coated tablets versus enteric-coated microtablets. The advantage of their study, besides measurement of pancreatic enzyme secretion, antral and duodenal motility, was recorded. Thus, the liquid test meal could be applied either alone or together with pancreatic enzymes exactly 30 min after an interdigestive migrating motor complex phase. With microtablets only, the authors observed an inhibition of pancreatic elastase secretion. One may postulate that the enteric-coated tablets either did not pass into the duodenum or that their proteases were not released in the duodenum within the time period studied. However, this study also has some drawbacks: the authors do not provide us with plasma CCK data. They observed no changes in bile acid secretion. Thus, one must speculate that plasma CCK was not changed, since an inhibition of CCK release should alter gallbladder contraction after application of a test meal. If feedback inhibition is not mediated by CCK in humans, the authors should have provided us with data confirming the theory that feedback inhibition in humans is mediated by an atropine-sensitive pathway. Furthermore, they observed an inhibition of pancreatic elastase secretion by application of only 2000 units of proteases. None of the studies published so far has demonstrated a negative feedback inhibition in humans at such low concentrations of proteases[27,40]. Thus, there remains a controversial discussion as to whether inhibition or stimulation of pancreatic enzyme secretion is caused by application of porcine pancreatic extracts, and whether this function depends on the brand tested.

NEGATIVE FEEDBACK INHIBITION OF PANCREATIC ENZYME SECRETION: STUDIES IN PATIENTS WITH CHRONIC PANCREATITIS

Some studies in patients with chronic pancreatitis have supported the concept that negative feedback regulation exists. In this disease, which leads to a decrease of pancreatic protease secretion, elevated plasma CCK levels have been reported[41,42]. However, we and others could not confirm that CCK levels are elevated in advanced chronic pancreatitis[43–47]. There are reports claiming that plasma CCK is elevated only in patients having chronic pancreatitis and pain[48–50] and that pain is directly correlated to low intraduodenal bile acid and trypsin concentrations[49,50] supporting the concept. In patients with chronic pancreatitis we and others demonstrated that application of pancreatic extracts to food caused higher plasma CCK levels than food alone[45,46] which could be explained by CCK release due to improvement of fat digestion. In severe pancreatic insufficiency lipase levels in the duodenum must be low. Thus, one is faced with a similar situation as compared to the Swiss study[37] in which lipase activity was inhibited in healthy controls by tetrahydrolipostatin: under both conditions fat digestion is altered and one should expect low plasma CCK levels and a decrease in pancreatic enzyme secretion. In another study just the opposite of our observations has been published, i.e. a decrease of CCK response in patients with chronic pancreatitis treated with pancreatic enzymes[49,50]. These data are difficult to interpret. According to the negative feedback concept, patients with advanced chronic pancreatitis, i.e. severe pancreatic insufficiency with steatorrhoea, should have elevated basal plasma CCK values. As in our studies the authors did not find elevated basal plasma CCK values. However, the authors report a decrease in food-stimulated plasma CCK response after 45 and 90 days of enzyme therapy, even after 3 days of therapy withdrawal. These data cannot be explained by the concept that CCK is rapidly released by protease-sensitive proteins present either in the pancreatic secretions or in the duodenal mucosa[16,17,19]. To complete the controversies, a Japanese group reported that patients with chronic pancreatitis showed identical plasma CCK profiles as compared to healthy controls irrespective of whether pancreatic porcine extracts were added or not[46].

Assuming that this negative feedback mechanism exists in humans, one is faced with two opposite mechanisms in pancreatic insufficiency: stimulation of pancreatic enzyme secretion due to low intraduodenal protease concentrations and inhibition of secretion due to altered fat digestion. It is completely unknown which mechanism is leading at which stage of the disease. At early stages without severe pancreatic insufficiency putative protease-mediated inhibition of secretion is clearly overplayed by stimulation of secretion due to sufficient fat digestion. At late stages with severe pancreatic insufficiency plasma CCK levels should be high due to low trypsin concentrations in the duodenum. However, meal-stimulated CCK release is hampered by maldigestion of fat. Pain can be present at all stages of chronic pancreatitis. However, it is generally accepted that pain is more a leading symptom at earlier stages when the exocrine tissue has not been substituted by fibrous tissue.

EFFECT OF ORAL PANCREATIC ENZYME ADMINISTRATION ON PAIN IN PATIENTS WITH CHRONIC PANCREATITIS

In two older studies treatment with pancreatic enzymes caused a reduction of pain which was considered to be due to lowering the intraductal pressure by intraluminal trypsin[25,52]. However, it is not generally accepted that treatment with pancreatic extracts leads to a reduction of pain[53].

After exclusion of biliary or duodenal obstruction, expanding pseudocysts or extrapancreatic diseases such as peptic ulcers as frequent causes of pain, an increased pressure of pancreatic ducts is considered to be a major pathogenetic factor, which causes pain[54]. Consequently, various therapeutic procedures such as drugs, endoscopic stents, disintegration of pancreatic stones via extracorporeal shock waves[55–63], drainage procedures or pancreatic resections[64] are offered to treat pain by lowering elevated pancreatic duct pressures.

Our studies in normal healthy volunteers did not support the concept that one can inhibit pancreatic enzyme secretion by oral application of porcine pancreatic extracts. However, pancreatic extracts may amelioriate pain in chronic pancreatitis via other mechanisms. Thus, we conducted a double-blind placebo-controlled multicentre study to see whether treatment with pancreatic extracts has a beneficial effect on pain in chronic pancreatitis. Forty-three patients with proven chronic pancreatitis were included. About 70% of all patients confirmed alcohol abuse in their history. Only patients with acute or chronic pain most likely due to chronic pancreatitis were included. Patients received either placebo or pancreatic extracts in a double-blind randomized manner for 14 days. This was followed by crossover treatment for another 14 days with either verum or placebo. Patients received acid-protected commercially available porcine pancreatic enzymes which were applied together with meals in a higher dosage than commonly used for treatment of pancreatic insufficiency (5×2 capsules/day; Panzytrat® 20000, Knoll AG, Ludwigshafen, Germany; capsules with microtablets, containing per capsule triacylglycerollipase 20000 Ph.Eur.-U., amylase 18000 Ph.Eur.-U., proteases 1000 Ph.Eur.-U.).

This dosage ensured the application of 10 000 Ph.Eur.-U. of proteases/day. For comparison with porcine pancreatic extracts used outside Europe, 1 Ph.Eur. unit corresponds to 1 F.I.P. unit.

At initial examination most patients had moderate pain. When pain score was evaluated by interview after 14 days of treatment the total number of patients with moderate and severe pain decreased irrespective of whether patients received verum or placebo. With regards to other symptoms such as diarrhoea, nausea, vomitus, and flatulence, again there was no difference whether patients were treated with either verum or placebo. If one compared each patient intraindividually whether the pain score improved on either treatment with porcine pancreatic extracts or with placebo, 14 out of 18 patients whose pain score improved under placebo improved when placebo was applied after verum. Similar results were seen in those patients whose pain score improved better under verum as compared to placebo. Eighteen out of 25 of this group received verum during the last 2 weeks of the 4-week study period[38]. Our observations were confirmed by another placebo-controlled study[65]. Several questions need clarification:

1. Does negative feedback regulation of pancreatic secretion play a physiological role in humans? There are more studies confirming this kind of regulation in humans than studies which neglect its existence. However, the high concentrations of trypsin needed to suppress pancreatic secretion in humans must raise some concerns.

2. Is pancreatic function really related to pain in the majority of patients or, vice-versa, does inhibition of pancreatic secretion decrease pain? The generally accepted clinical observation that pain decreases with 'burning out' of the pancreas does not imply that pain is directly related to a stimulation of pancreatic function because, with further destruction of acinar tissue, acute infiltration of the pancreas by inflammatory cells also becomes less likely. Thus, we believe that only in some patients with chronic pancreatitis is pain clearly related to stimulation of pancreatic function.

3. Does treatment with porcine pancreatic extracts influence pain? In the studies by Slaff et al. who observed a pain-relieving effect after treatment with porcine pancreatic extracts, it is surprising that many patients were women with idiopathic chronic pancreatitis[25]. In our studies most patients were males with alcoholic chronic pancreatitis. It has been suggested that a pain-relieving effect after treatment with pancreatic enzymes can be simulated due to the improvement of meteorism in patients with steatorhoea[53]. Thus, in our studies, severe steatorrhoea was an exclusion criterion. In our studies both porcine pancreatic extracts and placebo caused a similar pain-relieving effect within the first 2 weeks of treatment. Furthermore, porcine pancreatic extracts did not lower the use of analgesics. We interpreted these results as a spontaneous improvement. Thus, with improvement of acute inflammation pain improves.

4. How important is the choice of the pancreatic enzyme formulation if one wants to treat pain? For treatment of pancreatic insufficiency modern galenic formulas are preferred where lipase is acid-protected and extracts are packed in microtablets or micropellets. We used a modern acid-protected porcine pancreatic extract whose enzymes are rapidly released from microtablets at a pH of 6.6. Thus, one may argue that, for treatment of pain, it would be preferable to use conventional porcine extracts rich in proteases. However, the brand we used is rich not only in lipase but also in trypsin. According to our study design we applied a rather high dosage of trypsin, i.e. 10 000 Ph.E.U./day. In a study which is published only as an abstract[48] an acid-protected brand of porcine pancreatic extracts had no pain-relieving effect. Since plasma CCK was elevated in these patients, the authors argue that these acid-protected enzymes did not inhibit pancreatic secretion because their proteases are released not in the duodenum but in the jejunum. The five trials using porcine pancreatic extracts as acid-protected microtablets or microspheres reported no benefit[40,48,53,65,66], the two older trials using pancreatic enzymes as tablets showed a pain-relieving effect[25,52]. We may suggest that, for any further studies on this topic, it would be better to use pure trypsin preparations.

There are some drawbacks of all studies: exact grading of pain score is an important issue[67]. However, most of our patients were alcoholics and many of them were not able to give an exact description of their pain. The ideal patient for our studies would have been a patient with constant chronic pain; however, those patients are very rare. According to patient protocols most of them had chronic pain but pain intensity varied from day to day. Thus, many patients in our studies came to the hospital because their pain score deteriorated. We have evaluated pain behaviour in different subclassifications of patients: patients with true chronic pain; patients with either acute pain after a pain-free interval and/or elevations of serum amylase/lipase above 3 times the upper limit, which may be regarded as an acute attack; and patients with signs of slight cholestasis. There were no obvious differences between these groups. In patients with constant chronic pain, treatment studies may be more valid if one has a run-in period for 14 days and a wash-out period for another 14 days between switching to the other treatment regimen.

In a meta-analysis, Brown et al.[68] evaluated six randomized, double-blind, placebo-controlled trials (including our study) in which pancreatic enzymes were used to treat pain in chronic pancreatitis. Their statistical analysis revealed no significant benefit of pancreatic enzyme therapy to relieve pain. The study was criticized by protagonists of the concept that enzymes ameliorite pain by the statement that the studies used for the meta-analysis could not be compared since one cannot compare apples with oranges[69]. Our study does not encourage treating pain in chronic pancreatitis with porcine pancreatic extracts. However, to answer this question definitively, we suggested studies with even more strict inclusion and exclusion criteria with patients demonstrating the following characteristics[70]: pain has to be chronic for many weeks and has to be rather constant. An ERCP has to be performed immediately before study entrance that demonstrates only minimal pancreatic duct changes. If one has severe duct changes one already has advanced chronic pancreatitis, which may not respond to a therapy whose basis ought to be inhibition of pancreatic secretion. Patients with elevations of serum amylase or lipase have to be excluded because pain may be caused by an acute attack of the disease or by chronic active inflammation. Patients with narrowing of the bile duct or elevations of alkaline phosphatase have to be excluded because pain may be due to cholestasis. Patients with even minimal steatorrhoea should be excluded because steatorrhoea is a sign of advanced chronic pancreatitis, or pain may be due to meteorism. Certainly, patients with complications of the disease, such as pseudocysts, have to be excluded. Patients with stones in the main pancreatic duct should be excluded because these stones may already be a sign of advanced chronic pancreatitis. Patients should not be allowed to take analgesics in addition to treatment with the study medication. Proteases instead of acid-protected mixtures of pancreatic extracts should be used. Patients should be able to undergo a more sophisticated evaluation of measuring the degree of pain. Finally, one has to decide whether one includes only patients who stopped drinking alcohol or not, or only patients with idiopathic chronic pancreatitis. This study will probably never be conducted because of the complexity of the disease.

TREATMENT OF PAIN BY CONVENTIONAL PAIN-RELIEVING DRUGS

In treatment of pain due to acute pancreatitis or an acute relapse of chronic pancreatitis continuous intravenous application of procaine is recommended. However, recent studies have clearly demonstrated that opiods are more efficient[71–73]. There are only a few controlled trials studying medical treatment of chronic pain, especially in chronic pancreatitis. All treatment recommendations rely on the suggestions provided by the WHO for general treatment of chronic pain such as in tumours[74]. One starts with monotherapy. Lack of efficiency should lead to combination therapy. Analgesics which act at the periphery are combined with central-acting drugs such as metamizol in combination with tramadol. Tramadol has been shown to be very effective with fewer side-effects as compared to opioids when its dose is titrated individually[75]. Bupivacain (0.125–0.5%) applied via a peridural catheter, or epidural buprenoprhine injection[76] may be an alternative in severe pain. Percutaneous application of fentanyl offers the potential advantage of stable concentrations of this opioid. However, in a comparative trial transdermal fentanyl was not superior to sustained-release morphine tablets[77]. A rather high percentage of patients needed immediate-release morphine tablets as rescue medication. Furthermore, transdermal fentanyl causes skin side-effects. Regular application of analgesics is superior to application on demand; however, one should consider drug dependence and potentiation of drug side-effects when alcohol abuse is continued.

Blockage of the coeliac plexus by transcutaneous CT- or endosonography-guided injection of ethanol, anaesthetics or steroids may be an alternative in severe pain[78]. However, this option has to be compared with surgery[79].

PAIN DUE TO COMPLICATIONS OF CHRONIC PANCREATITIS

Treatment of pain due to pancreatic complications such as pseudocysts, compression of the duodenum, bile duct stenosis, or pancreatic duct stenosis is an interdisciplinary approach. Up to now there are almost no comparative prospective trials between medical treatment, surgery, or interventional endoscopy[80]. Most centres use, whenever feasible, an endoscopic approach[81] such as transgastric or transduodenal drainage of pseudocysts[82], stenting of the main pancreatic duct[83–85] or the distal bile duct[84]. Distal bile duct stenosis alone may not be responsible for pain[73]. Pain due to duodenal scarring by an inflammatory mass of the pancreatic head can certainly only be treated by surgical options such as duodenum-preserving pancreatic head resection.

ANTIOXIDATIVE THERAPY

Free radicals are thought to play a major role in pathogenesis of both acute and chronic pancreatitis. Furthermore, oxygen-derived radicals could mediate pain. However, there are no convincing randomized prospective comparative trials which prove that radical scavenging improves pain. In a single-centre study patients with chronic pancreatitis have been treated by an antioxidative combination consisting of L-methionine, beta-carotene, vitamin C, vitamin E and organic selenium. The authors claim that pain scores decreased[87]. Similar findings were seen in a crossover study running for 20 weeks[88]. Allopurinol, an inhibitor of xanthine oxidase, inhibits formation of free radicals. However, in a randomized double-blind crossover study, allopurinol did not reveal any pain-decreasing effect[89] in contrast to an earlier study[90].

References

1. Lankisch PG. Enzyme treatment of exocrine pancreatic insufficiency in chronic pancreatitis. Digestion. 1993;54(Suppl. 2):21–9.
2. Warshaw AL, Banks PA, Fernandez-Del Castillo C. AGA technical review: treatment of pain in chronic pancreatitis. Gastroenterology. 1998;115:765–76.
3. Malfertheiner P, Mayer D, Büchler M, Dominguez-Munoz JE, Schiefer B, Ditschuneit H. Treatment of pain in chronic pancreatitis by inhibition of pancreatic secretion with octreotide. Gut. 1995;36:450–4.
4. Shiratori K, Takeuchi T, Satake K, Matsuno S – Study Group of Loxiglumide in Japan. Clinical evaluation of oral administration of a cholecystokinin-A receptor antagonist (loxiglumide) to patients with acute, painful attacks of chronic pancreatitis: a multicenter dose–response study in Japan. Pancreas. 2002;25:1–5.
5. Green GM, Lyman RL. Feedback regulation of pancreatic enzyme secretion as a mechanism for trypsin inhibitor-induced hypersecretion in rats. Proc Soc Exp Biol Med. 1972;140:6–12.
6. Hara H, Narakino H, Kiriyama S. Enhancement of pancreatic secretion by dietary protein in rats with chronic diversion of bile–pancreatic juice from the proximal small intestine. Pancreas. 1994;9:275–9.
7. Ihse I, Lilja P, Lundquist I. Trypsin as a regulator of pancreatic secretion in the rat. Scand J Gastroenterol. 1979;13:873–80.
8. Li P, Lee KY, Ren XS, Chang TM, Chey WY. Effect of pancreatic proteases on plasma cholecystokinin, secretin, and pancreatic exocrine secretion in response to sodium oleate. Gastroenterology. 1990;98:1642–8.

9. Louie DS, May D, Miller P, Owyang C. Cholecystokinin mediates feedback regulation of pancreatic enzyme secretion in rats. Am J Physiol. 1986;G250:252–9.
10. Rausch U, Adler G, Weidenbach H et al. Stimulation of pancreatic secretory process in the rat by low-molecular weight proteinase inhibitor. I. Dose–response study on enzyme content and secretion, cholecystokinin release and pancreatic fine structure. Cell Tissue Res. 1987;247:187–93.
11. Shiratori K, Chen YF, Chey WY, Lee KY, Chang T-M. Mechanism of increased exocrine pancreatic secretion in pancreatic juice-diverted rats. Gastroenterology. 1986;91:1171–8.
12. Chernick SS, Lepkovsky S, Chaikoff IL. A dietary factor regulating the enzyme content of the pancreas: changes induced in size and proteolytic activity of the chick pancreas by ingestion of raw soybean meal. Am J Physiol. 1948;155:33–41.
13. Corring T. Mechanisme de la secretion pancréatique exocrine chez le porc: regulation par retro inhibition. Ann Biol Anim Biochim Biophys. 1973;13:755–6.
14. Fölsch UR, Cantor P, Wilms HM, Schafmayer A, Becker HD, Creutzfeldt W. Role of cholecystokinin in the negative feedback control of pancreatic enzyme secretion in conscious rats. Gastroenterology. 1987;92:449–58.
15. Lee PC, Newman BM, Praissman M, Cooney DR, Lebenthal E. Cholecystokinin: a factor responsible for the enteral feedback control of pancreatic hypertrophy. Pancreas. 1986;1:335–40.
16. Herzig KH, Schon I, Tatemoto K et al. Diazepam binding inhibitor is a potent cholecystokinin-releasing peptide in the intestine. Proc Natl Acad Sci USA. 1996;93:7927–32.
17. Herzig KH. Cholecystokinin- and secretin-releasing peptides in the intestine – a new regulatory interendocrine mechanism in the gastrointestinal tract. Regul Pept 1998;73:89–94.
18. Lu L, Louie D, Owyang C. A cholecystokinin releasing peptide mediates feedback regulation of pancreatic secretion. Am J Physiol. 1989;256:G430–5.
19. Fukuoka S-I, Kawajiri H, Fushiki T, Takahashi K, Iwai K. Localization of pancreatic enzyme secretion-stimulating activity and trypsin inhibitory activity in zymogen granule of the rat pancreas. Biochim Biophys Acta. 1986;84:18–24.
20. Jin HO, Song CW, Chang TM, Chey WY. Roles of gut hormones in negative-feedback regulation of pancreatic exocrine secretion in humans. Gastroenterology. 1994;107:1828–34.
21. Owyang C. Negative feedback control of exocrine pancreatic secretion: role of cholecystokinin and cholinergic pathway. J Nutr. 1994;124(Suppl. 8):S1321–6.
22. Dlugosz J, Fölsch UR, Czajkowski A, Gabryelewicz A. Feedback regulation of stimulated pancreatic enzyme secretion during intraduodenal perfusion or trypsin in man. Eur J Clin Invest. 1988;18:267–72.
23. Ihse I, Lilja P, Lundquist I. Feedback regulation of pancreatic enzyme secretion by intestinal trypsin in man. Digestion. 1977;15:303–8.
24. Liener IE, Goodale RL, Deshmukh A et al. Effect of a trypsin inhibitor from soybeans (Bowman-Birk) on the secretory activity of the human pancreas. Gastroenterology. 1984;94:419–27.
25. Slaff J, Jacobson D, Tillman CR, Curington C, Toskes P. Protease-specific suppression of pancreatic exocrine secretion. Gastroenterology. 1984;87:44–52.
26. Mizutani S, Miyata M, Izukura M, Tanaka Y, Matsuda H. Role of bile and trypsin in the release of cholecystokinin in humans. Pancreas. 1995;10:194–9.
27. Owyang C, Louie DS, Tatum D. Feedback regulation of pancreatic enzyme secretion. Suppression of cholecystokinin release by trypsin. J Clin Invest. 1986;77:2042–7.
28. Owyang C, May D, Louie DS. Trypsin suppression of pancreatic enzyme secretion. Differential effect of cholecystokinin release and the enteropancreatic reflex. Gastroenterology. 1986;91:637–43.
29. Adler G, Müllenhoff A, Koop I et al. Stimulation of pancreatic secretion in man by a protease inhibitor. Eur J Clin Invest. 1988;18:98–104.
30. Adler G, Reinshagen M, Koop I et al Differential effects of atropine and a cholecystokinin receptor antagonist on pancreatic secretion. Gastroenterology. 1989;96:1158–64.
31. Layer P, Jansen JBMJ, Cherian L, Lamers CBHW, Goebell H. Feedback regulation of human pancreatic secretion. Effects of protease inhibition on duodenal delivery and small intestinal transit of pancreatic enzymes. Gastroenterology. 1990;98:1311–19.

32. Krawisz BR, Miller LJ, DiMagno EP, Go VLW. In the absence of nutrients, pancreatic-biliary secretions in the jejunum do not exert feedback control of human pancreatic or gastric function. J Lab Clin Med. 1980;95:13–18.

33. Dlugosz J, Fölsch UR, Creutzfeldt W. Inhibition of intraduodenal trypsin does not stimulate exocrine pancreatic secretion in man. Digestion. 1983;26:197–204.

34. Mössner J, Back T, Regner U, Fischbach W. Plasma cholecystokinin in chronic pancreatitis. Z Gastroenterol. 1989;27:401–5.

35. Mössner J, Stange J, Ewald M, Kestel W, Fischbach W. Influence of exogenous application of pancreatic extracts on endogenous pancreatic enzyme secretion. Pancreas. 1991;6:637–44.

36. Jansen JB, Jebbink MC, Mulders HJ, Lamers CB. Effect of pancreatic enzyme supplementation on postprandial plasma cholecystokinin secretion in patients with pancreatic insufficiency. Regul Pept 1989;25:333–42.

37. Hildebrand P, Petrig C, Burckhardt B et al. Hydrolysis of dietary fat by pancreatic lipase stimulates cholecystokinin release. Gastroenterology. 1998;114:123–9.

38. Burton FR, Burton MS, Garvin PJ, Joshi SN. Enteral pancreatic enzyme feedback inhibition of the exocrine secretion of the human transplanted pancreas. Transplantation. 1992;54:988–92.

39. Dominguez-Munoz JE, Birckelbach U, Glasbrenner B, Sauerbruch T, Malfertheiner P. Effect of oral pancreatic enzyme administration on digestive function in healthy subjects: comparison between two enzyme preparations. Aliment Pharmacol Ther. 1997;11:403–8.

40. Mössner J, Secknus R, Meyer J, Niederau C, Adler G. Treatment of pain with pancreatic extracts in chronic pancreatitis: results of a prospective placebo controlled multicenter trial. Digestion. 1992;53:54–66.

41. Funakoshi A, Nakano I, Shinozaki H, Tateishi K, Hamaoka T, Ibayashi H: High plasma cholecystokinin levels in patients with chronic pancreatitis having abdominal pain. Am J Gastroenterol. 1986;81:1174–8.

42. Schafmayer A, Becker HD, Werner M, Fölsch UR, Creutzfeldt W. Plasma cholecystokinin levels in patients with chronic pancreatitis. Digestion. 1985;32:136–9.

43. Bozkurt T, Adler G, Koop I, Koop H, Türmer W, Arnold R. Plasma CCK levels in patients with pancreatic insufficiency. Dig Dis Sci. 1988;33:276–81.

44. Cantor P, Petronijevic L, Worning H. Plasma cholecystokinin concentrations in patients with advanced chronic pancreatitis. Pancreas. 1986;1:488–93.

45. Mössner J, Wresky H-P, Kestel W, Zeeh J, Regner U, Fischbach W. Influence of treatment with pancreatic enzymes on pancreatic enzyme secretion. Gut. 1989;30:1143–9.

46. Nakamura T, Takebe K, Kudoh K et al. No negative feedback regulation between plasma CCK levels and luminal tryptic activities in patients with pancreatic insufficiency. Int J Pancreatol. 1995;17:29–35.

47. Olsen O, Schaffalitzky de Muckadell OB, Cantor P, Erlanson-Albertsson C, Palnaes-Hansen C, Worning H. Effect of trypsin on the hormonal regulation of the fat-stimulated human exocrine pancreas. Scand J Gastroenterol. 1988;23:875–81.

48. Campbell D, Jadunandan I, Curington C, Liddle R, Solomon T, Toskes P. Alcoholic and idiopathic patients with painful chronic pancreatitis do not experience suppression of CCK levels or pain relief following treatment with enteric-coated pancreatin. Gastroenterology. 1992;102:A259.

49. Garces MC, Gomez-Cerezo J, Alba D et al Relationship of basal and postprandial intraduodenal bile acid concentrations and plasma cholecystokinin levels with abdominal pain in patients with chronic pancreatitis. Pancreas. 1998;17:397–401.

50. Garces MC, Gomez-Cerezo J, Codoceo R, Grande C, Barbado J, Vazquez JJ. Postprandial cholecystokinin response in patients with chronic pancreatitis in treatment with oral substitutive pancreatic enzymes. Dig Dis Sci. 1998;43:562–6.

51. Gomez Cerezo J, Codoceo R, Fernandez Calle P, Molina F, Tenias JM, Vazquez JJ. Basal and postprandial cholecystokinin values in chronic pancreatitis with and without abdominal pain. Digestion. 1991;48:134–40.

52. Isaksson G, Ihse I. Pain reduction by an oral pancreatic enzyme preparation in chronic pancreatitis. Dig Dis Sci. 1983;28:97–102.

53. Halgreen H, Pedersen TN, Worning H. Symptomatic effect of pancreatic enzyme therapy in patients with chronic pancreatitis. Scand J Gastroenterol. 1986;21:104–8.

54. Ebbehoj N, Borly L, Buelow J, Rasmussen SG, Madsen P. Evaluation of pancreatic tissue fluid pressure and pain in chronic pancreatitis. A longitudinal study. Scand J Gastroenterol. 1990;25:462–6.
55. Adamek HE, Jakobs R, Buttmann A, Adamek MU, Schneider AR, Riemann JF. Long term follow up of patients with chronic pancreatitis and pancreatic stones treated with extracorporeal shock wave lithotripsy. Gut. 1999;45:402–5.
56. Costamagna G, Gabbrielli A, Mutignani M et al. Extracorporeal shock wave lithotripsy of pancreatic stones in chronic pancreatitis: immediate and medium-term results. Gastrointest Endosc. 1997;46:231–6.
57. Delhaye M, Vandermeeren A, Baize M, Cremer M. Extracorporeal shock-wave lithotripsy of pancreatic calculi. Gastroenterology. 1992;102:610–20.
58. Kozarek RA, Brandabur JJ, Ball TJ et al. Clinical outcomes in patients who undergo extracorporeal shock wave lithotripsy for chronic calcific pancreatitis. Gastrointest Endosc. 2002;56:496–500.
59. Ohara H, Hoshino M, Hayakawa T et al. Single application extracorporeal shock wave lithotripsy is the first choice for patients with pancreatic duct stones. Am J Gastroenterol. 1996;91:1388–94.
60. Sauerbruch T, Holl J, Sackmann M, Paumgartner G. Extracorporeal shock wave lithotripsy of pancreatic stones. Gut. 1989;30:1406–11.
61. Sauerbruch T, Holl J, Sackmann M, Paumgartner G. Extracorporeal lithotripsy of pancreatic stones in patients with chronic pancreatitis and pain: a prospective follow up study. Gut. 1992;33:969–72.
62. Schreiber F, Gurakuqi GC, Pristautz H, Trauner M, Schnedl W. Sonographically-guided extracorporeal shockwave lithotripsy for pancreatic stones in patients with chronic pancreatitis. J Gastroenterol Hepatol. 1996;11:247–51.
63. van der Hul R, Plaisier P, Jeekel J, Terpstra O, den Toom R, Bruining H. Extracorporeal shock-wave lithotripsy of pancreatic duct stones: immediate and long-term results. Endoscopy. 1994;26:573–8.
64. Beger HG, Büchler M, Bittner RR, Oettinger W, Roscher R. Duodenum-preserving resection of the head of the pancreas in severe chronic pancreatitis. Ann Surg. 1989;209:273–8.
65. Malesci A, Gaia E, Fioretta A et al. No effect of long-term treatment with pancreatic extract on recurrent abdominal pain in patients with chronic pancreatitis. Scand J Gastroenterol. 1995;30:392–8.
66. Larvin M, McMahon MJ, Thomas WEG, Puntis MCA. Creon (enteric coated pancreatin microspheres) for the treatment of pain in chronic pancreatitis: a double blind randomised placebo-controlled crossover study. Gastroenterology. 1991;100:A283 (Abstract).
67. Seicean A, Grigorescu M, Tantau M, Dumitrascu DL, Pop D, Mocan T. Pain in chronic pancreatitis: assessment and relief through treatment. Rom J Gastroenterol. 2004;13:9–15.
68. Brown A, Hughes M, Tenner S, Banks PA. Does pancreatic enzyme supplementation reduce pain in patients with chronic pancreatitis: a meta-analysis. Am J Gastroenterol. 1997;92:2032–5.
69. Somogyi L, Toskes PP. Can a meta-analysis that mixes apples with oranges be used to demonstrate that pancreatic enzymes do not decrease abdominal pain in patients with chronic pancreatitis? Am J Gastroenterol. 1998;93:1396–8.
70. Mössner J. Is there a place for pancreatic enzymes in the treatment of pain in chronic pancreatitis? Digestion. 1993;54(Suppl. 2):35–9.
71. Jakobs R, Adamek MU, von Bubnoff AC, Riemann JF. Buprenorphine or procaine for pain relief in acute pancreatitis. A prospective randomized study. Scand J Gastroenterol. 2000;35:1319–23.
72. Kahl S, Zimmermann S, Pross M, Schulz HU, Schmidt U, Malfertheiner P. Procaine hydrochloride fails to relieve pain in patients with acute pancreatitis. Digestion. 2004;69:5–9.
73. Kahl S, Zimmermann S, Genz I et al. Biliary strictures are not the cause of pain in patients with chronic pancreatitis. Pancreas. 2004;28:387–90.
74. World Health Organization. Cancer Pain Relief and Palliative Care: Report of a WHO Expert Committee. Geneva: World Health Organization, 1990, Technical report series 804.

75. Wilder-Smith CH, Hill L, Osler W, O'Keefe S. Effect of tramadol and morphine on pain and gastrointestinal motor function in patients with chronic pancreatitis. Dig Dis Sci. 1999;44:1107–16.
76. Desai PM. Pain relief in chronic pancreatitis with epidural buprenorphine injection. Indian J Gastroenterol. 1997;16:12–13.
77. Niemann T, Madsen LG, Larsen S, Thorsgaard N. Opioid treatment of painful chronic pancreatitis. Int J Pancreatol. 2000;27:235–40.
78. Gress F, Schmitt C, Sherman S, Ikenberry S, Lehman G. A prospective randomized comparison of endoscopic ultrasound- and computed tomography-guided celiac plexus block for managing chronic pancreatitis pain. Am J Gastroenterol. 1999;94:900–5.
79. Madsen P, Hansen E: Coeliac plexus block versus pancreaticogastrostomy for pain in chronic pancreatitis. A controlled randomized trial. Scand J Gastroenterol. 1985;20:1217–20.
80. Dite P, Ruzicka M, Zboril V, Novotny I. A prospective, randomized trial comparing endoscopic and surgical therapy for chronic pancreatitis. Endoscopy. 2003;35:553–8.
81. Rösch T, Daniel S, Scholz M et al. for the European Society of Gastrointestinal Endoscopy Research Group. Endoscopic treatment of chronic pancreatitis: a multicenter study of 1000 patients with long-term follow-up. Endoscopy. 2002;34:765–71.
82. Barthet M, Sahel J, Bodiou-Bertei C, Bernard JP. Endoscopic transpapillary drainage of pancreatic pseudocysts. Gastrointest Endosc. 1995;42:208–13.
83. Cremer M, Deviere J, Delhaye M, Baize M, Vandermeeren A. Stenting in severe chronic pancreatitis: results of medium-term follow-up in seventy-six patients. Endoscopy. 1991;23:171–6.
84. Ell C, Rabenstein T, Schneider HT, Ruppert T, Nicklas M, Bulling D. Safety and efficacy of pancreatic sphincterotomy in chronic pancreatitis. Gastrointest Endosc. 1998;48:244–9.
85. Kozarek RA, Traverso LW. Endoscopic treatment of chronic pancreatitis. An alternative to surgery. Dig Surg. 1996;13:90–100.
86. O'Brien SM, Hatfield AR, Craig PI, Williams SP. A 5-year follow-up of self-expanding metal stents in the endoscopic management of patients with benign bile duct strictures. Eur J Gastroenterol Hepatol. 1998;10:141–5.
87. De las Heras Castano G, Garcia de la Paz A, Fernandez MD, Fernandez Forcelledo JL. Use of antioxidants to treat pain in chronic pancreatitis. Rev Esp Enferm Dig. 2000;92:375–85.
88. Uden S, Bilton D, Nathan L, Hunt LP, Main C, Braganza JM. Antioxidant therapy for recurrent pancreatitis: placebo-controlled trial. Aliment Pharmacol Ther. 1990;4:357–71.
89. Banks PA, Hughes M, Ferrante M, Noordhoek EC, Ramagopal V, Slivka A. Does allopurinol reduce pain of chronic pancreatitis? Int J Pancreatol. 1997;22:171–6.
90. Salim AS. Role of oxygen-derived free radical scavengers in the treatment of recurrent pain produced by chronic pancreatitis. A new approach. Arch Surg. 1991;126:1109–14.

19
Chronic pancreatitis: endoscopic versus surgical procedures for pain relief

N. ALEXAKIS and J. P. NEOPTOLEMOS

INTRODUCTION

The prevalence of chronic pancreatitis varies enormously from 20 to 200 per 10^5 per general population, and there is strong evidence that it is increasing secondary to environmental factors and in particular the rising consumption of alcohol[1-5]. Chronic pancreatitis is a progressive inflammatory process of the pancreas that leads to an irreversible destruction of the gland. Intractable disabling pain is the commonest symptom with a difficult and challenging management[6].

Pain in chronic pancreatitis is highly variable and can be severe, often requiring opioids. In the Mayo Clinic series pain was the predominant symptom in 77% of patients with chronic pancreatitis due to alcohol, 96% in early-onset and 54% in late-onset idiopathic pancreatitis[7]. In the Luneburg series pain persisted in 85% of patients treated conservatively 5 years after diagnosis and in 55% after 10 years follow-up[8]. A study by Amman et al. in the 1980s found that the progressive loss of exocrine function led to a decrease or even complete resolution of the pain in chronic pancreatitis[9], but in the Luneburg study pain relief was not obtained in the majority of patients, even after a long-term observation of more than 10 years[8], so the issue remains controversial.

CAUSES OF PAIN IN CHRONIC PANCREATITIS

The cause of pain is multifactorial, but considerable evidence exists that a major component of the pain syndrome in chronic pancreatitis is due to neural alterations, damage to the perineurium, an increase in neurotransmitters and neuroimmune interactions of inflammatory cells with the damaged nerves[10]. The number and diameter of intralobular and interlobular nerve bundles is increased in pancreatic tissue from patients with chronic pancreatitis[11].

Neurotransmitters such as calcitonin gene-related peptide and substance P are overexpressed in fibres contained in these nerves[12]. In chronic pancreatitis, GAP-43 (growth-associated protein 43, a marker of neural plasticity) is significantly increased in pancreatic nerve fibres and intrinsic neurons, and correlates with individual pain scores[13]. The infiltration of pancreatic nerves by immune cells is significantly correlated with the intensity of pain[13]. Nerve growth factor (NGF) and tyrosine kinase receptor A (TrkA) mRNA expression are increased 13-fold and 5.5-fold respectively in chronic pancreatitis, and there is a significant relation between (TrkA) mRNA and pain intensity[14].

Older theories include increased intraductal pressure[15], whilst the compartment syndrome hypothesis (that pain is due to increased ductal and parenchymal pressure that induces ischaemia) is supported in only one experimental study in cats[16]. Pain may also be due to pseudocysts, biliary tract or duodenal obstruction and malabsorption, although a study from Germany found that successful endoscopic drainage of biliary obstruction had no influence on the pain in these patients[17]. An issue further complicating pain management was raised by DiMagno, i.e. that differences in pain patterns may affect response to pain management: patients with intermittent pain appeared to have a favourable course without surgery[18].

GENERAL MANAGEMENT OF PAIN IN CHRONIC PANCREATITIS

Before endoscopic or surgical intervention is considered in chronic pancreatitis it is important that there is optimum medical therapy including enzyme supplements, treatment of diabetes mellitus (almost invariably needing insulin), proton pump-blockade, mild to moderate analgesia and psychosocial support. An American Gastroenterological Association technical review in 1998 concluded that a variety of medical treatments – including high-dose pancreas enzyme supplements, antioxidants, allopurinol, and octreotide – had no benefit in controlling pain in chronic pancreatitis[19].

Percutaneous coeliac plexus block

Busch et al. evaluated 16 patients with chronic pancreatitis in whom percutaneous coeliac plexus block with depot steroid was used to treat pain. Only four patients reported pain relief with the procedure. Of the 12 patients who did not obtain relief, narcotic dependence was present in 11, whereas no patient who obtained pain relief group was narcotic-dependent. Prior pancreatic surgery was present in nine of the 12 patients without relief and in only one of the four patients with relief. These results underscored the poor results experienced using neural blockade for the relief of chronic pain when narcotic dependence was present[20]. Leung et al. performed percutaneous coeliac plexus block for disabling pain in 36 patients – 13 with cancer and 23 with chronic pancreatitis. While 11 of the cancer patients had complete pain relief initially, and seven remained pain-free at the time of death, only 12 of the patients with chronic pancreatitis had complete pain relief, six had partial relief and there was no effect in five patients. The mean pain-free period in the chronic pancreatitis patients was only 2 months, and the longest 4 months. The benefit was least in patients with previous pancreatic surgery, and repeat blocks were unhelpful. Transient postural hypotension occurred in most patients; two had nerve root pain and one developed persistent weakness and anaesthesia of the left leg, with bladder disturbance. The authors concluded that coeliac plexus block was rarely indicated in chronic pancreatitis[21].

The American Gastroenterological Association in 1998 has proposed an algorithm[22] that may serve as a guideline for the management of pain in chronic pancreatitis (Figure 1).

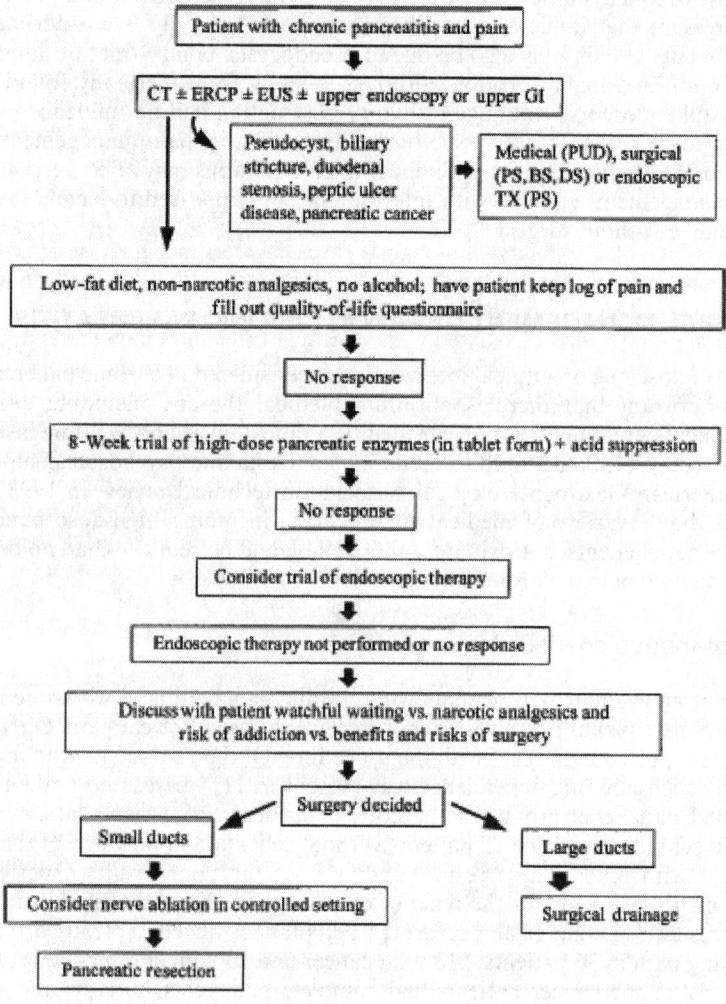

Figure 1 Management of pain in chronic pancreatitis from the American Gastroenterological Association medical position statement[22]

ENDOSCOPIC PROCEDURES FOR PAIN RELIEF

Endoscopy may be used to effect treatment: (a) by relieving main pancreatic duct obstruction caused by stones and/or strictures, (b) by drainage of the biliary tree, (c) by drainage of pancreatic pseudocysts and (c) for coeliac plexus block under endoluminal ultrasound guidance.

Endoscopic treatment of pancreatic stones and strictures

The main endoscopic approaches include pancreatic sphincterotomy, stone removal from the pancreatic duct, extracorporeal shockwave lithotripsy and pancreatic duct stenting of strictures. Many of the earlier endoscopic studies reported pain relief after pancreatic stone removal, but were uncontrolled, not always successful, with a high rate of complications, patients often had pain relapse and the follow-up was short. Endoscopic pancreatic sphincterotomy in chronic pancreatitis is relatively safe and has a high success rate[23]. Jakobs et al. successfully performed endoscopic pancreatic sphincterotomy in 167 (97.7%) of 171 patients. In 24 (14%) patients a precut technique was necessary using a needle-knife sphincterotome. Sphincterotomy-related complications occurred in only seven (4.1%) patients, including three cases of bleeding, three patients with mild pancreatitis and one with retroduodenal perforation, all of whom were managed medically; there was no treatment-related mortality.

The main problems associated with stenting of the main pancreatic duct are the need for frequent stent changes due to occlusion and the stent-induced parenchymal and ductal changes[24]. In a study from the University of Alabama 25 patients had 40 stent placement episodes. In 28 (70%) of the 40 episodes the main pancreatic duct calibre increased or was unchanged after stenting, and pain improved after 20 (71%) of these 28 procedures. Pain improved in six (50%) 12 patients with smaller ducts after stenting. Unfortunately most pancreatic stents were occluded upon retrieval and stent-induced strictures developed in 18%[24]. In addition, the cost of the repeated hospitalizations was substantive.

Binmoeller et al. treated 93 patients (65 men, mean age 49 years) with narcotic-dependent pain (mean history of 5.6 years) due to chronic pancreatitis and with a dominant pancreatic duct stricture visualized by endoscopic retrograde cholangiopancreatography by stent drainage over a 9-year period[25]. Sixty-nine (74%) patients reported complete (46 patients) or partial (23 patients) pain relief at 6 months. In this group of early responders, 60 patients experienced sustained improvement during a mean follow-up of 4.9 years and the other nine had recurrent pain after a mean of 1.2 years[25]. Stents were removed in 49 patients after a mean of 15.7 months, of whom 36 remained pain-free during a mean follow-up of 3.8 years[25]. Eleven of the 13 patients who relapsed were retreated by endoscopic drainage and subsequently became pain-free[25]. Procedure-related complications included mild pancreatitis in four and abscess formation secondary to stent blockage in two others[25].

Smits et al. evaluated the long-term results of endoscopic pancreatic stone removal in 53 patients with chronic pancreatitis, 33 with multiple and 20 with single stone with proximal dilation of the pancreatic duct (1984–1993)[26]. Thirty patients presented with pain and 23 with an exacerbation of chronic pancreatitis. A sphincterotomy was performed in 41 patients and a nasopancreatic drain was left *in situ* for saline flushing in six patients. A pancreatic stent was inserted beyond the stones in 28 patients. Fragmentation of stones was performed by mechanical lithotripsy in four patients or by extracorporeal shockwave lithotripsy in eight patients. Stone removal was successful in 42 (79%) patients, complete in 39 and partial in three patients. At a median (range) follow-up of 33 (4–131) months there was relief of symptoms in 38 (90%) and the remaining four patients had pancreatic surgery. Stone removal failed in 11 patients but three of these patients had symptomatic improvement. Of the remaining patients four needed pancreatic surgery and four continued conservative treatment. Thirteen of the 53 patients (25%) had recurrent stones, which could be removed endoscopically in 10 of 13. Procedure-related complications occurred in five (9%) patients, and seven (25%) of the 28 stented patients had stent-related complications[26].

Dumonceau et al. evaluated pancreatic sphincterotomy and attempted stone removal in 70 patients with chronic pancreatitis[27]. Complete ductal clearance of calculi was obtained in 50% of cases and immediate clinical improvement occurred in 95% of patients with painful attacks. No severe complications or mortality occurred. Fifty-four per cent of all patients with painful chronic pancreatitis did not experience any pain recurrence within 2 years. Statistically significant associations were ductal clearance and extracorporeal shockwave lithotripsy, pain disappearance and ductal clearance, pain recurrence and long history and severe disease before treatment and presence of a ductal substenosis. It was concluded that the best results were obtained when endoscopic treatment was performed early in the course of chronic calcifying pancreatitis[27].

In a study from Germany, extracorporeal shockwave lithotripsy had little effect on pain relief in chronic pancreatitis[28]. Only 43 of 80 patients were treated successfully with extracorporeal shockwave lithotripsy and 37 patients were not. The only feature associated with treatment success was the presence of a single stone rather than multiple stones. Successfully treated patients tended to experience less pain, although this did not reach statistical significance. A slight increase in weight was noted in our patients; however, there was no notable improvement in steatorrhoea or diabetes mellitus. Five patients died due to extrapancreatic reasons. No pancreatic carcinomas developed. It was concluded that pancreatic drainage by endoscopy and extracorporeal shockwave lithotripsy had almost no effect on pain in chronic pancreatitis. Furthermore, endoscopic management and extracorporeal shockwave lithotripsy did not prevent or postpone the development of pancreatic insufficiency[28].

The European Society of Gastrointestinal Endoscopy Research Group published in 2002 the results of a multicentre study of 1018 patients with painful chronic pancreatitis with ductal obstruction due to either strictures and/or stones treated endoscopically[29]. Endotherapy consisted of pancreatic sphincterotomy and stenting and/or extracorporeal shockwave lithotripsy. Follow-up data were obtained from 1018 of 1211 patients treated (84%) with mainly strictures (47%), stones (18%), or strictures plus stones (32%). After a mean (range) of 4.9 (2–12) years of follow-up, 60% of the patients had completed endotherapy, 16% were still receiving some form of endoscopic treatment, and 238 (24%) had undergone surgery. The long-term success of endotherapy was 86% in the entire group, but only 65% in an intention-to-treat analysis and pancreatic function was not improved by endoscopic therapy.

Endoscopic drainage of the biliary tree

Endoscopic therapy is relatively unsuccessful in the treatment of symptomatic main bile duct strictures caused by chronic pancreatitis. In a study from the University of Magdeburg, 61 patients with symptomatic strictures of the main bile duct caused by alcoholic chronic pancreatitis were treated by endoscopic stent insertion for 1 year with scheduled stent changes every 3 months[30]. Initial endoscopic drainage was successful in all cases, with complete resolution of the obstructive jaundice. After 1 year from the initial stent insertion the obstruction had resolved in 19 patients (31.1%) and stents were removed without any need of additional procedures. During a median (range) follow-up of 40 (18–66) months, 16 patients had no symptomatic recurrence of the bile duct stricture, giving a long term success rate 26.2%[30]. Of the 45 patients who needed definitive therapy, 12 (19.7%) were treated with repeated plastic stent insertion, three (4.9%) with insertion of a metal stent and 30 (49.2%) patients underwent surgery[17]. Calcification of the pancreatic head was the only factor that was found to be of prognostic value. Of 39 patients with calcification of the pancreatic head, only three (7.7%) were successfully treated, whereas in 13 (59.1%) of 22 patients without calcification, this treatment was successful[30]. Patients with calcification had a 17-fold increased risk of failure at 12 months from endoscopic stenting[30]. It was concluded that endoscopic drainage of biliary obstruction provided excellent short-term but only moderate long-term results, and it was patients without calcification of the pancreatic head who largely benefited from biliary stenting[30]. Similarly in a study from the University of Amsterdam the success rate of biliary stenting was only 28% after 49 months[26].

Endoscopic drainage of pancreatic pseudocysts

The results for endoscopic drainage are generally good, with a technical success rate between 80% and 90% for transmural pseudocystgastrostomy and pseudocystduodenostomy, and almost 85% for transpapillary methods[31]. In a recent review[31] of 17 endoscopic series comprising a total of 466 patients, 327 (70.2%) had a transmural approach, 111 (23.8%) had a transpapillary (transgastric or transduodenal) and 25 (5.4%) had a combined transmural and transpapillary approach with overall morbidity in 62 (13.3%) patients and only one death (0.2%)[32–48]. Complications may require emergency surgery; thus an experienced pancreatic surgical team and expert interventional radiology should always be available at short notice when these techniques are being undertaken. Although the published mortality rate is now less than 1% this appears biased in favour of experienced endoscopic teams and highly selected cases[31]. The endoscopic approach failed or surgery was needed in only 72 (15.4%) patients and recurrence occurred in 50 (10.7%) patients[31].

Endoluminal ultrasound-guided coeliac plexus block

A randomized trial of coeliac plexus neurolysis for controlling chronic abdominal pain associated with intra-abdominal malignancy and chronic pancreatitis compared computed tomography with endoluminal ultrasound to guide the block[49]. The endoluminal ultrasound coeliac block was performed with a 22-gauge sterile needle inserted into the coeliac region with guidance of real-time linear array endosonography followed by injection of 10 ml of bupivacaine (0.75%) and 3 ml (40 mg) of triamcinolone on both sides of the coeliac area. Four out of 22 consecutive patients (10 men, 12 women) randomized were excluded for protocol violations: endoluminal ultrasound-guided coeliac block was performed in 10 patients and computed tomography-guided coeliac block in eight. A significant improvement in pain scores with reduction in pain medication usage occurred in five (50%) of 10 of patients having the endoluminal ultrasound block. The mean (range) post-procedure follow-up was 15 (8–24) weeks. Persistent benefit was experienced by 40% of patients at 8 weeks and by 30% at 24 weeks. In the patients with computed tomography block, however, only two (25%) of eight had relief. The mean follow-up was 4 (2–6) weeks. Only one (12%) of eight patients had some relief at 12 weeks of follow-up. There were no complications. Endoluminal ultrasound-guided coeliac block was the preferred technique among patients who experienced both techniques. A cost comparison between the two techniques showed endoluminal ultrasound to be less costly than computed tomography[49].

The same group subsequently evaluated endoluminal ultrasound-guided coeliac plexus block in the treatment of abdominal pain associated with chronic pancreatitis in 90 patients (40 men and 50 women) with a mean (range) age of 45 (17–76) years[50]. Endoluminal ultrasound was performed by linear array endosonography using a 22-gauge needle (GIP, Mediglobe Inc., Tempe, AZ) inserted on each side of the coeliac area, followed by injection of 10 ml bupivacaine (0.25%) and 3 ml (40 mg) triamcinolone on each side of the coeliac plexus[50]. A significant improvement in overall pain scores occurred in 50 (55%) of the patients with a mean pain score decrease from 8 to 2 post-endoluminal ultrasound coeliac block at both 4 and 8 weeks follow-up[25]. In 26% of patients there was persistent benefit beyond 12 weeks but only 10% had a persistent benefit at 24 weeks; only three patients were pain-free between 35 and 48 weeks[50]. Younger patients, less than 45 years of age, and those having previous pancreatic surgery for chronic pancreatitis were unlikely to respond to the endoluminal ultrasound-guided coeliac block[50].

SURGICAL PROCEDURES FOR PAIN RELIEF

Approximately half of the patients with chronic pancreatitis will undergo some form of surgery. In the Mayo series 40% of the patients with alcoholic chronic pancreatitis and 42% with idiopathic chronic pancreatitis required surgery for pain relief[7], and in the Liverpool series 48% of the referred patients underwent pancreas resection[51]. The two main indications for surgery are chronic intractable abdominal pain and complications from chronic pancreatitis itself, including pseudocyst, biliary and duodenal obstruction, pancreatic ascites, pancreatic fistula, hepatic portal venous compression or occlusion, sinistral portal hypertension and pseudoaneurysm[31,52–54]. Another indication is suspicion of pancreatic malignancy because there is a 10–25-fold increased incidence of pancreatic ductal adenocarcinoma in sporadic forms of chronic pancreatitis and a 40–70-fold risk in hereditary pancreatitis[55–58]. Surgery may be used to: (a) divide the sympathetic nerves that carry afferent nerve fibres from the pancreas in the chest, (b) drain the main pancreatic duct, (c) drain pancreatic pseudocysts, (d) bypass of duodenal or biliary obstruction and (e) remove part or all of the pancreas.

Bilateral thoracoscopic splanchnicectomy

In 1990 Stone and Chauvin evaluated 15 patients with intractable pain of chronic alcohol-induced pancreatitis who underwent left transthoracic splanchnicectomy with concomitant bilateral truncal vagotomy[59]. All were malnourished, 11 were addicted to opiates and no respite had been obtained from 33 previous operative procedures. Each patient experienced almost immediate pain relief. Five, however, later had return of pain, but only to the right epigastrium. These five then underwent right transthoracic splanchnicectomy, after which four noted complete and apparently permanent disappearance of pain. At a mean follow-up of 16 months there was a 29% mean increase in body weight in those 14 with a successful outcome, elimination of strong opiate usage in 10 of the 11 patients and a return to gainful work or a relatively normal lifestyle in all 14. Although 11 of the 14 patients had delayed gastric emptying, only one has required a drainage procedure and there have been no other late complications[59].

This open transthoracic approach was subsequently superseded by a minimally invasive technique called bilateral thoracoscopic splanchnicectomy, that divides the greater, lesser and least splanchnic nerves in the chest and can be performed as an outpatient procedure. Bilateral thoracoscopic splanchnicectomy provides good short-term pain relief in about 50% of patients – especially in those with no prior intervention (Table 1). The benefit reduces in the long term[60–63], although there are a few reports of around 50% success at 43 and 48 months[64,65], but benefit continues to decline thereafter[63]. Patients with 'sympathetic'-type pain have pain improvement which is maintained in the mid-term but patients with 'somatic'-type pain have no benefit at all[66].

Pancreatic duct drainage procedures

Lateral pancreatojejunostomy is generally associated with low mortality (0–5%) and morbidity, but requires dilated ducts of at least 6–7 mm diameter to effect[67]. A review of 599 patients who underwent lateral pancreatojejunostomy from collected series showed a good to moderate result for pain relief in 478 (80%) patients in the short and medium term[67]. Unfortunately the long-term results are unsatisfactory, with only 50–66% of patients remaining pain-free at 5 years after operation[68–71].

Table 1   Results of thoracoscopic sympathectomy in patients with chronic pancreatitis

Series	Year	No. of patients	Unilateral/ bilateral	Opioid use	Success	Follow-up
Stone and Chauvin[59]	1988	15	10/5	11 (73%)	93%	16 months
Bradley et al.[66]	1998	16	5/11	16 (100%)	8 (50%)	23 months
Ihse et al.[64]	1999	21	0/21	14 (67%)	50%	42 months
Leksowski[61]	2001	20	16/4	20 (100%)	16 (80%)	6 months
Maher et al.[63]	2001	15	9/6	11 (73%)	0%	5.7 years
Howard et al.[60]	2002	55	0/55	NA	17 (31%)	12 months
Buscher et al.[65]	2002	44	0/44	36 (82%)	46%	36 months
Hammond et al.[62]	2004	20	0/20	20 (100%)	12 (60%)	15 months

Nealon and Thompson reported a small randomized trial of 17 patients with a dilated main pancreatic duct and mild to moderate chronic pancreatitis, nine of whom had lateral pancreatojejunostomy and eight being treated medically[72]. After a mean follow-up of 39 months, seven (78%) of nine operated patients retained their functional status and two (22%) developed severe chronic pancreatitis, whereas only two (25%) of eight patients randomized to medical treatment preserved their functional grade and six (75%) developed severe chronic pancreatitis[72].

In a separate evaluation of 143 patients followed up for a mean of 47.3 months there were 83 with mild to moderate chronic pancreatitis at initial evaluation and 60 with severe chronic pancreatitis. Eighty-seven patients underwent lateral pancreatojejunostomy to relieve abdominal pain, of whom 47 were in the mild to moderate group and 40 were in the severe group; the remainder were treated medically. No patient with severe chronic pancreatitis improved during follow-up, namely 40 treated by lateral pancreatojejunostomy and 20 medically. In contrast in patients with mild to moderate chronic pancreatitis this grade was preserved in 41 (87%) of 47 operated patients (six or 13% became severe) but in only eight (22%) of the 36 non-operated patients (28 or 78% became severe). These data support a policy of early operative drainage before the development of irreversible functional impairment in patients with chronic pancreatitis and associated dilation of the main pancreatic duct[72].

Drainage of pancreatic pseudocysts

The indications for surgical internal drainage of pancreatic pseudocysts include: contraindication or failure of endoscopic and radiological methods, pseudocysts with complex or multiple main pancreatic duct strictures, associated complex pathology such as an inflammatory mass in the head of the pancreas, pseudocysts with a main bile duct stricture, venous occlusive disease, multiple pseudocysts and most pseudocysts of the pancreatic tail[31]. In a recent collective review[31] of the surgical drainage of pancreatic pseudocysts in 321 patients the morbidity was 16% (complications in 25 out of 157 patients with data) and a mortality of 2.5% (eight deaths). The techniques included pseudocystjejunostomy with a 92% success rate (186 out of 172 patients treated), pseudocystgastrostomy with a 90% success rate (96 out of 107 patients treated) and pseudocystduodenostomy with 100% success rate (28 out of 28 patients treated). The long-term recurrence rates were also very low, being 8.5% (3/153), 12% (10/82) and 0% (0/28) respectively[73–80].

Bypass of biliary or duodenal obstruction

According to a recent collective review, in hospitalized patients with chronic pancreatitis the incidence of biliary stricture and duodenal obstruction is reported to be about 6% (based on 4497 patients) and 1.2% (based on 3729 patients), respectively, rising to 35% for biliary stricture and 12% for duodenal obstruction for patients requiring an operation[81]. The incidence of acute cholangitis and biliary cirrhosis in these patients is about 10% in each case (based on 777 and 256 patients, respectively). Operation is indicated in patients with common bile duct strictures secondary to chronic pancreatitis when there is evidence of cholangitis, biliary cirrhosis, common duct stones, progression of stricture, elevation of alkaline phosphatase and/or bilirubin for over a month and an inability to rule out cancer. The operation of choice is either choledochoduodenostomy or choledochojejunostomy with failure rates of only 2.5% and 2.1%, respectively. A cholecystenterostomy is less favoured because of its much higher failure rate in 23%. For duodenal obstruction, failure to resolve the obstruction after 2 weeks of conservative therapy is an indication for bypass, a gastrojejunostomy. Not uncommonly there is combined obstruction of the pancreatic duct, main bile duct and duodenum when combined drainage procedures or resection are used[81].

Pancreatic resection

During the past decade there have been major changes in the surgical management of chronic pancreatitis: (a) surgical techniques had undergone refinement[82–96], (b) mortality from surgical resection is low (1–5%)[82–96], (c) limited resection of the dominant focus of the disease may help break the cycle of pain[83] and (d) there is a move towards preservation of the adjacent structures during pancreatic resection: duodenum, spleen, stomach[82,83,95,97]. Pancreatic resection is now generally recognized as achieving the best results for intractable pain (long-term pain relief 70–95% of patients) and the local complications of chronic pancreatitis[53,54,68,69,82–96,98].

There is level I evidence that 'lesser' operations (duodenum-preserving pancreatic head resection) have replaced the major resections as surgical standards in the majority of cases. These procedures allow the preservation of exocrine and endocrine pancreatic function, provide pain relief in up to 90% of patients, and contribute to an improvement in the quality of life. Radical operations such as the Kausch–Whipple procedure have lost ground to organ-preserving operations.

In a randomized controlled trial from Hamburg, longitudinal pancreatojejunostomy with local pancreatic head excision (the Frey procedure) and the pylorus-preserving pancreatoduodenectomy provided the same pain relief (94–95%) and equal control of complications to adjacent organs, but the Frey procedure was better with regard to hospital morbidity (19% versus 53%) and quality of life (71% versus 43%)[90]. Studies further suggest that the duodenum-preserving pancreatic head resection (Beger operation) is better than the pylorus-preserving pancreatoduodenectomy. In the Berne trial the Beger operation had less morbidity (15% vs 20%) and, after 6 months, patients in the Beger group had less pain, greater weight gain, a better glucose tolerance and a higher insulin secretion capacity[84,99]. Data from a recent prospective study also found that the Beger procedure provided better results in the treatment of chronic pancreatitis than pancreatoduodenectomy in terms of quality of life, pain intensity as self-assessed by the patients, nutritional status, and length of hospital stay[100]. A randomized controlled trial from Hamburg comparing the Beger with the Frey operation found that the two procedures were equally effective in terms of pain relief, control of local complications and quality of life[89]. Resection but not drainage is also beneficial in the restoration of normal venous blood flow in the splenic–portal axis in cases of segmental portal hypertension[101]. Surgery in patients with intractable pain and vascular complications is high-risk but worthwhile[102,103]. Although there is an increase in morbidity, and indeed operative mortality, the long-term results are similar between those with and without vascular complications[102,103].

Total pancreatectomy (preferably with preservation of the duodenum and spleen) is indicated for patients with disabling pain for whom partial resection has failed, or for those with total endocrine and exocrine pancreatic failure[82]. The operation is also indicated as prophylaxis against cancer in hereditary pancreatitis. A contraindication is the presence or fear of pancreatic malignancy. The operation has acceptable morbidity and mortality with a reduction in pain and analgesic use after surgery, and weight gain[82]. Simultaneous islet autotransplantation during total pancreatectomy has a moderate success in rendering the patients insulin-independent[104,105].

Surgery is also beneficial in patients with prior narcotic use. In a study from the University of Liverpool, 21 (46%) patients with opioid use had a total pancreatectomy compared to nine (13.6%) without, and they had a higher frequency of postoperative bleeding and early reoperation. Mortality and overall morbidity, however, were not significantly different between the two groups. There was pain improvement in both groups (78% and 93%, respectively) during a median follow-up of 12 months. Twenty per cent of patients who used preoperative opioids, however, reverted to morphine use, compared to only 6% of patients who had not used opioids[51].

Randomized controlled trial of surgery versus endoscopic treatment for chronic pancreatitis

There has been only one prospective randomized trial of endoscopic versus surgical procedures; this was published in 2003[106]. This Czech group randomized 72 patients with painful obstructive chronic pancreatitis to either surgery (36 patients) or endoscopic therapy (36 patients). Surgery consisted mainly of resections for localized disease and drainage procedures for disease with ductal dilation. Endoscopic therapy consisted of pancreatic sphincterotomy, dilation of strictures, stenting and/or stone extraction. After 5 years of follow-up there was a significant difference with regard to pain (complete relief in 33.8% of the surgery group versus 15% in the endoscopy group) and body weight (increase in 47.2% in the surgery group versus 28.6% in the endoscopy group) between groups. The rate of development of new-onset diabetes mellitus was similar between the groups, 38.8% in the surgery group versus 34.2% in the endoscopy group. The conclusion was that surgery was superior to endoscopic therapy, and it is noteworthy that this paper was written by gastroenterologists.

CONCLUSIONS

The management of pain in chronic pancreatitis still represents a major challenge, and endoscopic measures have a limited role to play, particularly in patients with relatively simple problems such as a dilated main pancreatic duct with a simple stricture or single stone and uncomplicated pseudocysts. Although surgical approaches have the best long-term results these are still less than satisfactory, as the procedures continue to have a high morbidity and a small but not insignificant mortality. The optimum results are obtained in a multidisciplinary setting, including gastroenterologists, radiologists and pain specialists, as well as dedicated surgeons.

References

1. Dite P, Stary K, Novotny I et al. Incidence of chronic pancreatitis in the Czech Republic. Eur J Gastroenterol Hepatol. 2001;13:749–50.
2. Dufour M, Adamson M. The epidemiology of alcohol-induced pancreatitis. Pancreas. 2003;27:286.
3. Garg P, Tandon R. Survey on chronic pancreatitis in the Asia-Pacific region. J Gastroenterol Hepatol. 2004;19:998–1004.
4. Otsuki M. Chronic pancreatitis in Japan: epidemiology, prognosis, diagnostic criteria, and future problems. J Gastroenterol. 2003;38:315–26.
5. Tinto A, Lloyd D, Kang J et al. Acute and chronic pancreatitis – diseases on the rise: a study of hospital admissions in England 1989/90–1999/2000. Aliment Pharmacol Ther. 2002;16:2097–105.
6. Etemad B, Whitcomb D. Chronic pancreatitis: diagnosis, classification and new genetic developments. Gastroenterology. 2001;120:682–707.
7. Layer P, Yamamoto H, Kalthoff L, Clain J, Bakken L, DiMagno E. The different courses of early- and late-onset idiopathic and alcoholic chronic pancreatitis. Gastroenterology. 1994; 107:1481–7.
8. Lankisch P, Lohr-Happe A, Otto J, Creutzfeldt W. Natural course in chronic pancreatitis. Pain, exocrine and endocrine pancreatic insufficiency and prognosis of the disease. Digestion. 1993;54:148–55.
9. Ammann R, Akovbiantz A, Largiader F, Schueler G. Course and outcome of chronic pancreatitis. Longitudinal study of a mixed medical–surgical series of 245 patients. Gastroenterology. 1984;86:820–8.
10. Friess H, Shrikhande M, Martignoni M et al. Neural alterations in surgical stage chronic pancreatitis are independent of the underlying aetiology. Gut. 2002;50:682–6.
11. Bockman D, Büchler M, Malfertheiner P, Beger H. Analysis of nerves in chronic pancreatitis. Gastroenterology. 1988;94:1459–69.
12. Büchler M, Weihe E, Friess H et al. Changes in peptidergic innervation in chronic pancreatitis. Pancreas. 1992;7:183–92.
13. Di Sebastiano P, Fink T, Weihe E et al. Immune cell infiltration and growth- associated protein 43 expression correlate with pain in chronic pancreatitis. Gastroenterology. 1997; 112:1649–55.

14. Friess H, Zhou Z, di Mola F et al. Nerve growth factor and its high affinity receptor in chronic pancreatitis. Ann Surg. 1999;230:615–24.
15. Okazaki K, Yamamoto Y, Kagiyama S et al. Pressure of papillary sphincter zone and pancreatic main duct in patients with chronic pancreatitis in the early stage. Scand J Gastroenterol. 1988;23:501–7.
16. Karanjia N, Widdison A, Leung F, Alvarez C, Lutrin F, Reber H. Compartment syndrome in experimental chronic obstructive pancreatitis: effect of decompressing the main pancreatic duct. Br J Surg. 1994;81:259–64.
17. Kahl S, Zimmermann S, Genz I et al. Biliary strictures are not the cause of pain in patients with chronic pancreatitis. Pancreas. 2004;28:387–90.
18. DiMagno E. Towards understanding (and management) of painful chronic pancreatitis. Gastroenterology. 1999;116:1252–7.
19. Warshaw A, Banks P, Fernandez-Del Castillo P. AGA technical review: Treatment of pain in chronic pancreatitis. Gastroenterology. 1998;115:765–76.
20. Busch E, Atchison S. Steroid celiac plexus block for chronic pancreatitis: results in 16 cases. J Clin Anesth. 1989;1:431–3.
21. Leung J, Bowen-Wright M, Aveling W, Shorvon P, Cotton P. Celiac plexus block for pain in pancreatic cancer and chronic pancreatitis. Br J Surg. 1983;70:730–2.
22. Anonymous. American Gastroenterological Association medical position statement: treatment of pain in chronic pancreatitis. Gastroenterology. 1998;115:763–4.
23. Jakobs R, Benz C, Leonhardt A, Schilling D, Pereira-Lima J, Riemann J. Pancreatic endoscopic sphincterotomy in patients with chronic pancreatitis: a single-center experience in 171 consecutive patients. Endoscopy. 2002;34:551–4.
24. Morgan D, Smith J, Wilcox C. Endoscopic stent therapy in advanced chronic pancreatitis: relationships between ductal changes, clinical response, and stent patency. Am J Gastroenterol. 2003;98:821–6.
25. Binmoeller K, Jue P, Seifert H, Nam W, Izbicki J, Soehendra N. Endoscopic pancreatic stent drainage in chronic pancreatitis and a dominant stricture: long-term results. Endoscopy. 1995;27:638–44.
26. Smits M, Rauws A, Tytgat N, Huibregtse K. Endoscopic treatment of pancreatic stones in patients with chronic pancreatitis. Gastrointest Endosc. 1996;43:556–60.
27. Dumonceau J, Deviere J, Le Moine O et al. Endoscopic pancreatic drainage in chronic pancreatitis associated with ductal stones: long-term results. Gastrointest Endosc. 1996;43: 547–55.
28. Adamek H, Jakobs R, Buttmann A, Adamek M, Schneider A, Riemann J. Long term follow up of patients with chronic pancreatitis and pancreatic stones treated with extracorporeal shock wave lithotripsy. Gut. 1999;45:402–5.
29. Rosch T, Daniel S, Scholz M et al. Endoscopic treatment of chronic pancreatitis: a multicenter study of 1000 patients with long-term follow-up. Endoscopy. 2002;34:765–71.
30. Kahl S, Zimmermann S, Genz I et al. Risk factors for failure of endoscopic stenting of biliary strictures in chronic pancreatitis: a prospective follow-up study. Am J Gastroenterol. 2003;98:2448–53.
31. Rosso E, Alexakis N, Ghaneh P et al. Pancreatic pseudocyst in chronic pancreatitis: endoscopic and surgical treatment. Dig Surg. 2003;20:397–406.
32. Baron T, Harewood G, Morgan D, Yates M. Outcome differences after endoscopic drainage of pancreatic necrosis, acute pancreatic pseudocysts, and chronic pancreatic pseudocysts. Gastrointest Endosc. 2002;56:7–17.
33. Barthet M, Bugallo M, Moreira L, Bastid C, Sastre B, Sahel J. Traitements des pseudokystes de pancreatique aigue. Etude retrospective de 45 patients. Gastroenterol Clin Biol. 1992;16:853–9.
34. Bejanin H, Liguory C, Ink O. Endoscopic drainage of pseudocysts of the pancreas. Study of 26 cases. Gastroenterol Clin Biol. 1993;17:804–10.
35. Binmoeller K, Seifert H, Walter A, Soehendra N. Transpapillary and transmural drainage of pancreatic pseudocysts. Gastrointest Endosc. 1995;42:219–24.
36. Cremer M, Deviere J, Engelholm L. Endoscopic management of cysts and pseudocysts in chronic pancreatitis: long-term follow-up after 7 years of experience. Gastrointest Endosc. 1989;35:1–9.
37. Deviere J, Bueso H, Baize M et al. Complete disruption of the main pancreatic duct: endoscopic management. Gastrointest Endosc. 1995;42:445–51.

38. Funnell I, Bornmann P, Krige J, Beningfield S, Terblanche J. Endoscopic drainage of traumatic pseudocyst. Br J Surg. 1994;81:879–81.
39. Giovannini M, Pesenti C, Rolland A, Moutardier V, Delpero J. Endoscopic ultrasound-guided drainage of pancreatic pseudocysts or pancreatic abscesses using a therapeutic echo endoscope. Endoscopy. 2001;33:473–7.
40. Kozarek R, Brakyo C, Harlan J, Sanowski R, Cintora I, Kovac A. Endoscopic drainage of pancreatic pseudocysts. Gastrointest Endosc. 1985;31:322-328.
41. Kozarek R, Ball T, Patterson D, Freeny P, Ryan J, Traverso L. Endoscopic transpapillary therapy for disrupted pancreatic duct and peripancreatic fluid collections. Gastroenterology. 1991;100:1362-1370.
42. Libera E, Siqueira E, Morais M et al. Pancreatic pseudocysts transpapillary and transmural drainage. HPB Surg. 2000;11:333–8.
43. Norton I, Clain J, Wiersema M, DiMagno E, Petersen B, Gostout C. Utility of endoscopic ultrasonography in endoscopic drainage of pancreatic pseudocysts in selected patients. Mayo Clin Proc. 2001;76:794–8.
44. Sahel J, Bastid C, Pellat P, Schurgers P, Sarles H. Endoscopic cystoduodenostomy of cysts of chronic calcifying pancreatitis. Report of 20 cases. Pancreas. 1987;2:447–53.
45. Sharma S, Bhargawa N, Govil A. Endoscopic management of pancreatic pseudocyst: a long-term follow up. Endoscopy. 2002;34:203–7.
46. Smits M, Rauws E, Tygat G, Huibregtse K. The efficacy of endoscopic treatment of pancreatic pseudocysts. Gastrointest Endosc. 1995;42:202–7.
47. Vitale G, Lawhon J, Larson G, Harrel D, Reed D, MacLeod S. Endoscopic drainage of the pancreatic pseudocysts. Surgery. 1999;126:616–23.
48. White S, Sutton C, Berry D, Chillistone D, Rees Y, Dennison A. Experience of combined endoscopic percutaneous stenting with ultrasound guidance for drainage of pancreatic pseudocysts. Ann R Coll Surg Engl. 2000;82:11–15.
49. Gress F, Schmitt C, Sherman S, Ikenberry S, Lehman G. A prospective randomized comparison of endoscopic ultrasound- and computed tomography-guided celiac plexus block for managing chronic pancreatitis pain. Am J Gastroenterol. 1999;94:900–5.
50. Gress F, Schmitt C, Sherman S, Ciaccia D, Ikenberry S, Lehman G. Endoscopic ultrasound-guided celiac plexus block for managing abdominal pain associated with chronic pancreatitis: a prospective single center experience. Am J Gastroenterol. 2001;96:409–16.
51. Alexakis N, Connor S, Ghaneh P et al. Influence of opioid use on surgical and long term outcome following resection for chronic pancreatitis. Surgery. 2004;136:600–8.
52. Neoptolemos J, Winslet M. Pancreatic ascites. In Beger H, Büchler M, Ditschuneit H, Malfertheiner P, editors. Chronic Pancreatitis. Berlin: Springer-Verlag, 1990:268–79.
53. Neoptolemos J, Ghaneh P, Sutton R et al. Integrated radiology for surgical resection in chronic pancreatitis. In: Büchler M, Friess H, Malfertheiner P, editors. Chronic Pancreatitis: Novel Concepts in Biology and Therapy. Oxford: Blackwell, 2002:277–95.
54. Russell R. Indications of surgery. In: Beger H, Warshaw A, Büchler M et al., editors. The Pancreas. Oxford: Blackwell, 1998:815–23.
55. Lowenfels A, Maisonneuve P, Cavallini G, Ammann R, Lankisch P, Anderson J. Pancreatitis and the risk of pancreatic cancer. N Engl J Med. 1993;328:1433–7.
56. Finch M, Howes N, Ellis I et al. Hereditary pancreatitis and familial pancreatic cancer. Digestion. 1997;58:564–9.
57. Lowenfels A, Maisonneuve P, DiMagno E et al. Hereditary Pancreatitis and the risk of pancreatic cancer. J Natl Cancer Inst. 1997;89:442–6.
58. Howes N, Neoptolemos J. Risk of pancreatic ductal adenocarcinoma in chronic pancreatitis. Gut. 2002;51:765–6.
59. Stone H, Chauvin E. Pancreatic denervation for pain relief in chronic alcohol associated pancreatitis. Br J Surg. 1990;77:303–5.
60. Howard T, Swofford J, Wagner D, Sherman S, Lehman G. Quality of life after bilateral thoracoscopic splanchnicectomy: long-term evaluation in patients with chronic pancreatitis. J Gastrointest Surg. 2002;6:845–52.
61. Leksowski K. Thoracoscopic splanchnicectomy for the relief of pain due to chronic pancreatitis. Surg Endosc. 2001;15:592–6.
62. Hammond B, Vitale G, Rangnekar N, Vitale E, Binford J. Bilateral thoracoscopic splanchnicectomy for pain control in chronic pancreatitis. Am Surg. 2004;70:546–9.

63. Maher J, Johlin F, Heitshusen D. Long-term follow-up of thoracoscopic splanchnicectomy for chronic pancreatitis pain. Surg Endosc. 2001;15:706–9.
64. Ihse I, Zoucas E, Gyllstedt E et al. Bilateral thoracoscopic splanchnicectomy: effects on pancreatic pain and function. Ann Surg. 1999;230:785–90.
65. Buscher H, Jansen J, van Dongen R, Bleichrodt R, van Goor H. Long-term results of bilateral thoracoscopic splanchnicectomy in patients with chronic pancreatitis. Br J Surg. 2002;89:158–62.
66. Bradley E3, Reynhout J, Peer G. Thoracoscopic splanchnicectomy for 'small duct' chronic pancreatitis: case selection by differential epidural analgesia. J Gastrointest Surg. 1998;2:88–94.
67. Frey C, Suzuki M, Isaji S, Zhu Y. Pancreatic resection for chronic pancreatitis. Surg Clin N Am. 1989;69:499–528.
68. Sakorafas G, Farnell M, Farley D, Rowland C, Sarr M. Long-term results after surgery for chronic pancreatitis. Int J Pancreatol. 2000;27:131–42.
69. Sohn T, Kampbell K, Pitt H et al. Quality of life and long-term survival after surgery for chronic pancreatitis. J Gastrointest Surg. 2000;4:355–65.
70. Bradley E. Long-term results of pancreatojejunostomy in patients with chronic pancreatitis. Am J Surg. 1987;153:207–13.
71. Markowitz J, Rattner D, Warshaw A. Failure of symptomatic relief after pancreaticojejunal decompression for chronic pancreatitis. Strategies for salvage. Arch Surg. 1994;129:374–9.
72. Nealon W, Thompson J. Progressive loss of pancreatic function in chronic pancreatitis is delayed by main pancreatic duct decompression. A longitudinal prospective analysis of the modified puestow procedure. Ann Surg. 1993;217:458–66.
73. Altimari A, Aranha G, Greenlee H, Prinz R. Results of cystoduodenostomy for treatment of pancreatic pseudocysts. Am Surg. 1986;52:439–41.
74. Heider R, Meyer A, Galanko J, Behrns K. Percutaneous drainage of pancreatic pseudocysts is associated with a higher failure rate than surgical treatment in unselected patients. Ann Surg. 1999;229:781–9.
75. Nealon W, Townsend C, Thompson J. Preoperative endoscopic retrograde cholangiopancreatography (ERCP) in patients with pancreatic pseudocysts associated with resolving acute pancreatitis and chronic pancreatitis. Ann Surg. 1989;209:532–7.
76. Newell K, Liu T, Arancha G, Prinz R. Are cystogastrostomy and cystoduodenostomy equivalent operations for pancreatic pseudocysts? Surgery. 1990;108:635–9.
77. Sankaran S, Walt A. The natural and unnatural history of pancreatic pseudocysts. Br J Surg. 1975;62:37–44.
78. Spivack H, Galloway J, Amerson J et al. Management of pancreatic pseudocysts. J Am Coll Surg. 1998;186:507–11.
79. Usatoff V, Brancatisano R, Williamson R. Operative treatment of pseudocysts in patients with chronic pancreatitis. Br J Surg. 2000;87:1494–9.
80. Vitas G, Sarr M. Selected management of pancreatic pseudocysts: operative versus expectant management. Surgery. 1992;111:123–30.
81. Vijungco J, Prinz R. Management of biliary and duodenal complications of chronic pancreatitis. World J Surg. 2003;27:1258–70.
82. Alexakis N, Ghaneh P, Connor S, Raraty M, Sutton R, Neoptolemos J. Duodenum- and spleen-preserving total pancreatectomy for end-stage chronic pancreatitis. Br J Surg. 2003;90:1401–8.
83. Beger H, Schlosser W, Friess H, Büchler M. Duodenum-preserving head resection in chronic pancreatitis changes the natural course of the disease. Ann Surg. 1999;230:512–23.
84. Büchler M, Friess H, Muller M, Wheatley A, Beger H. Randomized trial of duodenum-preserving pancreatic head resection versus pylorus-preserving Whipple in chronic pancreatitis. Am J Surg. 1995;169:65–70.
85. Evans J, Wilson P, Carver C et al. Outcome of surgery for chronic pancreatitis. Br J Surg. 1997;84:624–9.
86. Fleming W, Williamson R. Role of total pancreatectomy in the treatment of patients with end-stage chronic pancreatitis. Br J Surg. 1995;82:1409–12.
87. Frey C, Amikura K. Local resection of the head of the pancreas combined with longitudinal pancreaticojejunostomy in the management of patients with chronic pancreatitis. Ann Surg. 1994;220:492–504.

88. Hutchins R, Hart R, Pacifico M, Bradley N, Williamson R. Long-term results of distal pancreatectomy for chronic pancreatitis in 90 patients. Ann Surg. 2002;236:612–18.
89. Izbicki J, Bloechle C, Knoefel W, Kuechler T, Binmoeller K, Broelsch C. Duodenum-preserving resection of the head of the pancreas in chronic pancreatitis. A prospective, randomized trial. Ann Surg. 1995;221:350–8.
90. Izbicki J, Bloechle C, Broering D, Knoefel W, Kuechler T, Broelsch C. Extended drainage versus resection in surgery for chronic pancreatitis: a prospective randomized trial comparing the longitudinal pancreaticojejunostomy combined with local pancreatic head excision with the pylorus-preserving pancreatoduodenectomy. Ann Surg. 1998;228:771–9.
91. Izbicki J, Bloechle C, Broering D, Kuechler T, Broelsch C. Longitudinal V-shaped excision of the ventral pancreas for small duct disease in severe chronic pancreatitis: prospective evaluation of a new surgical procedure. Ann Surg. 1998;227:213–19.
92. Jimenez R, Fernandez-del Castillo C, Rattner D, Chang Y, Warshaw A. Outcome of pancreatoduodenectomy with pylorus preservation or with antrectomy in the treatment of chronic pancreatitis. Ann Surg. 2000;231:293–300.
93. Linehan I, Lambert M, Brown D, Kurtz A, Cotton P, Russell R. Total pancreatectomy for chronic pancreatitis. Gut. 1988;29:358–65.
94. Stone W, Sarr M, Nagorney D, McIlrath D. Chronic pancreatitis. Results of Whipple's resection and total pancreatectomy. Arch Surg. 1988;123:815–19.
95. White S, Sutton C, Weymss-Holden S et al. The feasibility of spleen-preserving pancreatectomy for end-stage chronic pancreatitis. Am J Surg. 2000;179:294–7.
96. Schafer M, Mullhaupt B, Clavien P. Evidence based pancreatic head resection for pancreatic cancer and chronic pancreatitis. Ann Surg. 2002;236:137–48.
97. Lambert M, Linehan I, Russell R. Duodenum-preserving total pancreatectomy for end stage chronic pancreatitis. Br J Surg. 1987;74:35–9.
98. Traverso L, Kozarek R. Pancreatoduodenectomy for chronic pancreatitis: anatomic selection criteria and subsequent long-term outcome analysis. Ann Surg. 1997;226:429–35.
99. Muller M, Friess H, Beger H et al. Gastric emptying following pylorus-preserving Whipple and duodenum-preserving pancreatic head resection in patients with chronic pancreatitis. Am J Surg. 1997;173:257–63.
100. Witzigmann H, Max D, Uhlmann D et al. Outcome after duodenum-preserving pancreatic head resection is improved compared with classic Whipple procedure in the treatment of chronic pancreatitis. Surgery. 2003;134:53–62.
101. Bloechle C, Busch C, Tesch C et al. Prospective randomized study of drainage and resection on non-occlusive segmental portal hypertension in chronic pancreatitis. Br J Surg. 1997;84:477–82.
102. Izbicki J, Yekebas E, Strate T et al. Extrahepatic portal hypertension in chronic pancreatitis: an old problem revisited. Ann Surg. 2002;236:82–9.
103. Alexakis N, Sutton R, Raraty M et al. Major resection for chronic pancreatitis in patients with vascular involvement is associated with increased risk of postoperative mortality. Br J Surg. 2004;91:1020–4.
104. Rodriguez Rilo H, Ahmad S, D'Alessio D et al. Total pancreatectomy and autologous islet cell transplantation as a means to treat severe chronic pancreatitis. J Gastrointest Surg. 2003;7:978–89.
105. Clayton H, Davies J, Pollard C, White S, Musto P, Dennison A. Pancreatectomy with islet autotransplantation for the treatment of severe chronic pancreatitis: the first 40 patients at the leicester general hospital. Transplantation. 2003;76:92–8.
106. Dite P, Ruzicka M, Zboril V, Novotny I. A prospective, randomized trial comparing endoscopic and surgical therapy for chronic pancreatitis. Endoscopy. 2003;35:553–8.

Chronic pancreatitis II

Section VIII
Treatment of complications and outcome

Chair: G. ADLER and P.G. LANKISCH

20
Pancreatic exocrine insufficiency: rational treatment and its pathophysiological basis

P. LAYER

INTRODUCTION

Intraluminal hydrolysis and breakdown of macronutrients into smaller, absorbable metabolites is crucially dependent on the action of pancreatic enzymes. Brush border enzymes and several extrapancreatic enzymes participate in the digestive process but cannot prevent detrimental malabsorption, which invariably occurs as a result of untreated pancreatic exocrine insufficiency[1,2].

Recent scientific advances have helped to provide a rational basis for efficient treatment, by improving our understanding of secretion and luminal fate of pancreatic enzymes and their effects on nutrient digestion under physiological and pathophysiological conditions, and have led to rational therapeutic recommendations[3]. Moreover, options and future developments of enzyme replacement therapy will be discussed in this chapter.

PHYSIOLOGY OF PANCREATIC EXOCRINE REPONSES IN HUMANS

Under physiological conditions postprandial cumulative enzyme outputs exceed more than 10-fold the quantity required for digestion. Thus, in exocrine pancreatic insufficiency less than 10% of normal prandial secretory rates may be enough to prevent steatorrhea[4,5]. Experimental studies using specific enzyme inhibitors yielded similar results[6]. The most powerful stimulus of human pancreatic exocrine secretion is exposure of the duodenal mucosa to nutrients. There is experimental evidence that digestive products (such as free fatty acids) rather than intact macromolecules (such as triglycerides) induce neurohormonal stimulation of the prandial enzyme response[7,8]. In humans, digestion and absorption of normal chyme nutrient contents are incomplete even under physiological conditions; rather, substantial nutrient quantities regularly escape intestinal absorption, pass the ileocaecal junction and contribute to upper gastrointestinal secretory and motor inhibitory regulation[9-13]. Moreover, pancreatic exocrine function is coupled with gastrointestinal motility both in the fasting (interdigestive) state and following a meal, i.e. in response to endogenous stimulation[14,15].

After its secretion, intraluminal pancreatic enzyme activities decrease during transit along the small intestine. However, the rate of inactivation differs between enzymes because they have different stability against degradation[16,17]. Thus, pancreatic amylase is rather stable, not easily proteolysed and has a high duodeno-ileal survival rate. About 60% of duodenal protease activities reach the jejunum, and between 20% and 30% the ileum[17-21]. It should be noted that trypsin's hydrolytic activity survives better than its immunoeactivity, which suggests that its structural integrity may not be required for its enzymatic action[17,18]. Lipase is inactivated very rapidly in the absence of triglycerides, and only a small proportion reaches the distal small bowel[17,18]. Survival of lipase activity is greater in the presence of its substrate[18-22]. Chymotrypsin appears to be of particular importance for decreasing lipase activity and incomplete fat digestion[19,21,23,24].

PANCREATIC EXOCRINE INSUFFICIENCY IN CHRONIC PANCREATITIS

Insufficiency of exocrine pancreatic function occurs late in the course in the vast majority of cases of chronic pancreatitis, due to the large functional reserve of the gland[1,9,25]. In patients with alcoholic pancreatitis its manifestation usually develops within the second decade of clinical disease, but may also appear more rapidly[2,9,26]. Exocrine secretions including enzyme output decrease in the course of chronic pancreatitis, and clinically overt malabsorption usually develops in the second decade after onset of symptomatic disease[27]. During this process the site of maxial digestion and absorption is shifted from the duodenum to the more distal small intestine[28].

As a result, increased amounts of nutrients may be delivered to the distal ileum which result in disturbed reguation of motor and secretory function of upper gastrointestinal organs[9-13]. Moreover, gastroduodenal and small intestinal transit is significantly accelerated, and the available time for digestion and absorption is markedly decreased in patients with pancreatic insufficiency[28], which may further contribute to nutrient malabsorption. This further explains the effects of pancreatic enzyme supplementation on pain in certain patients[28,29].

Steatorrhoea as a clinical symptom and diagnostic and therapeutic problem is the most important digestive malfunction in pancreatic exocrine insufficiency, and may be associated with malabsorption of the lipid-soluble vitamins A, D, E, and K. It usually develops prior to manifest malabsorption of other nutrients[26], because protein digestion is induced by gastric proteolytic activity and intestinal brush-border peptidases, and is maintained even in the absence of pancreatic proteolytic activity[20]. Similarly, with lacking pancreatic amylase, starch digestion reaches about 80% due to salivary amylase and brush-border oligosaccharidases[6]. Since quantitative faecal fat excretion also depends on dietary lipid intake, the coefficient of fat absorption indicates efficacy of luminal fat digestion in different populations[30].

Malabsorption of lipids and protein results in steatorrhoea and creatorrhoea. By contrast, faecal carbohydrate measurements do not represent the extent of starch malabsorption[31-34] because carbohydrates are metabolized by the intracolonic flora. On the other hand, this can be used as a measure of starch malabsorption by determining hydrogen breath concentrations[8,35-37]. Earlier fat (compared to protein and carbohydrate) malabsorption is due to an interaction of mechanisms:

1. Acinar production and secretion of lipase decreases earlier and more markedly compared with proteases[1,9,26].

2. Pancreatic bicarbonate secretion, which protects enzymes intraduodenally from denaturation by gastric acid, is diminished in exocrine pancreatic insufficiency. In consequence intraluminal pH may decrease below 4, which may result in lipase inactivation[9,38].

3. Lipase as a protein is not only an enzyme for lipid digestion, but also a substrate for the action of proteases, and is hydrolysed during small intestinal transit more rapidly than other enzymes[17,19,21,27].

4. Potentially compensatory mechanisms, in particular extrapancreatic lipolysis (e.g. lingual and gastric lipase), contribute only marginally to cumulative fat digestion[39].

As a result, progressive chronic pancreatitis is characterized by a rapid decrease in the secretion of lipase, which also has shorter intraluminal survival and has virtually exclusive digestive action in the lumen, uncompensated by extrapancreatic enzymes. In consequence steatorrhoea is an early and severe exocrine malfunction in chronic pancreatitis.

BASIS AND PRACTICAL USE OF ENZYME SUPPLEMENTATION

Normalized nutrient digestion in exocrine pancreatic insufficiency requires that sufficient enzymatic activity must be delivered into the duodenal lumen simultaneously with the meal. Intraluminal lipase in postprandial chyme requires a minimum activity of 40–60 IU/ml throughout the digestive period. This translates into cumulative amounts between 25 000 and 40 000 IU of lipase for digestion of a regular meal[1,27].

However, because ingestion of unprotected enzymes preparations leads to rapid lipase inactivation due to acid and proteolytic destruction[19,27,38,40], it is necessary to administer up to 10-fold more lipase orally to correct steatorrhoea[14]. Enteric coating of entire pancreatin tablets or capsules, which prevents acidic destruction of lipase, does not result in superior preparations compared with unprotected pancreatin. This is explained by the physiology of gastric emptying: resistant particles of >2 mm in size are not emptied by the stomach with the meal, i.e. the substrate[41–43], which leads to a dissociation of duodenal passage of nutrients and enzymes[27]. Modern preparations contain pancreatin protected within acid-resistant, pH-sensitive microspheres, which mix intragastrically with the meal. They are emptied intact into the duodenum within chyme. Subsequently, increasing pH causes release of enzyme content. These preparations have been shown to be superior compared with unprotected pancreatin extracts in controlled studies[44,45]. Recent data suggest that a further decrease in sphere size may not be associated with greater clinical benefit[46]. Moreover, enzyme release from micropreparations takes several minutes after exposure to the intestinal milieu, which may additionally delay digestive action[26]. Hence, the site of maximal absorption is probably shifted distally[47], in particular in the presence of accelerated gastrointestinal transit characteristic for pancreatic exocrine insufficiency[28]. In consequence, the physicochemical properties of microsphere coating of an individual preparation are crucial for the efficacy of enzyme therapy[48].

Steatorrhoea

The majority of patients with exocrine pancreatic insufficiency are treated with pH-sensitive pancreatin microspheres taken with each meal. In order to reduce steatorrhoea to < 15 g of fat per day, 25 000–50 000 IU of lipase per meal are required. Four or five meals per day need to be administered. In many cases these doses must be doubled due to insufficient lipolytic action, as outlined above. Efficacy of treatment is checked clinically, mainly by monitoring body weight and consistency of faeces.

In cases of treatment failure, doses should be increased, and/or the patient should distribute his/her nutrient intake across five or six smaller meals[9]. If steatorrhoea still does not respond, the compliance of the patient needs be checked by faecal chymotrypsin measurement: low activities suggest an insufficient intake of enzymes. Whether in the compliant patient pancreatin doses should be increased further is controversial, because ultra-high doses have been associated with a dose-dependent risk of stenotic fibrosing colonopathy in patients with cystic fibrosis[49,50]. Recently it has been shown that the risk correlates directly with the amount of enzymes administered. On the other hand there is no evidence that analogous complications may occur in chronic pancreatitis.

Against the background of this still-controversial evidence we do not generally recommend dosages of more than 75 000 IU of lipase per meal. In refractory cases, pathophysiological and therapeutic alternatives should be considered: addition of an acid blocker (proton pump inhibitor, H2-blocker) may have beneficial effects when combined with an unprotected pancreatin preparation[1,51–53]. After previous gastric and/or intestinal resections, bacterial overgrowth[55] or intestinal infections such as *Giardia lamblia*, or other intestinal absorption disorders, may further compromise absorption and require specific medical or surgical intervention.

Patients with accelerated gastric emptying due to gastric resections or gastro-enterostomies should be treated with pancreatin granule or powder preparations, and achlorhydric patients, including those continuously receiving acid blockers, are treated successfully with conventional unprotected pancreatin preparations. In the presence of enzyme supplementation, medium-chain triglycerides do not further improve lipid absorption[54].

Enzyme treatment for pain?

A protease-dependent, luminal, negative feedback system has been shown to be operative in humans, but it has remained controversial whether this mechanism contributes to the pathogenesis of pain[1,9,19,29,56–61]. Moreover, from controlled therapeutic studies in patients with chronic pancreatitis, conflicting results have been reported[29,62–65]. Experimental evidence suggests that hormonally induced inhibition of pancreatic secretion alone is ineffective in painful pancreatitis[66].

We assume that amelioration of pain following enzyme administration may originate from correction of pathological maldigestion-induced ileal brake effects[11–15,28] by increasing and accelerating digestion and thus reverting the luminal site of major nutrient exposure from the distal to the proximal intestine.

Acknowledgements

Our own studies cited in this chapter were supported by the German Research Foundation (DFG, grants La 483/5-3) and the Esther-Christiansen Foundation.

References

1. Di Magno EP, Clain JE, Layer P. Chronic pancreatitis. In: Go VLW, DiMagno EP, Gardner JD et al., editors. The Pancreas: Biology, Pathobiology, and Diseases, 2nd edn. New York: Raven Press, 1993:665–706.
2. Layer P, DiMagno EP. Natural histories of alcoholic and idiopathic chronic pancreatitis. Pancreas. 1996;12:318–19.
3. Layer P, Keller J. Pancreatic enzymes: secretion and luminal nutrient digestion in health and disease. J Clin Gastroenterol. 1999;28:3–10.
4. DiMagno EP, Go VLW, Summerskill WHJ. Relations between pancreatic enzyme outputs and malabsorption in severe pancreatic insufficiency. N Engl J Med. 1973;288:813–15.
5. Hiele M, Ghoos Y, Rutgeerts P, Vantrappen G. Starch digestion in normal subjects and patients with pancreatic diseases, using a $^{13}CO_2$ breath test. Gastroenterology. 1989;96:503.
6. Layer P, Zinsmeister AR, DiMagno EP. Effects of decreasing intraluminal amylase activity on starch digestion and postprandial gastrointestinal function in humans. Gastroenterology. 1986;91:41–8.
7. Guimbaud R, Moreau JA, Bouisson M et al. Intraduodenal free fatty acids rather than triglycerides are responsible for the release of CCK in humans. Pancreas. 1997;14:76–82.
8. Layer P, Holtmann G. Pancreatic enzymes in chronic pancreatitis (State-of-the-Art). Int J Pancreatol. 1994;15:1–11.
9. Read NW, McFarlane A, Kinsman RJ et al. Effect of infusion of nutrient solutions into the ileum on gastrointestinal transit and plasma levels of neurotensin and enteroglucagon. Gastroenterology. 1984;86:274–80.
10. Spiller RC, Trotman IF, Higgins BE et al. The ileal brake–inhibition of jejunal motility after ileal fat perfusion in man. Gut. 1984;25:365–74.
11. Layer P, Peschel S, Schlesinger T, Goebell H. Human pancreatic secretion and intestinal motility: effects of ileal nutrient perfusion. Am J Physiol 1990;258:G196–201.
12. Layer P, Schlesinger T, Goebell H. Modulation of periodic interdigestive gastrointestinal motor and pancreatic function by the ileum. Pancreas. 1993;8:426–32.

13. Keller J, Rünzi M, Goebell H, Layer P. Duodenal and ileal nutrient deliveries regulate human intestinal motor and pancreatic responses to a meal. Am J Physiol. 1997;272:G632–7.
14. DiMagno EP, Layer P. Human exocrine pancreatic enzyme secretion. In: Go VLW, DiMagno EP, Gardner JD et al., editors. The Pancreas: Biology, Pathobiology, and Diseases, 2nd edn. New York: Raven Press, 1993:275–300.
15. Layer P, Chan ATH, Go VLW, DiMagno EP. Human pancreatic secretion during phase II antral motility of the interdigestive cycle. Am J Physiol. 1988;254:G249–53.
16. Borgström B, Dahlqvist A, Lundh G, Sjövall J. Studies of intestinal digestion and aborption in the human. J Clin Invest. 1957;36:1521–36.
17. Layer P, Go VLW, DiMagno EP. Fate of pancreatic enzymes during aboral small intestinal transit in humans. Am J Physiol. 1986;251:G475–80.
18. Granger M, Abadie B, Marchis-Mouren G. Limited action of trypsin on porcine pancreatic amylase: characterization of the fragments. FEBS Lett. 1975;56:189–93.
19. Layer P, Jansen JBMJ, Cherian L, Lamers CBHW, Goebell H. Feedback regulation of human pancreatic secretion: effects of protease inhibition on duodenal delivery and small intestinal transit of pancreatic enzymes. Gastroenterology. 1990;98:1311–19.
20. Layer P, Baumann J, Hellmann C, v d Ohe M, Gröger G, Goebell H. Effect of luminal protease inhibition on prandial nutrient digestion during small intestinal chyme transit. Pancreas. 1990;5:718.
21. Holtmann G, Kelly DG, Sternby B, DiMagno EP. Survival of human pancreatic enzymes during small bowel transit: effect of nutrients, bile acids, and enzymes. Am J Physiol. 1997; 273:G553–8.
22. Kelly DG, Sternby B, DiMagno EP. How to protect human pancreatic enzyme activities in frozen duodenal juice. Gastroenterology. 1991;100:189–95.
23. Thiruvengadam R, DiMagno EP. Inactivation of human lipase by proteases. Am J Physiol. 1988;255:G476–81.
24. Layer P, Hellmann C, Baumann J, v.d. Ohe M, Gröger G, Goebell H. Modulation of physiologic fat malabsorption in humans. Digestion. 1990; 46:153.
25. DiMagno EP, Go VLW, Summerskill WHJ. Relations between pancreatic enzyme outputs and malabsorption in severe pancreatic insufficiency. N Engl J Med. 1973;288:813–15.
26. DiMagno EP, Malagelada JR, Go VLW. Relationship between alcoholism and pancreatic insufficiency. Ann NY Acad Sci. 1975;252:200–7.
27. Layer P, Yamamoto H, Kalthoff L, Clain JE, Bakken LJ, DiMagno EP. The different courses of early- and late-onset idiopathic and alcoholic chronic pancreatitis. Gastroenterology. 1994;107:1481–7.
28. Layer P, von der Ohe MR, Holst JJ et al. Altered postprandial motility in chronic pancreatitis: role of malabsorption. Gastroenterology. 1997;112:1624–34.
29. Slaff J, Jacobson D, Tillmann CR, Curington C, Toskes PP. Protease-specific suppression of pancreatic exocrine secretion. Gastroenterology. 1984;87:44–52.
30. Nakamura T, Takeuchi T. Pancreatic steatorrhea, malabsorption, and nutrition biochemistry: a comparison of Japanese, European and American patients with chronic pancreatitis. Pancreas. 1997;14:323–33.
31. Bond JH, MD. Fate of soluble carbohydrate in the colon of rats and man. J Clin Invest. 1976;57:1158–64.
32. Bond JH, Currier BE, Buchwald H, Levitt MD. Colonic conservation of malabsorbed carbohydrate. Gastroenterology. 1980;78:444–7.
33. Stephen AM, Haddad AC, Phillips SF. Passage of carbohydrate into the colon. Gastroenterology. 1983;85:589–95.
34. Flourie B, Florent C, Jouany JP et al. Colonic breakdown of 50 g wheat starch in healthy man: effect on symptoms and fecal outputs. Gastroenterology. 1986;90:111–19.
35. Mackie RD, Levine AS, Levitt MD. Malabsorption of starch in pancreatic insufficiency. Gastroenterology. 1981;80:1220.
36. Patel VP, Jain NK, Agarwal N, GeeVarghese PJ, Pitchumoni CS. Comparisons of bentiromide test and rice flour breath hydrogen test in the detection of exocrine pancreatic insufficiency. Pancreas. 1986;1:172.
37. Kerlin P, Wong L, Harris B, Capra S. Rice flour, breath hydrogen, and malabsorption. Gastroenterology. 1984;87:578.

38. DiMagno EP, Malagelada JR, Go VLW, Moertel CG. Fate of orally ingested enzymes in pancreatic insufficiency: comparison of two dosage schedules. N Engl J Med. 1977;296: 1318–22.
39. Sternby B, Holtmann G, Kelly DG, DiMagno EP. Effect of gastric or duodenal nutrient infusion on gastric and pancreatic lipase secretion. Gastroenterology. 1992:102:A292.
40. Heizer WD, Cleaveland CR, Iber FL. Gastric inactivation of pancreatic supplements. Bull Johns Hopkins Hosp. 1965;116:261–70.
41. Goebell H, Klotz U, Nehlsen B, Layer P. Oroileal transit of slow release 5-ASA. Gut. 1993; 34:669–75.
42. Code CF, Schlegel JF. The gastrointestinal interdigestive housekeeper: motor correlates of the interdigestive myoelectric complex of the dog. In: EE Daniel, editor. Proceedings of the 4th International Symposium on GI Motility, Vancouver: Mitchell Press, 1973:631–4.
43. Schlegel JF, Code CF. The gastric peristalsis of the interdigestive housekeeper. In: G. Vantrappen, editor. Proceedings of the 5th International Symposium on GI Motility. Leuven: Typoff-Press, 1975:321.
44. Kölbel C, Layer P, Hotz J, Goebell H. Der Einfluss2 eines säuregeschützten, mikroverkapselten Pankreatinpräparats auf die pankreatogene Steatorrhö. Med Klin. 1986;81:85–6.
45. Lankisch PG, Lembcke B, Göke B, Creutzfeldt W. Therapie der pankreatogenen Steatorrhoe: Bietet der Säureschutz für Pankreasenzyme Vorteile? Verh dtsch Ges Inn Med. 1983; 89:864–7.
46. Meyer JH, Lake R. Mismatch of duodenal deliveries of dietary fat and pancreatin from enterically coated microspheres. Pancreas. 1997;15:226–35.
47. Dutta SK, Rubin J, Harvey J. Comparative evaluation of the therapeutic efficacy of a pH-sensitive enteric-coated pancreatic enzyme preparation with conventional pancreatic enzyme therapy in the treatment of exocrine pancreatic insufficiency. Gastroenterology. 1983;84:476–82.
48. Hendeles L, Dorf A, Stecenko A, Weinberger M. Treatment failure after substitution of generic pancrelipase capsules. Correlation with in vitro lipase activity. J Am Med Assoc. 1990;263:2459–61.
49. FitzSimmons SC, Burkhart GA, Borowitz D et al. High-dose pancreatic enzyme supplements and fibrosing colonopathy in children with cystic fibrosis. N Engl J Med. 1997;336: 1283–9.
50. MacSweeney EJ, Oades PJ, Buchdahl R, Rosenthal M, Bush A. Relation of thickening of colon wall to pancreatic-enzyme treatment in cystic fibrosis. Lancet. 1995;345:752–6.
51. Regan PT, Malagelada JR, DiMagno EP, Glanzman SL, Go VLW. Comparative effects of antacids, cimetidine, and enteric coating on the therapeutic response to oral enzymes in severe pancreatic insufficiency. N Engl J Med. 1977;297:854–8.
52. Carroccio A, Pardo F, Montalto G et al. Use of famotidine in severe exocrine pancreatic insufficiency with persistent maldigestion on enzymatic replacement therapy. Dig Dis Sci. 1992;37:1441–6.
53. Heijerman HG, Lamers CB, Bakker W. Omeprazole enhances the efficacy of pancreatin (Pancrease) in cystic fibrosis. Ann Intern Med. 1991;114:200–10.
54. Caliari S, Benini L, Sembenini C, Gregori B, Carnielli V, Vantini I. Medium-chain triglyceride absorption in patients with pancreatic insufficiency. Scand J Gastroenterol. 1996;31:90–4.
55. Casellas F, Guarner L, Vaquero E, Antolin M, de Gracia X, Malagelada JR. Hydrogen breath test with glucose in exocrine pancreatic insufficiency. Pancreas. 1998;16:481–6.
56. Krawisz BR, Miller LJ, DiMagno EP, Go VLW. In the absence of nutrients pancreatic–biliary secretions in the jejunum do not exert feedback control of human pancreatic or gastric function. J Lab Clin Med. 1980;95:13–18.
57. Hotz J, Ho SB, Go VLW, DiMagno EP. Short-term inhibition of duodenal tryptic activity does not affect human pancreatic, biliary or gastric function. J Lab Clin Med. 1983;101: 488–95.
58. Owyang C, Louie DS, Tatus D. Feedback regulation of pancreatic enzyme secretion. Suppression of cholecystokinin release by trypsin. J Clin Invest. 1986;77:2042–7.
59. Owyang C, May D, Louie DS. Trypsin suppression of pancreatic enzyme secretion. Differential effect on cholecystokinin release and the enteropancreatic reflex. Gastroenterology. 1986;91:637–43.

60. Adler G, Reinshagen M, Koop I et al. Differential effects of atropine and a cholecystokinin receptor antagonist on pancreatic secretion. Gastroenterology. 1989;96:1158–64.
61. Ihse I, Lilja P, Lundquist I. Feedback regulation of pancreatic enzyme secretion by intestinal trypsin in man. Digestion. 1977;15:303–8.
62. Mössner J, Stange JH, Ewald M, Kestel W, Fischbach W. Influence of exogenous application of pancreatic extract on endogenous pancreatic enzyme secretion. Pancreas. 1991;6:637–44.
63. Isaksson F, Ihse I. Pain reduction by an oral pancreatic enzyme preparation in chronic pancreatitis. Dig Dis Sci. 1983;28:97–102.
64. Halgreen H, Thorsgaard Pedersen N, Worning H. Symptomatic effect of pancreatic enzyme therapy in patients with chronic pancreatitis. Scand J Gastroenterol. 1986;21:104–8.
65. Mössner J, Secknus R, Meyer J, Niederau C, Adler G. Treatment of pain with pancreatic extracts in chronic pancreatitis: results of a prospective placebo-controlled multicenter trial. Digestion. 1992;53:54–66.
66. Malfertheiner P, Mayer D, Büchler M, Dominguez-Munoz JE, Schiefer B, Ditschuneit H. Treatment of pain in chronic pancreatitis by inhibition of pancreatic secretion with octreotide. Gut. 1995;36:450–4.

21
Pancreatic enzyme therapy in cystic fibrosis

M. STERN and A. HOFMANN

INTRODUCTION

Cystic fibrosis (CF) is the most frequent cause of exocrine pancreatic insufficiency in childhood. Together with bile acid loss and intestinal malabsorption, pancreatic insufficiency contributes to malnutrition and growth failure. Pancreatic enzyme replacement therapy (PERT) is therefore an important part of the multidisciplinary approach to CF therapy, and it has a strong impact on long-term prognosis.

PATHOPHYSIOLOGY OF MALABSORPTION IN CF – NUTRITION AND PROGNOSIS

Cystic fibrosis is the most common lethal hereditary disease in Caucasians. Prevalence in Western Europe is 1:2500. More than 1000 different mutations have been identified in a single gene coding for the CF transmembrane conductance regulator (CFTR). The CFTR gene product is a membrane-bound chloride channel present in epithelial cells of many organs including the gastrointestinal tract[1]. CF is characterized by severe progressive lung disease and exocrine pancreatic insufficiency. However, exocrine pancreatic insufficiency is present only in 85% of CF patients, pancreatic sufficiency implying a better prognosis with regard to quality of life and survival[2,3]. Besides exocrine pancreatic insufficiency, other gastrontestinal factors contribute to malabsorption in CF; these are loss of bile salts and an incompletely defined intestinal component[4–6]. The complex pathophysiology of malabsorption in CF may explain why simple PERT still does not lead to complete correction of malabsorption and malnutrition in CF. In addition to this, higher enzyme doses have to be used in CF compared to exocrine pancreatic insufficiency of other causes in adult patients.

Malnutrition is still a major problem with a strong prognostic impact in CF. In Germany, in the year 2003, 27% of children and 34% of adult patients fulfilled criteria of malnutrition (weight for height less than 90%, BMI less than

19)[7]. Poor nutritional status and pancreatic insufficiency are on top of a list of factors associated with poor prognosis[8]. In her epidemiological classic, Mary Corey showed in 1988 that improved survival in CF patients treated in Toronto compared to Boston was due to an aggressive nutritional strategy including high-caloric food and adjusted PERT[9]. In this context of preventing and treating malnutrition[10,11] PERT is of paramount importance. Compared to the early years of pancreatic enzyme treatment[12] progress has been made. However, there are still limitations to therapy effectiveness in CF[6,13–16].

DIAGNOSIS OF PANCREATIC INSUFFICIENCY IN CF

Before PERT is instituted a clear diagnosis of exocrine pancreatic insufficiency has to be established in CF. Enzyme replacement based merely on a clinical diagnosis and sweat testing leads to malclassification of patients and over-treatment. In a recent multicentre series involving 33 US centres, 5.5% of patients had been misclassified and were in fact pancreatic sufficient[3]. The classical delta F508 mutation leads to pancreatic insufficiency, whereas less frequent mutations such as R117H and L334W are connected to pancreatic sufficiency not necessitating enzyme replacement. However, mutation analysis is not the appropriate tool for establishing pancreatic insufficiency in CF. An ideal test should be non-invasive, it should be highly sensitive and specific, it should be simple, reproducible and cheap. For diagnosis it should be independent of therapy; for monitoring therapy an additional test system would be required. It is obvious that no single test fulfils all these conditions[17,18]. The invasive secretin–pancreozymin test requires duodenal intubation and has served as a gold standard. More practical and feasible in children are indirect methods, namely the 72-h fat balance study which is also useful for therapy monitoring, stool elastase determination for diagnosis and stool chymotrypsin determination for monitoring[17,19–21]. Recently ^{13}C mixed triglyceride breath tests have been used for diagnosis and monitoring[22–24]. With wider availability and improved practical use ^{13}C breath tests may replace current test systems. At present, however, at least for diagnosis, stool elastase is a good practical tool to differentiate CF patients with pancreatic insufficiency and sufficiency[3,21]. Of course, limitations also apply to the determination of stool elastase, for example, if there are fluid stools, and also in cases with mild pancreatic insufficiency as well as in patients with Shwachman syndrome or short gut syndrome.

In patients initially classified as pancreatic sufficient, follow-up is necessary, since development of pancreatic insufficiency can occur gradually, usually in the first years of life[20,25]. Summarizing the diagnostic situation there should be a positive diagnosis of pancreatic insufficiency initially after diagnosis of CF, and later follow-up is required of pancreatic status in pancreatic-sufficient CF patients. Indirect pancreatic function tests are used for therapy monitoring.

PANCREATIC ENZYME REPLACEMENT THERAPY (PERT)

In pancreatic insufficiency caused by CF, the therapeutic aim is to increase fat absorption to 85–95% which can be achieved by pancreatic enzyme replacement in many cases. This is the basis for hypercaloric nutrition, rich in fat, to counterbalance increased energy expenditure in CF. Acid-resistant enteric-coated microsphere and mini-tablet preparations of porcine pancreatin effectively reduce steatorrhoea[6,11,13,14,16,26–28]. Different pancreatic enzyme preparations contain different relative activities of lipase, protease and amylase. Several preparations contain the polymer eudragit acrylic resin as an enteric coating. Dose adjustment is usually accomplished using lipase given per kilogram body weight or lipase given per gram fat ingested[11,13].

Only a very few studies of PERT have been carried out placebo-controlled[29]. It was shown that the fat absorption coefficient increased from 52% to 84% in paediatric patients and from 51% to 87% in adult CF patients. Most clinical studies have been carried out in a randomized double-blind fashion, but were not placebo-controlled in order not to put CF patients off treatment.

Depending on age, 500–4000 IU lipase per gram fat ingested are recommended[11]. After description of fibrosing colonopathy with high pancreatic enzyme dosage, the aim was set to keep lipase dose below 10 000 IU kg body weight per day.

In a practical survey of 81 CF patients (age 2–42 years) their status of PERT was checked. Therapy monitoring was achieved by fat balance studies. It could be shown that during PERT, in a considerable portion of these patients, fat absorption was not completely restored to normal (Figure 1). Lipase dose reached per kilogram body weight (Figure 2a) and lipase dose reached per gram fat ingested (Figure 2b) was clearly exceeding the current recommenda-

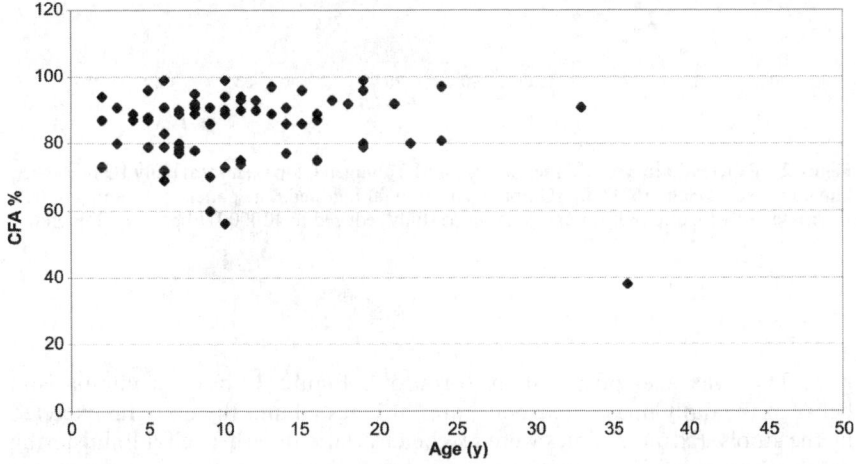

Figure 1 Coefficient of fat absorption (CFA) in 81 Tübingen CF patients on PERT. Fat absorption not completely restored to normal (85–95%) in a considerable proportion of patients

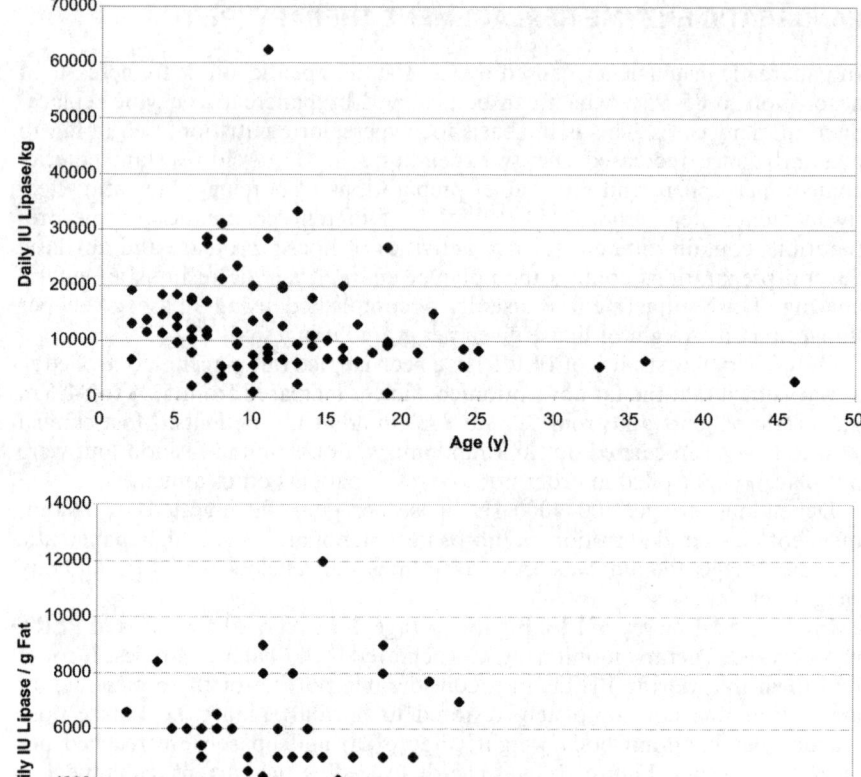

a

b

Figure 2 Pancreatic enzyme (lipase) dosage in 81 Tübingen CF patients. (**a**) daily IU lipase per kilogram body weight. (**b**) Daily IU lipase per gram fat ingested. The patient consuming 62 000 IU lipase per kilogram (self-dosage) was successfully reduced to 40 000 IU lipase per kilogram

tion. This was also observed in Toronto[14]. Figure 3 shows a comparison between the daily lipase dose per gram fat ingested and the daily fat excreted by the stools. Extreme values were reached by patients either self-administering an overdose or having stopped prescribed enzymes totally. Some were not able to ingest the recommended dietary fat. It is obvious from this survey that everyday PERT is far from ideal, and needs adjustment as well as substantial improvement according to current criteria[11,13,14].

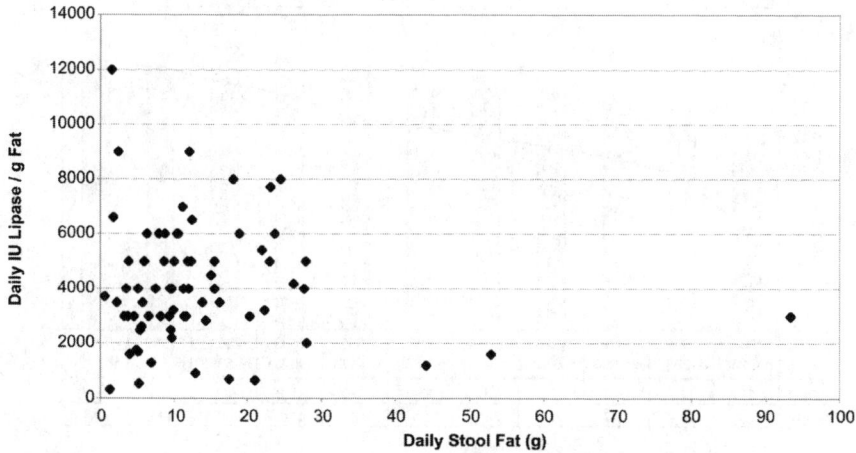

Figure 3 Pancreatic enzyme dosage in 81 Tübingen CF patients. Daily IU lipase per gram fat ingested versus daily stool fat excreted (normal below 3 g in infants, below 7 g from school age to adulthood)

Side-effects of PERT include hyperuricosaemia and hyperuricosuria, which are rare events with modern preparations. Allergic symptoms including oral and perianal irritation occur. Sometimes enzyme particles are visible in the faeces. The most severe but very rare side-effect of PERT is fibrosing colonopathy, which is characterized by colonic obstruction requiring surgery in patients usually on an excessively high pancreatic enzyme dose. After the initial description in 1994 several cases have been described in the UK and USA, but only extremely rarely in the rest of Europe[30,31]. In a careful epidemiological study[32] it was shown that the risk of fibrosing colonopathy increased 200-fold in patients receiving more than 50 000 U of lipase per kilogram body weight per day. Dose reductions have been introduced and recommendations have been made[11,13,33,34] and fibrosing colonopathy has almost disappeared today. However, there have been single cases on low-dose PERT. The role of eudragit has not been clearly established and there may also be a pre-existing CF-specific intestinal factor leading to fibrosing colonopathy in some patients who are on an excessively high pancreatic dosage.

Specific intestinal involvement with colonic wall thickening was found in many cases without any clinical symptoms and without fibrosing colonopathy. This colonic wall thickening was found to be maximal in the ascending colon; it was dependent on age and not on pancreatic enzyme dose[35,36]. In the Tübingen series[35] there was no progression of colonic wall thickening even with high-dose PERT (compare Figures 2a and 2b). Generally, fibrosing colonopathy has shed some light on the complexity of gastrointestinal CF manifestations with and without relation to PERT.

There are many factors causing failure to control symptoms in PERT despite proper enzyme dosage[4–6,11–13,37]. Enzyme factors such as reduced shelf-life, dietary factors such as insufficient fat intake and individual factors such as non-

221

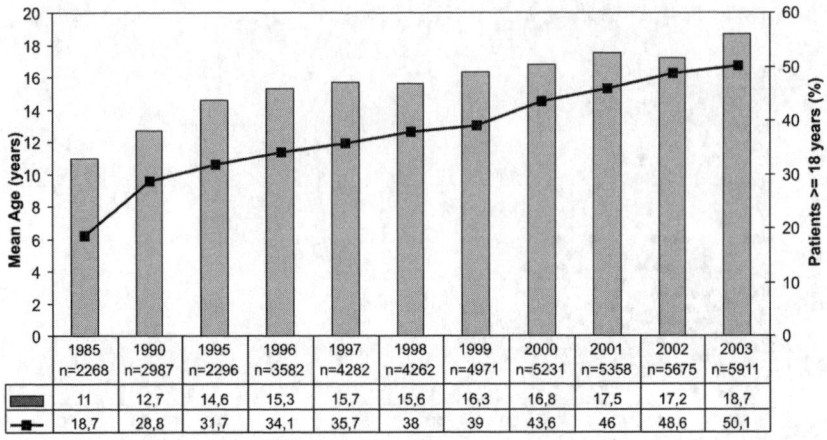

	1985 n=2268	1990 n=2987	1995 n=2296	1996 n=3582	1997 n=4282	1998 n=4262	1999 n=4971	2000 n=5231	2001 n=5358	2002 n=5675	2003 n=5911
▨	11	12,7	14,6	15,3	15,7	15,6	16,3	16,8	17,5	17,2	18,7
▬■	18,7	28,8	31,7	34,1	35,7	38	39	43,6	46	48,6	50,1

Figure 4   Age development of CF patients in Germany 1985–2003 (reprinted with permission)

compliance and self-dosage are contributory. Acid intestinal environment and enzyme degradation are specific problems in CF and may be overcome by agents such as ranitidine and omeprazole inhibiting acid secretion as an adjuvant therapy to PERT[38–40]. If failure to control symptoms of malabsorption persist, diagnostic work-up is necessary to identify any concurrent gastrointestinal disorder like enteritis, lactose malabsorption, coeliac disease, or Crohn's disease in order to find appropriate additional treatment[13]. Beyond this there should be dietary monitoring and nutritional counselling at regular intervals (yearly) in order to achieve dose adjustment and refinement. Educational aspects are very important with respect to the high degree of non-compliance with PERT, which has always to be expected if a direct benefit of the therapeutic regimen cannot be noticed by the patient[41–43]. The current therapeutic situation in PERT is far from ideal. Therapy monitoring, dose correction, dietary counselling and increased awareness of possible failure to control malabsorption in CF are mandatory.

PERT IN PERSPECTIVE

In perspective, new enzyme sources from fungi and bacteria may help to improve efficiency in PERT[44–46]. However, it should be kept in mind that porcine enzyme preparations contain many different enzymes, e.g. phospholipase, which may be difficult to add in newly composed enzyme mixtures based on enzymes produced by genetic engineering. A liquid enzyme preparation is eagerly awaited by CF specialists since high-caloric feeding frequently has to be achieved by tube feeding, including percutaneous endoscopic gastrostomy (PEG). The current situation requires discontinuous enzyme dosage by the oral route, since current solid enzyme preparations do not pass nasogastric and PEG tubes. Of course, improved PERT has to be seen in the context of improving nutritional status of CF patients and also in the context of patients growing into adulthood: 50.1% of patients registered in Germany in the year 2003 were 18 years of age or older. Thus, adult gastroenterology has to face the specific adult CF patient population posing many new therapeutic problems extending beyond PERT (Figure 4)[7].

References

1. Strong TV, Boehm K, Collins FS. Localization of cystic fibrosis transmembrane conductance regulator mRNA in the human gastrointestinal tract by *in situ* hybridization. J Clin Invest. 1994;93:347–54.
2. Shalon LB, Adelson JW. Cystic fibrosis: gastrointestinal complications and gene therapy. Pediatr Clin N Am. 1996;43:157–96.
3. Borowitz D, Baker SS, Duffy L et al. Use of fecal elastase-1 to classify pancreatic status in patients with cystic fibrosis. J Pediatr. 2004;145:322–6.
4. Gregory PC. Gastrointestinal pH, motility/transit and permeability in cystic fibrosis. J Pediatr Gastroenterol Nutr. 1996;23:513–23.
5. Kalivianakis M, Minich DM, Bijleveld CMA et al. Fat malabsorption in cystic fibrosis patients receiving enzyme replacement therapy is due to impaired intestinal uptake of long-chain fatty acids. Am J Clin Nutr. 1999;69:127–34.
6. Littlewood JM, Wolfe SP. Control of malabsorption in cystic fibrosis. Paediatr Drugs. 2000;2:205–22.
7. Stern M, Sens B, Wiedemann B, Busse O, Damm G, Wenzlaff P. editors. Qualitätssicherung Mukoviszidose 2003 – Überblick über den Gesundheitszustand der Patienten in Deutschland 2003. Hannover: Zentrum für Qualitätsmanagement im Gesundheitswesen, 2004.
8. Orenstein DV, Winnie GB, Altman W. Cystic fibrosis: a 2002 update. J Pediatr. 2002;140: 156–64.
9. Corey M, Laughlin FJ, Williams M, Levison H. A comparison of survival, growth, and pulmonary function in patients with cystic fibrosis in Boston and Toronto. J Clin Epidemiol. 1988;41:583–91.
10. Ramsey BW, Farrell PM, Pencharz P, Consensus Committee. Nutritional assessment and management in cystic fibrosis: a consensus report. Am J Clin Nutr. 1992;55:108–16.
11. Sinaasappel M, Stern M, Littlewood J et al. Nutrition in patients with cystic fibrosis: a European Consensus. J Cystic Fibrosis. 2002;1:51–75.
12. Guarner L, Rodríguez R, Guarner F, Malagelada JR. Fate of oral enzymes in pancreatic insufficiency. Gut. 1993;34:708–12.
13. Borowitz DS, Grand RJ, Durie PR, Consensus Committee. Use of pancreatic enzyme supplements for patients with cystic fibrosis in the context of fibrosing colonopathy. J Pediatr. 1995;127:681–4.
14. Durie P, Kalnins D, Ellis L. Uses and abuses of enzyme therapy in cystic fibrosis. J R Soc Med. 1998;91(Suppl. 34):2–13.
15. Benabdeslam H, Garcia I, Bellon G, Gilly R, Revol A. Biochemical assessment of the nutritional status of cystic fibrosis patients treated with pancreatic enzyme extracts. Am J Clin Nutr.1998;67:912–18.
16. Schibli S, Durie PR, Tullis ED. Proper usage of pancreatic enzymes. Curr Opin Pulm Med. 2002;8:542–6.
17. Walkowiak J, Cichy WK, Herzig K-H. Comparison of fecal elastase-1 determination with the secretin-cholecystokinin test in patients with cystic fibrosis. Scand J Gastroenterol. 1999;34:202–7.
18. Walkowiak J. Assessment of maldigestion in cystic fibrosis. J Pediatr. 2004;145,285–7.
19. Cade A, Walters MP, McGinley N et al. Evaluation of fecal pancreatic elastase-1 as a measure of pancreatic exocrine function in children with cystic fibrosis. Pediatr Pulmonol. 2000;29:172–6.
20. Leus J, Van Biervliet S, Robberecht E. Detection and follow up of exocrine pancreatic insufficiency in cystic fibrosis: a review. Eur J Pediatr. 2000;159:563–8.

21. Beharry S, Ellis L, Corey M, Marcon M, Durie P. How useful is fecal pancreatic elastase 1 as a marker of exocrine pancreatic disease? J Pediatr. 2002;141:84–90.
22. Amarri S, Harding M, Coward WA, Evans TJ, Weaver LT. [13]Carbon mixed triglyceride breath test and pancreatic enzyme supplementation in cystic fibrosis. Arch Dis Child. 1997; 76:349–51.
23. Swart GR, Baartman EA, Wattimena JLD, Rietveld T, Overbeek SE, van den Berg JWO. Evaluation studies of the ^{13}C-mixed triglyceride breath test in healthy controls and adult cystic fibrosis patients with exocrine pancreatic insufficiency. Digestion. 1997;58:415–20.
24. De Boeck K, Delbeke I, Eggermont E, Veereman-Wauters G, Ghoos Y. Lipid digestion in cystic fibrosis: comparison of conventional and high-lipase enzyme therapy using the mixed-triglyceride breath test. J Pediatr Gastroenterol Nutr. 1998;26:408–11.
25. Couper RTL, Corey M, Moore DJ, Fisher LJ, Forstner GG, Durie PR. Decline of exocrine pancreatic function in cystic fibrosis patients with pancreatic sufficiency. Pediatr Res. 1992; 32:179–82.
26. Brady MS, Rickard K, Yu PL, Eigen H. Effectiveness and safety of small vs. large doses of enteric coated pancreatic enzymes in reducing steatorrhea in children with cystic fibrosis: a prospective randomized study. Pediatr Pulmonol. 1991;10:79–85.
27. Lancellotti L, Cabrini G, Zanolla L, Mastella G. High- versus low-lipase acid-resistant enzyme preparations in cystic fibrosis: a crossover randomized clinical trial. J Pediatr Gastroenterol Nutr. 1996;22:73–8.
28. Regele S, Henker J, Münch R, Barbier Y, Stern M. Indirect parameters of pancreatic function in cystic fibrosis (CF) during a controlled double-blind trial of pancreatic supplementation. J Pediatr Gastroenterol Nutr. 1996;22:68–72.
29. Stern RC, Eisenberg JD, Wagener JS et al. A comparison of the efficacy and tolerance of pancrelipase and placebo in the treatment of steatorrhea in cystic fibrosis patients with clinical exocrine pancreatic insufficiency. Am J Gastroenterol. 2000;95:1932–8.
30. Smyth RL, Ashby D, O'Hea U et al. Fibrosing colonopathy in cystic fibrosis: results of a case-control study. Lancet. 1995;346:1247–51.
31. Littlewood JM, Hind CRK, editors. Fibrosing colonopathy in children with cystic fibrosis. Postgrad Med J. 1996;72(Suppl. 2):S2–64.
32. FitzSimmons SC, Burkhart GA, Borowitz D et al. High-dose pancreatic-enzyme supplements and fibrosing colonopathy in children with cystic fibrosis. N Engl J Med. 1997;336: 1283–9.
33. Stevens JC, Maguiness KM, Hollingsworth J, Heilman DK, Chong SK. Pancreatic enzyme supplementation in cystic fibrosis patients before and after fibrosing colonopathy. J Pediatr Gastroenterol Nutr. 1998;26:80–4.
34. Lowdon J, Goodchild MC, Ryley HC, Doull IJM. Maintenance of growth in cystic fibrosis despite reduction in pancreatic enzyme supplementation. Arch Dis Child. 1998;78:377–8.
35. Haber HP, Benda N, Fitzke G et al. Colonic wall thickness measured by ultrasound: striking differences in patients with cystic fibrosis versus healthy controls. Gut. 1997;40: 406–11.
36. Connett GJ, Lucas JS, Atchley TM, Fairhurst JJ, Rolles CJ. Colonic wall thickening is related to age and not dose of high strength pancreatin microspheres in children with cystic fibrosis. Eur J Gastroenterol Hepatol. 1999;11:181–3.
37. O'Hare MMT, McMaster C, Dodge JA. Stated versus actual lipase activity in pancreatic enzyme supplements: implications for clinical use. J Pediatr Gastroenterol Nutr. 1995;21: 59–63.
38. Heijerman HG, Lamers CB, Bakker W. Omeprazole enhances the efficacy of pancreatin (pancrease) in cystic fibrosis. Ann Intern Med. 1991;114:200–1.
39. Francisco MP, Wagner MH, Sherman JM, Theriaque D, Bowser E, Novak DA. Ranitidine and omeprazole as adjuvant therapy to pancrelipase to improve fat absorption in patients with cystic fibrosis. J Pediatr Gastroenterol Nutr. 2002;35:79–83.
40. Proesmans M, De Boeck K. Omeprazole, a proton pump inhibitor, improves residual steatorrhoea in cystic fibrosis patients treat with high dose pancreatic enzyme. Eur J Pediatr. 2003;162:760–3.
41. Anthony H, Collins C, Davidson G et al. Pancreatic enzyme replacement therapy in cystic fibrosis: Australian guidelines. J Paediatr Child Health. 1999;35:125–9.
42. Basketter HM, Sharples L, Bilton D. Knowledge of pancreatic enzyme supplementation in adult cystic fibrosis (CF) patients. J Hum Nutr Dietet. 2000;13:353–61.

43. Stapleton DR, Gurrin LC, Zubrick SR, Silburn SR, Sherriff JL, Sly PD. What do children with cystic fibrosis and their parents know about nutrition and pancreatic enzymes? J Am Diet Assoc. 2000;100:1494–500.
44. Zentler-Munro PL, Assoufi BA, Balasubramanian K et al. Therapeutic potential and clinical efficacy of acid-resistant fungal lipase in the treatment of pancreatic steatorrhoea due to cystic fibrosis. Pancreas. 1992;7:311–19.
45. Raimondo M, DiMagno EP. Lipolytic activity of bacterial lipase survives better than that of porcine lipase in human gastric and duodenal content. Gastroenterology. 1994;107:231–5.
46. Suzuki A, Mizumoto A, Sarr MG, DiMagno P. Bacterial lipase and high-fat diets in canine exocrine pancreatic insufficiency: a new therapy of steatorrhea? Gastroenterology. 1997;112:2048–55.

22
Optimal control of diabetes mellitus in pancreatitis

F. J. M. GÖKE and B. GÖKE

Patients with chronic pancreatitis (CP) often suffer from endocrine pancreatic dysfunction. This leads to a distinct clinical diabetes form regarded as a secondary type of diabetes[1]. Diabetes mellitus (DM) secondary to CP accounts for <1% of all diabetes cases, which is probably the reason why it is not of much interest for most diabetologists. On the other hand, 80% of patients with CP develop an overt DM in the long run, and DM is an independent risk factor for mortality in patients with CP[2-4]. This makes this form of DM highly relevant to the gastroenterologist.

The most frequent cause of secondary DM in patients with pancreatic diseases in the western hemisphere is chronic alcoholic pancreatitis[5]. Its occurrence is attributed to the close anatomical and functional links between exocrine and endocrine pancreas. It is believed that CP progressively developing fibrosis and sclerosis alters pancreatic capillary circulation and thereby reduces islet perfusion. This results in an impaired function of the insulin-producing beta cells and the glucagon-producing alpha cells.

Interestingly, in tropical countries and India, a special form of non-alcoholic tropical calcifying pancreatitis leads to DM. Although little is known about the exact aetiology of this form of diabetes it has been found that beta cell function is damaged whereas alpha cells are preserved[6,7]. This is in contrast to the non-tropical chronic pancreatitis in which both cell populations are altered. In any case, two different pathogenic mechanisms have been proposed, one eliciting CP and the other selective pancreatic beta cell impairment and subsequent DM. It is an open question whether such a selective hit on the beta cell also plays a role in non-tropical CP.

In acute pancreatitis up to 50% of patients show only transient hyperglycaemia with persistent DM developing in less than 5%, unless further attacks occur with permanent tissue damage[5]. Apparently the severity of inflammation is decisive for the impairment of glucose tolerance. Endocrine pancreatic impairment was found significantly more often in patients after severe acute pancreatitis compared with patients after mild pancreatitis attacks. However, the incidence of DM in connection with acute pancreatitis does not significantly exceed the reported values for the general population. This is quite in contrast to the situation in CP.

DM caused by chronic inflammation of the exocrine pancreas develops typically in 80% of patients within the first 10 years after the initial diagnosis of CP[8]. Chronic calcifying pancreatitis (60–70%) leads to diabetes more often than non-calcifying pancreatitis (15–30%)[2,9]. The duration of CP plays an important role: the continuing inflammatory–fibrotic disturbance of exocrine and endocrine tissue with a significant loss of beta cells, and hence a progressive decrease of insulin secretion, triggers overt DM. DM occurs when approximately 80% of beta cells are destroyed[10].

The subsequently developing hyperglycaemia probably adds an aditional glucotoxic action to the beta cell, causing further deterioration to the endocrine function.

The risk of DM manifestation in CP is sometimes influenced by pancreatic surgery[4]. However, only distal pancreatectomy is clearly associated with a higher rate of DM and insulin requirement as compared to other types of surgical procedures (e.g. pancreaticoduodenectomy). This is in accordance with the heterogeneous distribution of Langerhans islets along the pancreatic gland, prominently localized in the tail of the pancreas. Remarkably, DM appearing after pancreaticoduodenectomy performed for CP is almost always delayed for a minimum of 1 year after surgery, suggesting that disease progression prevails in the risk of DM as opposed to the surgery itself. This assumption is also supported by a definite correlation between the onset of calcification and endocrine insufficiency.

Pancreatic damage *per se* may not be the only factor leading to diabetes, since some patients show an endocrine dysfunction whereas others do not. Several concepts exist to shed more light on this issue.

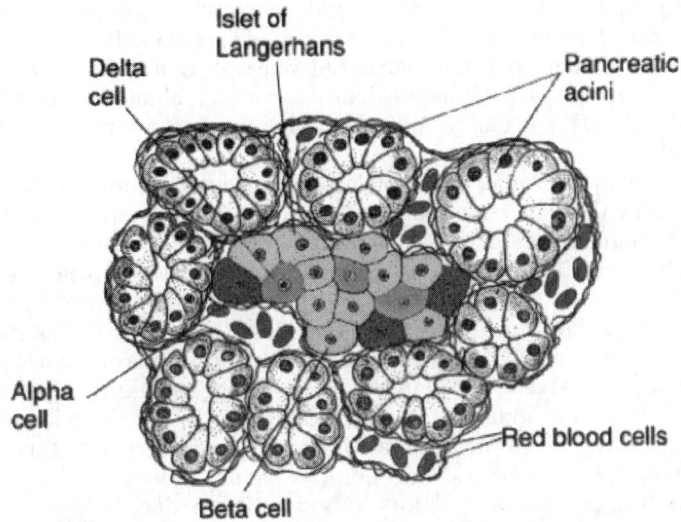

Figure 1 The endocrine islet of Langerhans is surrounded by exocrine pancreatic acini. The islet comprises insulin-producing beta cells, glucagon-producing alpha cells, and somatostatin-producing delta cells

One can try to explain the occurrence of pancreatic exocrine dysfunction as a complication of preexisting diabetes. However, only in a few patients do overt DM symptoms precede a later finding of CP. It is questionable whether DM is the reason for CP, rather than CP being oligosymptomatic and allowing DM to become overt somewhat earlier. Anyway, this may lead to an initial misclassification[11,12]. Overall, it seems unlikely that DM is a true risk factor of CP in the vast majority of patients. Whether newly developing concepts of the pathogenesis of CP will shed more light on this question is so far only speculative[13].

Several risk factors for the development of diabetes in CP have been defined[4]. Diabetes is more likely to occur at a younger age, and has a higher prevalence after surgery at that time. Younger patients are also more likely to show pancreatic calcifications and liver cirrhosis. The onset of pancreatic calcifications is significantly associated with the risk of DM; the earlier they appear, the greater the risk appears of DM and insulin requirement. A tight correlation between onset of pancreatic calcifications and pancreatic endocrine insufficiency is known. Alcoholic pancreatitis, especially with continuing alcohol abuse, is more likely associated with the development of DM. Further risk factors are severe exocrine pancreatic insufficiency and a family history of type 2 DM.

The clinical presentation of DM comes with symptoms like those in other diabetes forms. The suspicion that an impaired glucose tolerance or established diabetes is secondary to chronic pancreatitis is often based on a history of CP with a known cause. To confirm the diagnosis, fasting plasma glucose levels or 2 h glucose values during an oral glucose tolerance test may be used[11].

Diabetes and steatorrhoea are manifested only in the later stages of CP. This secondary form of DM is also accompanied by complications such as microangiopathic/macroangiopathic and neuropathic complications analogous to other diabetes types[14]. Here, the risk of such complications is similar. Less is known about the more advanced stages of diabetic complications in patients suffering from CP-based diabetes, such as blindness and end-stage kidney disease. This is due to the overall high mortality of patients with late-stage CP[14].

Patients with CP suffer from malabsorption and nutritional deficiencies, which makes the understanding of the relationship between endocrine and exocrine dysfunction in CP even more complicated. It was shown that ultimately all patients with severe dysfunction of the exocrine pancreas became glucose intolerant[15].

There are special clinical features in secondary DM during the course of CP: a glycaemic lability is typical with wide fluctuations in plasma glucose levels. More frequently, severe and unpredictable hypoglycaemic episodes occur[11]. Certain factors contribute to the increased risk of hypoglycaemia and metabolic instability: malabsorption, maldigestion, accelerated intestinal transit, low carbohydrate intake, alcohol, non-compliance, abnormalities in insulin secretion, lack of counterregulatory hormones (e.g. reduced glucagon plasma levels), a decrease in glucose utilization by peripheral tissues and fatty acid abnormalities[11,16,17]. Diabetic patients with CP have a smaller risk of ketoacidosis than do patients with type 1 diabetes[18]. Earlier studies have shown reduced plasma glucagon responses to a glucose challenge[9,11,12], although some patients even show increased glucagon plasma levels in response to an oral glucose load. In this context it is difficult to draw clear-cut conclusions concerning the role of glucagon in the relative ketosis resistance in CP-induced DM.

Besides treating CP and its consequences it is necessary to deal with the occurring impaired glucose tolerance, especially with an overt DM. Statistically, in the long run an estimated 10% of patients die because of endocrine dysfunction, diabetic late complications or severe hypoglycaemia resulting from insulin injections[11,14]. The coexistant exocrine deficiency makes a dietary regimen more challenging, especially under an insulin treatment schedule. If the diet therapy does not work properly hypoglycaemic episodes are more likely to occur.

Basically, diabetes therapy in chronic pancreatitis needs to take several problems into account: patients may lack appropriate compliance for an insulin treatment regimen, especially when a continuous alcohol consumption alters an appropiate diet and favours the occurrence of hypoglycaemia by its effect on liver metabolism. Furthermore, inadequate eating behaviour because of pain after meals leads to an unpredictable consumption of carbohydrates. Such problems induced by the diet may also occur at an accelerated intestinal transit following maldigestion (if the enzyme replacement therapy is not effective). A glucagon deficiency and/or blunted glucagon response may favour a reduced counterbalance in response to insulin injections, causing hypoglycaemia. Additionally, neuropathic disease, possibly coming with poorly controlled DM, may lead to a disturbance of gastric emptying and intestinal transit, making dietary regimens hard to follow. A too-aggressive insulin substitution regimen with too-high initial dosages can lead to rapid severe hypoglycaemia. HbA1c values ranging between 7% and 8% are often acceptable, and are associated with a decreased risk of severe hypoglycaemia.

When designing a therapy of DM in CP (Table 1), first one should consider lifestyle, eating habits, comorbidities, prognosis, age, and the metabolic stability of the patient. Therapy must be individually tailored and based upon an adequate nutritional status of the patient, sufficient enzyme substitution compensating exocrine insufficiency, and alcohol abstinence. This is the basis of a safer insulin-based DM therapy. If there is known incompliance, especially continuing alcohol consumption, insulin therapy is not indicated; 50% of patients with CP can be treated by diet. Oral antidiabetics are often problematic

Table 1 Treatment of diabetes mellitus in chronic pancreatitis

Basis of therapy
  Adequate nutritional status, sufficient enzyme substitutions, alcohol abstinence, comorbidities and overall prognosis, age, metabolic stability

Problem
  Severe hypoglycaemia

Target
  HbA1c values of 7–8%

Insulin requirement
  0.30–0.45 IU insulin/kg body weight per day

and only shortly-acting sulphonylureas may offer a treatment option, although only in a minority of patients. Metformin is often contraindicated, especially having alcoholic CP in mind. Insulin sensitizers such as the glitazones are without indication, since insulin deficiency rather than resistance is the key problem. Maldigestion comes with progressive CP and exocrine pancreatic failure, and decompensates when combined with glucosidase inhibitors. With a continuing endocrine insufficiency insulin therapy becomes indispensable[11]. Clearly, less insulin is needed than in the conventional treatment of DM type 1 or 2[14]. The patient is generally highly sensitive to insulin. A close follow-up on blood glucose levels is indicated, to decrease the risk of hypoglycaemia. An intensified insulin treatment regimen with multiple injections of small amounts of short-acting insulin[11] offers advantages. Combinations of normal and retarded insulins are possible only under a stable condition of metabolism, which is rarely the case. The daily insulin requirement is low, ranging daily between 0.30 and 0.45 IU/kg body weight. Initially, an insulin load of 0.8–1.4 IU/12 g carbohydrates can be tried. The insulin regimen then needs further individual tailoring. In highly motivated patients insulin pump therapy may become an option. Basal infusion rates of the insulin pump amount normally to 20–30% of the daily insulin needs, with meal-connected bolus infusions of 0.8–1.4 IU insulin/12 g carbohydrates. Insulin pumps are especially of interest for patients after total pancreatectomy.

References

1. Expert Committee on the Diagnosis and Classification: Report of the expert committee on the diagnosis and classification of diabetes mellitus. Diabetes Care. 1997;20:1183–97.
2. Ammann RW, Akovbiantz A, Largiader F, Schueler G. Course and outcome of chronic pancreatitis. Longitudinal study of a mixed medical–chirurgical series of 245 patients. Gastroenterology. 1984;86:820–8.
3. Levy P, Milan C, Pignon JP, Baetz A, Bernades P. Mortality factors associated with chronic pancreatitis. Unidimensional and multidimensional analysis of a medical–surgical series of 240 patients. Gastroenterology. 1989;96:1165–72.
4. Malka D, Hammel P, Sauvanet A et al. Risk factors for diabetes mellitus in chronic pancreatitis. Gastroenterology. 2000;119:1324–32.
5. Banks S. Chronic pancreatitis: clinical features and medical management. Am J Gastroenterol. 1986;81:153–67.
6. Rossi L, Parvin S, Hassan Z et al. Diabetes mellitus in tropical chronic pancreatitis is not just a secondary type of diabetes. Pancreatology. 2004;4:461–7.
7. Govindarajan M, Mohan V, Deepa R, Ashok S, Pitchumoni CS. Histopathology and immunhistochemistry of pancreatic islets in fibrocalculous pancreatic diabetes. Dig Res Clin Pract. 2001;51:29–38.
8. Lankisch PG, Löhr-Hoppe A, Otto J, Creutzfeldt W. Natural course in chronic pancreatitis. Digestion. 1993;54:148–55.
9. Larsen S. Diabetes mellitus secondary to chronic pancreatitis. Den Med Bull. 1993;40:153–62
10. Vinik AI. Insulin secretion in chronic pancreatitis. In: Tiengo A, Alberti KGMM, DelPrato S, Vranic M, editors. Diabetes Secondary to Pancreopathy. Amsterdam: Excerpta Medica, 1988:35–50.
11. Diem P. Pathogenesis and treatment of diabetes secondary to chronic pancreatis. In: Büchler MW, Friess H, Uhl W, Malfertheiner P, editors. Chronic Pancreatitis. Oxford: Blackwell, 2002:355–8.
12. Siegel EG, Jakobs R, Riemann JF. Pankreopriver und hepatogener Diabetes. Besondere Aspekte in Pathophysiologie und Behandlung. Internist. 2001;42(Suppl. 1):S8–S19.

13. Stevens T, Conwell DL, Zuccaro G. Pathogenesis of chronic pancreatitis: an evidence-based review of past theories and recent developments. Am J Gastroenterol. 2004;99:2256–70.
14. Del Prato S, Tiengo A. Pancreatic diabetes. Diab Rev. 1993;1:260–85.
15. Quereda AL, Orti SL, Chornet CJ et al. Early carbohydrate metabolism dysfunction in chronic pancreatitis. Relation with exocrine pancreatic function. Med Clin (Barc). 2001; 117:561–6.
16. Diaz-Rubio JL, Torre-Delgadillo A, Robles Diaz. Diabetes mellitus in acute pancreatitis. Rev Gastroenterol Mex. 2002;67:278–84.
17. Quillot D, Walters E, Böhme P et al. Fatty acid abnormalities in chronic pancreatitis: effect of concomitant diabetes mellitus. Eur J Clin Nutr. 2003;57:496–503.
18. Perusicova J. Diabetes mellitus in chronic pancreatitis. Vnitr Lek. 2004;50:375–8.

23
Chronic pancreatitis: precursor of carcinoma?

A. B. LOWENFELS and P. MAISONNEUVE

INTRODUCTION

The incidence of pancreas cancer is relatively low, but because of its highly lethal course this tumour is one of the commonest causes of cancer mortality. The high mortality rate from this tumour has stimulated a great deal of interest in searching for the underlying cause(s) of this cancer. Chronic pancreatitis has been proposed as a possible aetiological factor: this chapter will review the evidence linking chronic pancreatitis with pancreas cancer. Acute pancreatitis, a much more common disease than chronic pancreatitis, has never been linked to pancreatic cancer, unless there is progression of the acute process to chronic pancreatitis.

In the nineteenth century Virchow, an outstanding German pathologist, proposed that an inflammatory change in an organ might eventually lead to cancer. His observations were based mainly on careful autopsy records; in the twentieth century his hypothesis has been confirmed by numerous epidemiological studies. With respect to the digestive tract there are numerous examples in which cancer eventually develops many years after the diagnosis of a benign lesion. The process is a gradual one, usually taking decades, with the risk increasing as the duration of the underlying benign process increases (Table 1). For some organs the risk is exceptionally high: in the liver, for example, infection with hepatitis B or C is associated with a 100-fold increased risk of liver cancer – one of the strongest risks for any type of cancer[1]. About half of all cases of gallbladder cancer can be traced to pre-existing chronic cholecystitis and cholelithiasis[2]. Does pancreas cancer follow this same pattern? And if pre-existing benign pancreatitis lead to pancreatic cancer, how frequently does this occur?

232

Table 1 Association between pre-existing benign digestive tract disease and cancer in non-pancreatic organs

Organ	Pre-existing benign disease	Remarks
Esophagus	Reflux oesophagitis	Strong risk factor for adenocarcinoma in lower part of oesophagus; frequency rapidly increasing
Stomach	Atrophic gastritis	*H. pylori* induced atrophic gastritis is a precursor for gastric cancer
Colon	Benign polyps	Most intestinal cancers are thought to originate from underlying polyps; risk increases with increasing polyp diameter
Liver	Cirrhosis	Alcoholic, viral hepatitis precede most cases of hepatocellular cancer
Gallbladder	Chronic cholecystitis, cholelithiasis	Nearly all cases of gallbladder cancer occur in association with gallstones
Bile duct	Choledochal cyst, sclerosing cholangitis, bile duct stricture	Several benign bile duct lesions, usually causing bile stasis, are risk factors for bile duct cancer

CHRONIC PANCREATITIS AND PANCREATIC CANCER: ASSESSING THE EVIDENCE

Various methods have been used to assess the association between pancreatitis and pancreatic cancer. Case reports have linked chronic pancreatitis to pancreas cancer, but this type of evidence is unreliable, qualitative, and does not provide any reliable evidence for causality, or for the strength of the relationship (relative risk).

Case–control studies

Several case–control studies have been performed to determine whether patients who develop pancreas cancer are more likely to have had a prior history of pancreatitis than do control patients[3–6]. Most case–control studies do show an association; cases are four or five times more likely to report a history of antecedent pancreatitis than control subjects. Unfortunately, in these types of studies, there is a real possibility of bias because patients with pancreatic cancer might be more likely to remember or report pancreatitis than are control subjects. Another problem is that pancreatic cancer is such an aggressive disease that often a proper history must be obtained from a surrogate informant, rather than from the patient. Secondary information obtained in this manner is likely to be inaccurate.

Record linkage studies

In countries where there are large, electronically stored health records it is possible to perform record linkage studies. One could query a patient database, extract records for all patients with pancreatitis then, using the same or perhaps a supplementary database, obtain follow-up data. Record linkage studies have been performed looking at the pancreatitis–pancreatic cancer relationship in two countries. The Swedish national hospital database and the Swedish cancer registry have been linked together, revealing a significant but somewhat weak relationship between chronic pancreatitis and pancreas cancer[7,8]. The relationship became somewhat weaker as the interval from diagnosed pancreatitis to pancreas cancer increased. The authors speculated that, in some patients, occult pancreas cancer might have been present in patients who developed pancreas cancer soon after the onset of chronic pancreatitis.

In another study, based on the United States Veterans Association database[9], antecedent chronic pancreatitis was a significant risk factor for pancreas cancer. A high proportion of patients in this study had chronic alcoholic pancreatitis – the commonest type.

Record linkage studies provide valuable information, but their accuracy depends upon careful coding of patient diagnostic categories. Furthermore, changes in coding practices or categories can affect the results.

Cohort studies

Other than intervention studies, which would not be possible, cohort studies provide the strongest evidence to determine whether or not chronic pancreatitis leads to pancreatic cancer. Several such studies have been performed, with the evidence summarized in Table 2. The evidence supports the concept that chronic pancreatitis is a risk factor for pancreatic cancer.

The information available from cohort studies, as well as from all other study types, implies that chronic pancreatitis is indeed a risk factor for pancreatic cancer. This relationship holds true even after exclusion of patients who develop pancreatic cancer less than 2 years after symptoms of chronic pancreatitis.

CHRONIC PANCREATITIS AND PANCREATIC CANCER: IMPLICATIONS

As in other parts of the digestive tract, the evidence strongly suggests that prior inflammatory disease, culminating in chronic pancreatitis, leads to pancreatic cancer. How often does this occur? How much of the burden of pancreas cancer can be explained by pre-existing chronic pancreatitis?

In patients with alcoholic or idiopathic pancreatitis the cumulative incidence of pancreas cancer increases steadily over time, but even 20 years after the onset of chronic pancreatitis only about 4–5% of patients will have developed pancreas cancer. Thus, although the risk of pancreas cancer is much greater than the risk in persons without pancreatitis, only a small proportion of

Table 2 Pancreatitis–pancreatic cancer: results of cohort studies

Reference	Type of pancreatitis	Study population	No. pancreas cancer cases	Remarks
Lowenfels et al., 1993[24]	Chronic pancreatitis	Historical cohort, 2015 subjects with chronic pancreatitis	29 cases, 18 with at least 5 years follow-up	SMR = 16.5 for patients with >2 years follow-up; 14.4 for patients with >5 years follow-up
Talamini et al., 1999[25]	Chronic pancreatitis	715 chronic pancreatitis patients with median 10-year follow-up	14	13-fold increased risk of pancreas cancer
Malka et al., 2002[26]	Chronic pancreatitis	373 patients, median follow-up 9.2 years	4	19-fold increased risk of pancreas cancer
Lowenfels et al., 1997[11]	Hereditary pancreatitis	246 patients with hereditary pancreatitis	8	Greater than 50-fold increased risk of pancreas cancer
Howes et al., 2004[12]	Hereditary pancreatitis	418 patients	26	67-fold increased risk of pancreas cancer
Chari et al., 1994[13]	Tropical pancreatitis	185 patients with tropical calcifying pancreatitis	6	100-fold increased risk of pancreas cancer

235

patients with chronic pancreatitis will ever develop pancreatic cancer. This has important implications for screening (see below). The converse is also true: because chronic pancreatitis is a rare disease, few patients with pancreatic cancer will have had a prior history of pancreatitis.

RARE TYPES OF PANCREATITIS AND PANCREAS CANCER

Heavy consumption of alcohol is the commonest cause of chronic pancreatitis, accounting for more than two-thirds of all cases. Idiopathic pancreatitis is the second most frequent cause. However, the rarer types of pancreatitis, often beginning early in life, are usually associated with a high risk of pancreatic cancer.

Hereditary pancreatitis is an autosomal dominant disease caused by a mutation in the trypsinogen gene[10]. Usually, but not always, multiple generations are involved and patients develop symptoms before or soon after puberty. Hereditary pancreatitis provides strong evidence for the association between chronic pancreatitis and pancreas cancer because the lifetime risk of pancreatic cancer is at least 40%[11,12]. In most patients pancreatitis has been present for 30–50 years, and presumably this long exposure period is responsible for the exceptionally high risk of cancer.

Tropical pancreatitis is a common form of pancreatitis in southern India and parts of Africa. Calcification and diabetes are common, as is early onset of disease. The exact cause of this disease is unknown but, similar to hereditary pancreatitis, it carries a high risk of pancreatic cancer[13].

Cystic fibrosis is the commonest autosomal recessive disease of Caucasian populations. The lungs and multiple digestive organs are involved, and in most patients the disease results in massive destruction of the pancreas, occurring during gestation or in the neonatal period. The risk of early-onset pancreas cancer is high, although only a few such patients have been reported in Europe and North America over a period of more than 20 years[14–16].

CHRONIC PANCREATITIS AND PANCREAS CANCER: POSSIBLE PATHWAYS

The available evidence supports the hypothesis that pre-existing chronic pancreatitis can lead to pancreas cancer. The exact mechanism is still elusive, but the underlying pathways are becoming clearer. We know that inflammatory changes in many organs lead to increased cell turnover, increasing the possibility of coding errors and deleterious mutations. Injured tissues attract inflammatory cells which, in turn, can result in the formation of damaging free radical intermediate products. Using gene array analysis Farrow and co-workers have reported similar inflammatory components in both chronic pancreatitis and pancreatic cancer[17].

We now know that premalignant changes called panin lesions are seen in pancreata in association with or preceding overt malignancy. These same premalignant lesions have been detected in patients with chronic pancreatitis[18].

On the cellular level, K-ras changes have been found in patients with chronic pancreatitis[19]. Some, but not all, studies have noted that K-ras mutations in patients with chronic pancreatitis are associated with subsequent occurrence of pancreatic cancer[20,21]. In the study reported by Arvanitakis and co-workers 10% of 44 pancreatitis patients with a K-ras mutation developed pancreatic cancer over a 42-month period; in contrast, none of 68 patients without a K-ras mutation developed pancreas cancer[20].

The p16 tumour-suppressor gene is one of the most important genes involved in the aetiology of many types of tumour, and is altered in nearly all patients with pancreas cancer. Loss of expression of p16 has also been found in 6.5% of patients with chronic pancreatitis. In this subgroup the frequency of p16 loss increased with increasing degree of panin dysplasia[18]. Loss of p16 function could be a potential link between pancreatitis and pancreatic cancer.

SCREENING FOR PANCREAS CANCER IN PATIENTS WITH CHRONIC PANCREATITIS

To date, screening most groups of patients with chronic pancreatitis for pancreas cancer has not been feasible. For patients with either alcoholic or idiopathic pancreatitis – the commonest types – the cumulative risk of pancreas cancer over a period of two decades is only about 5%. The predictive value of a positive screening test assuming a sensitivity and specificity of 90% would not be high enough to justify such a programme.

Patients with hereditary pancreatitis have a lifetime risk of pancreas cancer that is 40% or higher. A consensus conference on screening held at the Third International Symposium on Hereditary Diseases of the Pancreas recommended that screening could be offered to these patients, especially if it was offered at a centre with considerable experience in the management of these patients and where optimal imaging technology was available[22]. Endoscopic ultrasound (EUS) was the suggested initial screening tool, along with collection of blood samples and pancreatic juice to be stored for future analysis.

In patients with hereditary pancreatitis, smoking lowers the age of onset of pancreas cancer[12,23]; these patients should be warned not to smoke or, if they are current smokers, they should be encouraged to enter a smoking cessation programme. Alcohol is known to damage the pancreas, so these patients should be advised not to drink.

SUMMARY

Over the past few decades evidence has accumulated linking chronic but not acute pancreatitis with the subsequent development of pancreas cancer. The time interval between the onset of chronic pancreatitis and the development of pancreas cancer is generally greater than 20 years. In the past there has been some aetiological confusion because pancreatitis can be an early manifestation of pancreas cancer. If the diagnosis of pancreas cancer is made within a year or two after the onset of pancreatitis, we can assume that pancreatitis was caused by ductal obstruction from the neoplastic process. All forms of chronic pancreatitis carry a risk of pancreas cancer, but the highest risk seems to be in persons with an early onset of pancreatitis, as seen in tropical pancreatitis, hereditary pancreatitis, or cystic fibrosis. Chronic pancreatitis causes only about 5% of the total burden of pancreatic cancer so, except for hereditary pancreatitis, screening pancreatitis patients for cancer is not recommended.

Acknowledgement

This work was supported in part by grants from the C.D. Smithers Foundation, Mill Neck, NY, Solvay Pharmaceuticals, Marietta, GA, USA.

References

1. Beasley RP. Hepatitis B virus. The major etiology of hepatocellular carcinoma. Cancer. 1988;61:1942–56.
2. Lowenfels AB, Lindstrom CG, Conway MJ. Gallstones and risk of gallbladder cancer. J Natl Cancer Inst. 1985;75:77–80.
3. Mack TM, Yu MC, Hanisch R, Henderson BE. Pancreas cancer and smoking, beverage consumption, and past medical history. J Natl Cancer Inst. 1986;76:49–60.
4. Farrow DC, Davis S. Diet and the risk of pancreatic cancer in men. Am J Epidemiol. 1990; 132:423–31.
5. Jain M, Howe GR, St Louis P, Miller AB. Coffee and alcohol as determinants of risk of pancreas cancer: a case–control study from Toronto. Int J Cancer. 1991;47:384–9.
6. Kalapothaki V, Tzonou A, Hsieh CC, Toupadaki N, Karakatsani A, Trichopoulos D. Tobacco, ethanol, coffee, pancreatitis, diabetes mellitus, and cholelithiasis as risk factors for pancreatic carcinoma. Cancer Causes Control. 1993;4:375–82.
7. Ekbom A, McLaughlin JK, Karlsson BM et al. Pancreatitis and pancreatic cancer: a population-based study. J Natl Cancer Inst. 1994;86:625–7.
8. Karlson BM, Ekbom A, Josefsson S, McLaughlin JK, Fraumeni JF Jr, Nyren O. The risk of pancreatic cancer following pancreatitis: an association due to confounding? Gastroenterology. 1997;113:587–92.
9. Bansal P, Sonnenberg A. Pancreatitis is a risk factor for pancreatic cancer. Gastronenterology. 1995;109:247–51.
10. Whitcomb DC, Gorry MC, Preston RA et al. Hereditary pancreatitis is caused by a mutation in the cationic trypsinogen gene [see comments]. Nat Genet. 1996;14:141–5.
11. Lowenfels AB, Maisonneuve P, DiMagno EP et al. Hereditary pancreatitis and the risk of pancreatic cancer. International Hereditary Pancreatitis Study Group. J Natl Cancer Inst. 1997;89:442–6.
12. Howes N, Lerch MM, Greenhalf W et al. Clinical and genetic characteristics of hereditary pancreatitis in Europe. Clin Gastroenterol Hepatol. 2004;2:252–61.
13. Chari ST, Mohan V, Pitchumoni CS, Viswanathan M, Madanagopalan N, Lowenfels AB. Risk of pancreatic carcinoma in tropical calcifying pancreatitis: an epidemiologic study. Pancreas. 1994;9:62–6.
14. Maisonneuve P, FitzSimmons SC, Neglia JP, Campbell PW, III, Lowenfels AB. Cancer risk in nontransplanted and transplanted cystic fibrosis patients: a 10-year study. J Natl Cancer Inst. 2003;95:381–7.
15. Neglia JP, FitzSimmons SC, Maisonneuve P et al. The risk of cancer among patients with cystic fibrosis. N Engl J Med. 1995;332:494–9.
16. Schoni MH, Maisonneuve P, Schoni-Affolter FS, Lowenfels AB. Cancer risk in patients with cystic fibrosis: the European data. J R Soc Med. 1996;27:38–43.
17. Farrow B, Sugiyama Y, Chen A, Uffort E, Nealon W, Mark EB. Inflammatory mechanisms contributing to pancreatic cancer development. Ann Surg. 2004;239:763–9.
18. Rosty C, Geradts J, Sato N et al. p16 Inactivation in pancreatic intraepithelial neoplasias (PanINs) arising in patients with chronic pancreatitis. Am J Surg Pathol. 2003;27:1495–501.

19. Lohr M, Maisonneuve P, Lowenfels AB. K-Ras mutations and benign pancreatic disease. Int J Pancreatol. 2000;27:93–103.
20. Arvanitakis M, Van Laethem JL, Parma J, De M, V, Delhaye M, Deviere J. Predictive factors for pancreatic cancer in patients with chronic pancreatitis in association with K-ras gene mutation. Endoscopy. 2004;36:535–42.
21. Tada M, Omata M, Ohto M. Clinical application of ras gene mutation for diagnosis of pancreatic adenocarcinoma. Gastroenterology. 1991;100:233–8.
22. Ulrich CD for the Consensus Committees of the European Registry of Hereditary Pancreatic Diseases, the Midwest Multi-Center Pancreatic Study Group and the International Association of Pancreatology. Pancreatic cancer in hereditary pancreatitis: consensus guidelines for prevention, screening and treatment. Pancreatology. 2001;1:416–22.
23. Lowenfels AB, Maisonneuve P, Whitcomb DC, Lerch MM, DiMagno EP. Cigarette smoking as a risk factor for pancreatic cancer in patients with hereditary pancreatitis. J Am Med Assoc. 2001;286:169–70.
24. Lowenfels AB, Maisonneuve P, Cavallini G et al. Pancreatitis and the risk of pancreatic cancer. International Pancreatitis Study Group. N Engl J Med. 1993;328:1433–7.
25. Talamini G, Falconi M, Bassi C et al. Incidence of cancer in the course of chronic pancreatitis. Am J Gastroenterol. 1999;94:1253–60.
26. Malka D, Hammel P, Maire F et al. Risk of pancreatic adenocarcinoma in chronic pancreatitis. Gut. 2002;51:849–52.

24
Mortality and survival in chronic pancreatitis: a personal and international study

S. BANK, N. POORAN, J. XIE and R. BRUNNER

INTRODUCTION

Longtidunal studies on the cause, treatment and prognosis of chronic pancreatitis have been carried out in a number of centres, notably by Ammann[1–4] (Ammann, personal communication) in Switzerland, Lankisch et al. in Germany[5], Marks and Bank and co-workers in South Africa[6–10], Sahel in Marseilles (personal communication), Dani et al. in Brazil[11], Hayakawa et al. in Japan[12,13], Geevarghese[14] and Tandon (personal communication) in India. Lowenfels et al.[15] in the USA collated a multicentre study on the mortality of chronic pancreatitis from various countries, mostly in Europe, and the USA, which showed an increased mortality over a 10–20-year period from the onset of the disease, compared to the expected mortality in the population. The variability in the mortality and survival prevalence in these studies can of course be contributed to a number of factors, which can be categorized into variations in geography, i.e. tropical vs western type of chronic pancreatitis; alcohol-related vs non-alcoholic; socioeconomic factors; access to treatment, mainly surgical, endoscopic, radiological expertise of the area; the inclusion of the number of severe cases in the series, i.e. those with calcification as compared to series with earlier disease, i.e. non-calcific, or pre-calcific disease; and finally what appears to be an increasing incidence of pancreatic and extra-pancreatic cancer in different series[16,17]. One of the difficulties in relating the mortality to the pancreatic disease is the mortality due to co-morbid disease. Various authors might include conditions such as infection, gastrointestinal haemorrhage, and maybe even cerebrovascular deaths under co-morbid causes, and others might attribute these to the precarious nutritional or immunological state of the patients with severe chronic pancreatitis – for example, failed metabolic reserve[8,9]. Thus there may be difficulty in categorizing these conditions related to the pancreatic disease or unrelated causes. In addition, with increased longevity of the population as a whole, earlier death from these conditions might well be related to the pancreatic disease even though the mean mortality age in various series ranges from 60 to 65 years[11] (Ammann, personal communication).

The virtually inevitable progression of the disease to pain, diabetes, steator-rhoea or a complication singly or in combination contributes to an earlier mortality. However, advances in the treatment of the complications, especially cysts and gastrointestinal bleeding, as well as improved diabetes and steator-rhoea control, have probably resulted in an increased longevity of some 10–20 years[18,19], especially in areas of poorer socioeconomic conditions which have since developed improved facilities. On the other hand, improved survival to a more advanced age appears to have resulted in an increased mortality from non-pancreatic causes, particularly extrapancreatic cancers and cerebrovascu-lar accidents[4] (Ammann, personal communication). This chapter will attempt to come to some consensus regarding: (a) the overall mortality and survival of chronic pancreatitis over a specific period of time; (b) whether factors such as inclusion of related or unrelated causes of death contribute to the variability in mortality prevalence from various geographic, socioeconomic or aetiological groups; (c) whether there has been improved survival over the past 20 years; and (d) whether we should be paying more attention to the quality of life with current therapy rather than being preoccupied with mortality.

MATERIAL AND METHODS

Two groups of series will be considered: (1) a personal series of 162 patients obtained for personal experience and hospital records seen at Long Island Jewish Medical Center in the USA and followed for 12 years from 1984 to 1996 and as far as possible thereafter, and (2) an international series consisting of a review of 36 published papers, abstracts and replies to a questionnaire sent to selected pancreatologists in the USA, Switzerland, Italy, Germany, Britain, Japan, India, Chile, South Africa, Brazil, Argentina, etc. Of these 21 were printed papers consisting mainly of medical series (five were largely surgical series and four from tropical areas). The remaining 15 were answers to a questionnaire sent out to selected pancreatologists worldwide. Table 1 shows an example of the questionnaire that was sent, in which special reference was made to whether there had been improvement in the survival of pancreatitis from the years before 1984 compared to the years after 1984, whether the deaths were definitively related to chronic pancreatitis or to 'so-called' co-morbid conditions, the length of follow-up and the possible reasons for improved survival over the past 20 years if indeed this is so. This resulted in an evaluation of a total of some 4800 cases (excluding Lowenfels' series). In addition, there were four papers related to the quality of life using the SF 36 or the EORTCQOL 30 or PAN 26 scales[19,20] (Doule et al., personal communica-tion). Although the time from clinical onset to death varied in the various series, and the exact cause was frequently not specified (for example, there were always a number of unknown causes or some labelled 'failed metabolic reserve' or 'miscellaneous' as well as 'lost to follow-up' in nearly every series). To conform as much as possible to our current series between 1984 and 1996 the mortality over a 12-year period (10–14 years), where stated in the literature and questionnaire, was taken as a workable number, and the cause of death, especially whether related to the pancreatic disease or not, often had to be

Table 1 Example of questionnaire sent to selected pancreatologists worldwide (present example from a personal communication from L. Gullo)

Please complete as best as possible

Mortality

1. Number of patients with alcoholic CP in your series: _____135_____
2. Number of patients who have died:__21____
3. Age at death (mean/range:___52___ YRS 29-76

Cause of Death

Number definitely related to CP: ____1___
Number probably related to CP: ___2___
Number of surgical deaths: ___2___
Number unrelated to CP (eg. Cardiac, Ca,) __16___
Number developing cancer: ___7__

Etiology of Pancreatitis/Mortality:

Number – Alcohol: ____135____
Number – Tropical: ____---____
Number – Idiopathic: ____---____
Number – Other: ____---____

Time of follow up before death (mean/range): ___12__ YRS 5-38

Survival:

Has there been an improvement in survival in the last 20 yrs.? YES (NO) Probably

If yes, due to interventional endoscopy?   YES   NO
Due to surgical technique?   YES   NO
Due to better diabetic care?   YES   NO
Due to better steatorrhea therapy?   YES   NO

Does social/economic status influence survival? (YES)   NO

Please enter any factors which you consider of importance with regard to mortality/survival that you would like included in a talk booklet – it would be acknowledged adequately.

inferred from the data. This led to a considered but inexact calculation in many instances[21,22].

RESULTS

Personal series

Table 2 shows that the 12-year mortality at Long Island Jewish Medical Center from 1984 to 1996 was 33%. However, the death rate that could be directly implicated to pancreatic disease and its complications was 18.4%. With the inclusion of infection, gastrointestinal bleeding and development of pancreatic cancer, the death rate due possibly to the effects of pancreatic disease and its consequences accounted for a 51% increase over and above the 18.4%. Even this did not include patients who died outside the hospital from miscellaneous causes or cardiovascular disease, or were lost to follow-up, in which the cause may have been indirectly related to the chronic pancreatitis, especially in older age groups. On the other hand, the age factor had to be considered in those patients with senile chronic pancreatitis with a high mortality who are, of course, prone to develop carcinoma of the pancreas *de novo* which may be incidental to the calcific pancreatitis. In the current series the mean age of onset of the disease was 60 years in the late-onset or senile group, and the mean age of deaths was 63 years for the whole group. As with many other series there was a relatively high incidence of pancreatic cancer, i.e. 4.3% for pancreatic cancer and 6% for all cancers.

Table 2 Twelve-year mortality in various aetiological groups in personal series of chronic pancreatitis from 1984 to 1966

	Alcohol	Idiopathic		Other	Total
		Juvenile	Senile		
Aetiology	73 (45%)	10 (6%)	27 (17%)	52 (32%)	162
Mortality	17 (23%)	3 (33%)	17 (63%)	17 (37%)	54 (33%)
Age at death	67 + 10	46 + 4	67 + 13	73 + 13	63 + 15

International series

Although the period of longitudal review in these 36 series varied quite considerably from 5 to 35 years, to conform with our personal series at ± 12 years the mean of the larger of the series were reviewed, especially taking into account those series pre- and post-1984. The largest of the series in Table 3 was the multicentre study from Lowenfels et al.[15] Ammann et al.'s personal experience[4] (Ammann, personal communication) and those from Marks and Bank[6,8]. In all medical series the 10–12-year mortality ranged from a low of

Table 3 Mortality of chronic pancreatitis in four series (percentages)

Years followed	Marks and Bank (1959–1977)	Bank (1984–1996)	Ammann (1981–2003)	Lowenfels* (1994)
0–5	6			
10–12	27	33	30	30
20	72			55
22			57	

*Lowenfels, Multicenter study.

13–18% in two Italian series[23] (Gullo, personal communication) to 30–50% in most series, and up to 70% at 20–30 years in the Ammann and the Marks and Bank series. Some of the increase in mortality in these latter series may of course be due to the inevitable ageing of many patients. Nevertheless, there does appear to have been a decrease in mortality, albeit slight, from ±30% over 12 years in 1984 to some 13–15% in most series thereafter. This appeared to be particularly true of series from tropical areas and patients with non-alcohol-induced pancreatitis, and may also reflect the inclusion of less severe cases of chronic pancreatitis. Thus, it should be noted that 80% of Ammann's patients were calcific, the mean age of onset was 33 years and the mean age at death 67 years. In the four surgical series reviewed the mortality ranged from 33% to 44% from France, Brazil and South Africa[11,19,22], but despite this Bornman had estimated from his surgical series[19] that survival had improved by some 10–20 years from pre-1984 to the more recent series. In his series the quality-of-life values on the EORTCQOL 30 and PAN 26 scales were improved by surgery for pain; however, postoperative diabetes and steatorrhoea still severely affected the quality of life. In two surgical series the incidence of cancer was 2.7–5%. In a further quality-of-life series from Germany in 265 patients all parameters of the SF 36 quality-of-life scores were severely affected by patients having chronic pancreatitis, perhaps not an unexpected finding[20]. In the five tropical and subtropical series from India and Brazil, and including an early series from South Africa, the 12-year mortality was 50%[11,14,15,24] in the Marks and Banks series[7] prior to 1984, and the 20-year mortality ranged from 43% to 70% in the various series. Tandon, from India, reports a 3% mortality after 3–5 years after 1984; however, of 171 patients 40 were lost to follow-up. In a 13-year surgical series Ramesh[24] reported an incidence of cancer of the pancreas developing in young Indians with calcific pancreatitis among 650 patients of 22%, whereas most medical series from western countries had a cancer incidence of between 2.7% and 8.3%. Table 4 shows the causes of death in chronic pancreatitis comparing a series from Cape Town between 1950 and 1977 to our personal series from 1984 to 1996 in the USA. It can be seen that in the South African series failed metabolic reserve, hypoglycaemia, and unknown causes predominated, whereas in the USA from 1984 to 1996 the striking differences were in malignancies and in particular pancreatic carcinoma. Table 5 compares the causes of death between the Ammann series from 1981 to 2003 and our personal series from 1984 to 1996, which really show a

Table 4 Causes of death in chronic pancreatitis in a pre-1984 series from Cape Town, South Africa to the current series in the USA

	Cape Town, 1950–1977*		USA, 1984–1996**
	Caucasian	Black/mixed	All ethnic groups
Frail metabolic reserve	5%	42%	20% (infection)
Hypoglycaemia	9.5%	8%	0%
Postsurgical	23%	5%	?
Cirrhosis	10%	2%	4%
Unknown	9.5%	32%	7%
Miscellaneous	43%	11%	11%
Cardiovascular			20%
Gastrointestinal bleeding			13%
Malignancy (lung)			24%
Cancer of pancreas		19%	13%
Mean age at death	49 years		67 years

*Marks and Bank.
**Bank et al. (our present series).

Table 5 Comparison of causes of death from Switzerland and USA + pancreatic cancer in Kerala, India

	Ammann* 1981–2003	Bank** 1984–1996	(Ramesh) (2003)
Mortality	197–343	54/162	(650 cases)
Malignancy	22%	24%	
(Pancreatic	?	13%)	(22%)
Cardiovascular	28%	13%	
Infection	15%	20%	
Gastrointestinal bleeding	5%	13%	
Cirrhosis	7%	4%	
Miscellaneous	22%	19%	
Unknown	1%	7%	
	100%	100%	

*Ammann et al. (Personal communication).
**Bank et al. (our present series).

remarkable similarity in causes of death; however, whether gastrointestinal bleeding, infection, and miscellaneous or unknown causes should be included in the mortality figures remains conjectural. Thus, although the mortality rates which are regarded as chronic pancreatitis-related were 14.6% in the Ammann series and 18% in our series, if one added diseases possibly related to chronic pancreatitis factors such as infection, bleeding, postoperative deaths and carcinoma, the total possible chronic pancreatitis-related mortality becomes 55% in the Ammann series and 51% in our personal series at 12 years. Lastly,

Table 6 Factors affecting survival in chronic pancreatitis. In earlier series compared to more current publications (percentages)

	Mortality	Then	Now
Cysts	↓	±13	0.3
Gastrointestinal bleeding	↓	±50	14
Hypoglycaemia	↓	±9	?0
Infection	↓	±?	?
Postoperative	↓	±5–10	±1–5
Pancreatic cancer	↑	±1–3	3–22
Age-related co-morbidity	↑	?50	?80
Suicide	↑	3	?

↓, Decreased mortality.

↑ Increased mortality.

Table 6 shows the factors affecting survival in chronic pancreatitis over the past 20 years. The mortality from cysts, gastrointestinal bleeding, hypoglycsemia, probably infection, and operation, have all contributed to decreased mortality, whereas pancreatic cancer and age-related co-morbidity appear to be the main factors that have prevented a further decrease in mortality[18,245]. In response to the question in the questionnaire as to whether there had been an improvement in survival over the past 20 years, mainly in the alcoholic group, 14 responses were received worldwide. Seven authors responded 'Yes', four responded 'No' and three were 'unsure'.

DISCUSSION

The findings in this study have confirmed that patients with chronic pancreatitis have a decreased survival compared to the expected survival in comparable lifetime tables for the population above the age of 35, as shown by Lowenfels et al., Ammann et al., Lankisch et al., Marks and Bank, and Bank[5,6] (Ammann, personal communication). The present study, perusal of the literature and personal communications with pancreatologists do, however, show a wide variety of percentages for mortality, because longitudinal studies have been rather uncommon and many authors report results from a variety of years ranging from 5 to 35 years. To try to obviate this problem, this chapter selected a group of papers in which a mortality rate could be induced from a 12-year[9–13] follow-up from the beginning of symptoms or presentation to death. In those studies the mortality was fairly consistent at between 30% and some 40% over the 12 years. In those few studies continuing for 20 years or more mortality rates were higher, ranging from 50% to 70% over 20–35 years. However, in these latter series it should be remembered that patients are drifting into an age group in which co-morbidities may be as important as the pancreatic disease. There seemed to be little difference between the medically treated patients and those who had received one or other form of surgery[26] for their chronic pancreatitis, although there had been some improvement in more recent years because of improved treatments for cysts, gastrointestinal bleeding and the surgery itself. Mortality rates were particularly high in early reports of tropical pancreatitis by Geevarghese[14] and Ramesh[24]. However, it would appear that with improved facilities and treatment even this latter group have shown improved survival, as reported by Tandon and Pitchumoni (personal communication). Thus, it may be concluded from these studies that there is still a considerable mortality in patients with chronic pancreatitis, particularly in those who continue to drink alcohol and who have developed endocrine and exocrine insufficiency.

Some of the difficulties that arise in arriving at a consensus of mortality and survival in chronic pancreatitis relate to differences in geographic and environmental issues and the method of reporting, but also in the type of patients who have been followed. For example, in the Ammann series 80% of patients had calcific pancreatitis (which obviously excludes some of the less advanced cases) and perhaps most of all, what the author considers to be the cause of death in these patients. Despite this still-high long-term mortality, the combined evidence suggests an improved survival in longevity over the past 20 years, and Bornman et al. in South Africa consider life expectancy for these patients to have increased by some 10–20 years. However, when the question was put to international authors as to whether they thought longevity had improved since 1984, there was only a slight majority who answered 'Yes' over 'No' or 'unsure', particularly for patients with alcohol-induced disease. In addition, when the question was put with regard to whether the mortalities were higher in poorer socioeconomic areas such as India and South Africa, in which the previous algorithm, 'Diabetes in their teens and death in the second decade of life', was often quoted, has changed substantially as in the latest report by Tandon, and our American experience of a 33% mortality in 12 years compared to our previous experience in Cape Town of a 60–70% mortality over 20 years and 50% in 12 years. It is of course difficult to understand the marked differences in reported mortality from western countries, i.e. 13–20% in Italy and considerably higher mortalities in Switzerland, England and France. The problem of reporting needs to be examined, and the question of whether reported co-morbid conditions contributing to the mortality are importantly affected by the underlying pancreatic disease. For example, in the Ammann series the deaths related directly to pancreatic disease were in the order of 14%, and in our own series 18%, but the question arises whether those deaths listed under the co-morbid causes such as infection, gastrointestinal bleeding, and perhaps even some cardiovascular disease, may be attributable secondarily to the underlying diabetes, steatorrhoea, chronic pain and weight loss, or possibly even poorer immune response that patients with chronic pancreatitis have to be taken into account. The Cape Town group included a large group of patients with failed metabolic reserve who developed tuberculosis and other infections; it thus behoves us in the future to perhaps include these as probable causes of mortality, rather than to relegate them to the area of co-morbid disease. One further problem is that nearly all the series have a large group of patients in whom the cause of death was unknown, or have miscellaneous causes of death, and an even larger group of patients who did not submit to follow-up; their future was thus unknown. Clearly, many patients die from the effects of alcohol, such as cirrhosis, and of smoking and extrapancreatic cancer. One of the disturbing features that appear to have occurred over the years is an increase in carcinoma of the pancreas in patients with chronic pancreatitis. This may of course be due to the fact that the patients are living 10 or 20 years longer, and creeping into the pancreatic carcinoma age group, but more recent studies appear to have a pancreatic cancer rate of anything from 4% to 22% on long-term follow-up, a disturbing number not only with regard to mortality but also with regard to the difficulties in diagnoses once cancer supervenes[27,28].

Finally, although there seems to have been only a modest improvement in life expectancy over the years, except for those with tropical pancreatitis, there are increasing numbers of papers relating to the quality of life with modern therapy. Clearly the quality of life as shown by Wehler et al.[20] and Bornman et al.[19] is certainly substantially curtailed, as measured by almost any of the quality-of-life measurements including the SF 36 and others. Tailored surgery, improved treatment of diabetes, improved pancreatic replacement enzymes for the treatment of steatorrhoea and in particular the treatment of cysts, bleeding and other complications, seem to have resulted in an improved quality of life for these patients; however, almost never reaching normal quality-of-life measures. In this regard it seems as though deaths from hypoglycaemia due to over-administration of insulin or other diabetic therapies seem to have completely disappeared since the recognition that, when these patients do become hypoglycaemic, they do not have glucagon reserve to stabilize the blood sugar; therefore more careful observations of patients on insulin and insulin-promoting drugs have been instituted[9].

In conclusion, it appears from our personal series, and an international review of over 4800 patients, that the mortality of chronic pancreatitis is still formidable, in the order of 33% over a 12-year period, but varying markedly in the literature depending on geographic areas, socioeconomic conditions and co-morbid conditions (in fact much of the mortality in recent years has been attributable to co-morbid disease). However, it behooves us to decide whether the co-morbid disease is obviously or peripherally related to the underlying pancreatic problem. Current data suggest that there has been an improvement in survival over the past 20 years compared to periods before 1984, but not all authors are in agreement with this result, especially concerning those patients with alcohol-induced pancreatitis. Lastly, it is important to consider quality of life in patients with chronic pancreatitis, to try to improve their rather dismal existence once calcification, diabetes, steatorrhoea or complication has occurred, and to be watchful for the development of pancreatic cancer on a long-term follow-up basis.

Acknowledgement

I would like to thank the following colleagues for replying to the questionnaire: R Ammann, P.Banks, G Barbezat, J Barkin, P Bornman, J Clain, G Gecelter, L Gullo, P Lankisch, AB Lowenfels, IN Marks, J Sahel, S Sherman, RK Tandon, J Velenzuela.

References

1. Ammann RW, Akovbiantz A, Largiader F, Schueler G. Course and outcome of chronic pancreatitis. Longitudinal study of a mixed medical–surgical series of 245 patients. Gastroenterology. 1984;86:820–8.
2. Ammann RW. Alcohol and non-alcohol induced pancreatitis: clinical aspects. In: Bank S, Burns, GP, editors. Disorders of the Pancreas. New York: McGraw-Hill, 1992:253–72.
3. Ammann RW, Muellhaupt B, Meyerberger C, Heitz PU. Alcololic non-progressive chronic pancreatitis. Prospective long-term study of a large cohort with alcohol acute pancreatitis (1976–1992). Pancreas. 1994;9:365–73.
4. Ammann RW, Heitz PU, Kloppel G. Course of alcoholic chronic pancreatitis. A prospective clinico-morphological long term study. Gastroenterology. 1996;111:224–51.
5. Lankisch PG, Lohr-Happe A, Otto J, Creutzfeldt W. Natural course in chronic pancreatitis – pain, exocrine and endocrine pancreatic insuffiency and prognosis of the disease. Digestion. 1993;54:148–55.
6. Marks IH, Bank S. The etiology, clinical features and diagnosis of chronic pancreatitis in the south western Cape. S African Med J. 1963;37:1039–42.
7. Marks IN, Girdwood AH, Bank S, Louw JH. The prognosis of alcohol-induced calcific pancreatitis. S African Med J. 1980;57:640–3.
8. Marks IN, Bank S. Chronic pancreatitis. In: Berk JE, editor. Bockus Gastroenterology. Philadelphia: WB Saunders, 1985:4020–39.
9. Bank S. Chronic pancreatitis; clinical features and medical management. Am J Gastroenterol. 1986;81:133–56.
10. Xie J, Pooran N, Huang C, Brunner R, Fernandes A, Bank S. Mortality and survival in chronic pancreatitis; has it changed over the last 20 years. Gastroenterology. 2004;126:A381.
11. Dani R, Penna FJ, Nogueira CED. Etiology of chronic calcifying pancreatitis in Brazil. A report of 329 consecutive cases. Int J Pancreatol. 1986;1:399–406.
12. Hayakawa T, Kondo T, Shibata T, Sugimoto Y, Kitagawa M. Chronic alcoholism and evolution of pain and prognosis in chronic pancreatitis. Dig Dis Sci. 1989;34:33–8.
13. Hayakawa T, Noda A, Kondo T. Medical treatment of chronic pancreatitis – a long term follow-up study. In: Sato T, Yamauchi H, editors. Pancreatitis: Its Physiology and Clinical Aspects. University of Tokyo Press, Tokyo, 1985:359–66.
14. Geevarghese PJ. Calcific pancreatitis. Causes and mechanisms in the tropics compared to the subtropics. Trivadrun (Kerala) India: St Josephs Press, 1986.
15. Lowenfels AB, Maisonneuve P, Cavallini G et al. Prognosis of chronic pancreatitis. An international multicenter study. International Pancreatitis Study Group. Am J Gastroenterol. 1994:89:1467–71.
16. Bank S, Marks IN, Lurie B. Pre-calcific pancreatitis. S African Med J. 1972;46:2093–7.
17. Bank S. Alcoholic and non-alcoholic chronic pancreatitis – differences in natural history? Pancreas. 1987;2:365–7.
18. Cremer M, Deviere J, Englehoim L. Endoscopic management of cysts and pseudocysts in chronic pancreatitis: long-term follow up after 7 years of experience. Gastrointest Endosc. 1989;35:1–5.
19. Bornman PC, Bechingham IJ. Chronic pancreatitis. Br Med J. 2001;322: 660–3.
20. Wehler M, Nichterlein R, Fischer B et al. Factors associated with health related quality of life in chronic pancreatitis. Am J Gastroenterol. 2004;99:138–46.
21. Miyake H, Harada H, Ochi K et al. Prognosis and prognostic factors in chronic pancreatitis. Dig Dis Sci. 1989;34:449–55.
22. Leger L, Lenriot JP, Lemaiere G. Five to twenty year follow up after surgery for chronic pancreatitis in 148 patients. Ann Surg. 1974;180:185–91.
23. Scuro LA, Vantini I, Piubello W et al. Evolution of pain in chronic relapsing pancreatitis. A study of operated and non-operated patients. Am J Gastroenterol. 1983;78:495–501.
24. Ramesh H. Proposal for a new grading system for chronic pancreatitis – the ABC system. J Clin Gastroenterol. 2002;35:67–70.
25. Thuluvath PJ, Imperio D, Nair S, Cameron JL. Chronic pancreatitis: long term pain relief with and without surgery, cancer risk and mortality. J Clin Gastroenterol. 2003;36:98–9.
26. Strate T, Knoefel W, Yekebas E, Izbicki JR. Chronic pancreatitis; etiology, pathogenesis, diagnosis and treatment. Int J Colorectal Dis. 2003;18:97–106.

27. Bank S, Singh P, Pooran N. The ABC system. Proposal for a new grading system for chronic pancreatitis. J Clin Gastroenterol. 2002;35:3–4.
28. Cavestro GM, Comparato G, Nouvenne A, Sianesi M, Dimorio F. The race from chronic pancreatitis to pancreatic cancer. J Pancreas (on line). 2003;4:165–81.

Index

Falk Symposium Series

43. Reutter W, Popper H, Arias IM, Heinrich PC, Keppler D, Landmann L, eds.: *Modulation of Liver Cell Expression*. Falk Symposium No. 43. 1987
ISBN: 0-85200-677-2*
44. Boyer JL, Bianchi L, eds.: *Liver Cirrhosis*. Falk Symposium No. 44. 1987
ISBN: 0-85200-993-3*
45. Paumgartner G, Stiehl A, Gerok W, eds.: *Bile Acids and the Liver*. Falk Symposium No. 45. 1987
ISBN: 0-85200-675-6*
46. Goebell H, Peskar BM, Malchow H, eds.: *Inflammatory Bowel Diseases – Basic Research & Clinical Implications*. Falk Symposium No. 46. 1988
ISBN: 0-7462-0067-6*
47. Bianchi L, Holt P, James OFW, Butler RN, eds.: *Aging in Liver and Gastrointestinal Tract*. Falk Symposium No. 47. 1988
ISBN: 0-7462-0066-8*
48. Heilmann C, ed.: *Calcium-Dependent Processes in the Liver*. Falk Symposium No. 48. 1988
ISBN: 0-7462-0075-7*
50. Singer MV, Goebell H, eds.: *Nerves and the Gastrointestinal Tract*. Falk Symposium No. 50. 1989
ISBN: 0-7462-0114-1
51. Bannasch P, Keppler D, Weber G, eds.: *Liver Cell Carcinoma*. Falk Symposium No. 51. 1989
ISBN: 0-7462-0111-7
52. Paumgartner G, Stiehl A, Gerok W, eds.: *Trends in Bile Acid Research*. Falk Symposium No. 52. 1989
ISBN: 0-7462-0112-5
53. Paumgartner G, Stiehl A, Barbara L, Roda E, eds.: *Strategies for the Treatment of Hepatobiliary Diseases*. Falk Symposium No. 53. 1990
ISBN: 0-7923-8903-4
54. Bianchi L, Gerok W, Maier K-P, Deinhardt F, eds.: *Infectious Diseases of the Liver*. Falk Symposium No. 54. 1990
ISBN: 0-7923-8902-6
55. Falk Symposium No. 55 not published
55B. Hadziselimovic F, Herzog B, Bürgin-Wolff A, eds.: *Inflammatory Bowel Disease and Coeliac Disease in Children*. International Falk Symposium. 1990
ISBN 0-7462-0125-7
56. Williams CN, eds.: *Trends in Inflammatory Bowel Disease Therapy*. Falk Symposium No. 56. 1990
ISBN: 0-7923-8952-2
57. Bock KW, Gerok W, Matern S, Schmid R, eds.: *Hepatic Metabolism and Disposition of Endo- and Xenobiotics*. Falk Symposium No. 57. 1991
ISBN: 0-7923-8953-0
58. Paumgartner G, Stiehl A, Gerok W, eds.: *Bile Acids as Therapeutic Agents: From Basic Science to Clinical Practice*. Falk Symposium No. 58. 1991
ISBN: 0-7923-8954-9
59. Halter F, Garner A, Tytgat GNJ, eds.: *Mechanisms of Peptic Ulcer Healing*. Falk Symposium No. 59. 1991
ISBN: 0-7923-8955-7
60. Goebell H, Ewe K, Malchow H, Koelbel Ch, eds.: *Inflammatory Bowel Diseases – Progress in Basic Research and Clinical Implications*. Falk Symposium No. 60. 1991
ISBN: 0-7923-8956-5
61. Falk Symposium No. 61 not published
62. Dowling RH, Folsch UR, Löser Ch, eds.: *Polyamines in the Gastrointestinal Tract*. Falk Symposium No. 62. 1992
ISBN: 0-7923-8976-X
63. Lentze MJ, Reichen J, eds.: *Paediatric Cholestasis: Novel Approaches to Treatment*. Falk Symposium No. 63. 1992
ISBN: 0-7923-8977-8
64. Demling L, Frühmorgen P, eds.: *Non-Neoplastic Diseases of the Anorectum*. Falk Symposium No. 64. 1992
ISBN: 0-7923-8979-4
64B. Gressner AM, Ramadori G, eds.: *Molecular and Cell Biology of Liver Fibrogenesis*. International Falk Symposium. 1992
ISBN: 0-7923-8980-8

*These titles were published under the MTP Press imprint.

Falk Symposium Series

65. Hadziselimovic F, Herzog B, eds.: *Inflammatory Bowel Diseases and Morbus Hirsch-prung.* Falk Symposium No. 65. 1992   ISBN: 0-7923-8995-6
66. Martin F, McLeod RS, Sutherland LR, Williams CN, eds.: *Trends in Inflammatory Bowel Disease Therapy.* Falk Symposium No. 66. 1993   ISBN: 0-7923-8827-5
67. Schölmerich J, Kruis W, Goebell H, Hohenberger W, Gross V, eds.: *Inflammatory Bowel Diseases – Pathophysiology as Basis of Treatment.* Falk Symposium No. 67. 1993   ISBN: 0-7923-8996-4
68. Paumgartner G, Stiehl A, Gerok W, eds.: *Bile Acids and The Hepatobiliary System: From Basic Science to Clinical Practice.* Falk Symposium No. 68. 1993   ISBN: 0-7923-8829-1
69. Schmid R, Bianchi L, Gerok W, Maier K-P, eds.: *Extrahepatic Manifestations in Liver Diseases.* Falk Symposium No. 69. 1993   ISBN: 0-7923-8821-6
70. Meyer zum Büschenfelde K-H, Hoofnagle J, Manns M, eds.: *Immunology and Liver.* Falk Symposium No. 70. 1993   ISBN: 0-7923-8830-5
71. Surrenti C, Casini A, Milani S, Pinzani M , eds.: *Fat-Storing Cells and Liver Fibrosis.* Falk Symposium No. 71. 1994   ISBN: 0-7923-8842-9
72. Rachmilewitz D, ed.: *Inflammatory Bowel Diseases – 1994.* Falk Symposium No. 72. 1994   ISBN: 0-7923-8845-3
73. Binder HJ, Cummings J, Soergel KH, eds.: *Short Chain Fatty Acids.* Falk Symposium No. 73. 1994   ISBN: 0-7923-8849-6
73B. Möllmann HW, May B, eds.: *Glucocorticoid Therapy in Chronic Inflammatory Bowel Disease: from basic principles to rational therapy.* International Falk Workshop. 1996   ISBN 0-7923-8708-2
74. Keppler D, Jungermann K, eds.: *Transport in the Liver.* Falk Symposium No. 74. 1994   ISBN: 0-7923-8858-5
74B. Stange EF, ed.: *Chronic Inflammatory Bowel Disease.* Falk Symposium. 1995   ISBN: 0-7923-8876-3
75. van Berge Henegouwen GP, van Hoek B, De Groote J, Matern S, Stockbrügger RW, eds.: *Cholestatic Liver Diseases: New Strategies for Prevention and Treatment of Hepatobiliary and Cholestatic Liver Diseases.* Falk Symposium 75. 1994.   ISBN: 0-7923-8867-4
76. Monteiro E, Tavarela Veloso F, eds.: *Inflammatory Bowel Diseases: New Insights into Mechanisms of Inflammation and Challenges in Diagnosis and Treatment.* Falk Symposium 76. 1995.   ISBN 0-7923-8884-4
77. Singer MV, Ziegler R, Rohr G, eds.: *Gastrointestinal Tract and Endocrine System.* Falk Symposium 77. 1995.   ISBN 0-7923-8877-1
78. Decker K, Gerok W, Andus T, Gross V, eds.: *Cytokines and the Liver.* Falk Symposium 78. 1995.   ISBN 0-7923-8878-X
79. Holstege A, Schölmerich J, Hahn EG, eds.: *Portal Hypertension.* Falk Symposium 79. 1995.   ISBN 0-7923-8879-8
80. Hofmann AF, Paumgartner G, Stiehl A, eds.: *Bile Acids in Gastroenterology: Basic and Clinical Aspects.* Falk Symposium 80. 1995   ISBN 0-7923-8880-1
81. Riecken EO, Stallmach A, Zeitz M, Heise W, eds.: *Malignancy and Chronic Inflammation in the Gastrointestinal Tract – New Concepts.* Falk Symposium 81. 1995   ISBN 0-7923-8889-5
82. Fleig WE, ed.: *Inflammatory Bowel Diseases: New Developments and Standards.* Falk Symposium 82. 1995   ISBN 0-7923-8890-6
82B. Paumgartner G, Beuers U, eds.: *Bile Acids in Liver Diseases.* International Falk Workshop. 1995   ISBN 0-7923-8891-7

Falk Symposium Series

Falk Symposium Series

Falk Symposium Series

117. Gerbes AL, Beuers U, Jüngst D, Pape GR, Sackmann M, Sauerbruch T, eds. *Hepatology 2000 – Symposium in Honour of Gustav Paumgartner.* Falk Symposium 117. 2000   ISBN 0-7923-8765-1

117A. Acalovschi M, Paumgartner G, eds. *Hepatobiliary Diseases: Cholestasis and Gallstones.* Falk Workshop. 2000   ISBN 0-7923-8770-8

118. Frühmorgen P, Bruch H-P, eds. *Non-Neoplastic Diseases of the Anorectum.* Falk Symposium 118. 2001   ISBN 0-7923-8766-X

119. Fellermann K, Jewell DP, Sandborn WJ, Schölmerich J, Stange EF, eds. *Immunosuppression in Inflammatory Bowel Diseases – Standards, New Developments, Future Trends.* Falk Symposium 119. 2001   ISBN 0-7923-8767-8

120. van Berge Henegouwen GP, Keppler D, Leuschner U, Paumgartner G, Stiehl A, eds. *Biology of Bile Acids in Health and Disease.* Falk Symposium 120. 2001
                    ISBN 0-7923-8768-6

121. Leuschner U, James OFW, Dancygier H, eds. *Steatohepatitis (NASH and ASH).* Falk Symposium 121. 2001   ISBN 0-7923-8769-4

121A. Matern S, Boyer JL, Keppler D, Meier-Abt PJ, eds. *Hepatobiliary Transport: From Bench to Bedside.* Falk Workshop. 2001   ISBN 0-7923-8771-6

122. Campieri M, Fiocchi C, Hanauer SB, Jewell DP, Rachmilewitz R, Schölmerich J, eds. *Inflammatory Bowel Disease – A Clinical Case Approach to Pathophysiology, Diagnosis, and Treatment.* Falk Symposium 122. 2002   ISBN 0-7923-8772-4

123. Rachmilewitz D, Modigliani R, Podolsky DK, Sachar DB, Tozun N, eds. *VI International Symposium on Inflammatory Bowel Diseases.* Falk Symposium 123. 2002   ISBN 0-7923-8773-2

124. Hagenmüller F, Manns MP, Musmann H-G, Riemann JF, eds. *Medical Imaging in Gastroenterology and Hepatology.* Falk Symposium 124. 2002 ISBN 0-7923-8774-0

125. Gressner AM, Heinrich PC, Matern S, eds. *Cytokines in Liver Injury and Repair.* Falk Symposium 125. 2002   ISBN 0-7923-8775-9

126. Gupta S, Jansen PLM, Klempnauer J, Manns MP, eds. *Hepatocyte Transplantation.* Falk Symposium 126. 2002   ISBN 0-7923-8776-7

127. Hadziselimovic F, ed. *Autoimmune Diseases in Paediatric Gastroenterology.* Falk Symposium 127. 2002   ISBN 0-7923-8778-3

127A. Berr F, Bruix J, Hauss J, Wands J, Wittekind Ch, eds. *Malignant Liver Tumours: Basic Concepts and Clinical Management.* Falk Workshop. 2002
                    ISBN 0-7923-8779-1

128. Scheppach W, Scheurlen M, eds. *Exogenous Factors in Colonic Carcinogenesis.* Falk Symposium 128. 2002   ISBN 0-7923-8780-5

129. Paumgartner G, Keppler D, Leuschner U, Stiehl A, eds. *Bile Acids: From Genomics to Disease and Therapy.* Falk Symposium 129. 2002   ISBN 0-7923-8781-3

129A. Leuschner U, Berg PA, Holtmeier J, eds. *Bile Acids and Pregnancy.* Falk Workshop. 2002   ISBN 0-7923-8782-1

130. Holtmann G, Talley NJ, eds. *Gastrointestinal Inflammation and Disturbed Gut Function: The Challenge of New Concepts.* Falk Symposium 130. 2003
                    ISBN 0-7923-8783-X

131. Herfarth H, Feagan BJ, Folsch UR, Schölmerich J, Vatn MH, Zeitz M, eds. *Targets of Treatment in Chronic Inflammatory Bowel Diseases.* Falk Symposium 131. 2003
                    ISBN 0-7923-8784-8

132. Galle PR, Gerken G, Schmidt WE, Wiedenmann B, eds. *Disease Progression and Carcinogenesis in the Gastrointestinal Tract.* Falk Symposium 132. 2003
                    ISBN 0-7923-8785-6

Falk Symposium Series

132A. Staritz M, Adler G, Knuth A, Schmiegel W, Schmoll H-J, eds. *Side-effects of Chemotherapy on the Gastrointestinal Tract*. Falk Workshop. 2003
ISBN 0-7923-8791-0

132B. Reutter W, Schuppan D, Tauber R, Zeitz M, eds. *Cell Adhesion Molecules in Health and Disease*. Falk Workshop. 2003   ISBN 0-7923-8786-4

133. Duchmann R, Blumberg R, Neurath M, Schölmerich J, Strober W, Zeitz M. *Mechanisms of Intestinal Inflammation: Implications for Therapeutic Intervention in IBD*. Falk Symposium 133. 2004   ISBN 0-7923-8787-2

134. Dignass A, Lochs H, Stange E. *Trends and Controversies in IBD – Evidence-Based Approach or Individual Management?* Falk Symposium 134. 2004
ISBN 0-7923-8788-0

134A. Dignass A, Gross HJ, Buhr V, James OFW. *Topical Steroids in Gastroenterology and Hepatology*. Falk Workshop. 2004   ISBN 0-7923-8789-9

135. Lukáš M, Manns MP, Špičák J, Stange EF, eds. *Immunological Diseases of Liver and Gut*. Falk Symposium 135. 2004   ISBN 0-7923-8792-9

136. Leuschner U, Broomé U, Stiehl A, eds. *Cholestatic Liver Diseases: Therapeutic Options and Perspectives*. Falk Symposium 136. 2004   ISBN 0-7923-8793-7

137. Blum HE, Maier KP, Rodés J, Sauerbruch T, eds. *Liver Diseases: Advances in Treatment and Prevention*. Falk Symposium 137. 2004   ISBN 0-7923-8794-5

138. Blum HE, Manns MP, eds. *State of the Art of Hepatology: Molecular and Cell Biology*. Falk Symposium 138. 2004   ISBN 0-7923-8795-3

138A. Hayashi N, Manns MP, eds. *Prevention of Progression in Chronic Liver Disease: An Update on SNMC (Stronger Neo-Minophagen C)*. Falk Workshop. 2004
ISBN 0-7923-8796-1

139. Adler G, Blum HE, Fuchs M, Stange EF, eds. *Gallstones: Pathogenesis and Treatment*. Falk Symposium 139. 2004   ISBN 0-7923-8798-8

140. Colombel J-F, Gasché C, Schölmerich J, Vucelic C, eds. *Inflammatory Bowel Disease: Translation from Basic Research to Clinical Practice*. Falk Symposium 140. 2005.   ISBN 1-4020-2847-4

141. Paumgartner G, Keppler D, Leuschner U, Stiehl A, eds. *Bile Acid Biology and its Therapeutic Implications*. Falk Symposium 141. 2005   ISBN 1-4020-2893-8

142. Dienes H-P, Leuschner U, Lohse AW, Manns MP, eds. *Autoimmune Liver Disease*. Falk Symposium 142. 2005   ISBN 1-4020-2894-6

143. Ammann RW, Büchler MW, Adler G, DiMagno EP, Sarner M, eds. *Pancreatitis: Advances in Pathobiology, Diagnosis and Treatment*. Falk Symposium 143. 2005
ISBN 1-4020-2895-4